暨南大学本科教材资助项目（港澳台侨学生使用教材资助项目）

简明医学机能学实验指导

Concise Guideline to the Medical Functional Experiment

（中英文双语版）

主　审　龚永生（温州医科大学）

主　编　王跃春（暨南大学）

副主编　牛海涛（暨南大学）　　　　肖　飞（暨南大学）
　　　　李红梅（暨南大学）

编　委　许戈阳（暨南大学）　　　　魏　伟（暨南大学）
　　　　彭　爽（广州体育学院）　　方梅霞（暨南大学）
　　　　赵　月（暨南大学）　　　　宋琳亮（暨南大学）
　　　　和　君（暨南大学）　　　　齐春丽（暨南大学）
　　　　廖薮祺（暨南大学）　　　　刘庭君（暨南大学）
　　　　张珂珂（暨南大学）　　　　樊晓娜（暨南大学）

北京大学医学出版社

JIANMING YIXUE JINENGXUE SHIYAN ZHIDAO

图书在版编目（CIP）数据

简明医学机能学实验指导：汉文、英文 / 王跃春主编 .
—北京：北京大学医学出版社，2023.2
　ISBN 978-7-5659-2682-2

　Ⅰ.①简…　Ⅱ.①王…　Ⅲ.①实验医学—教材—汉、英
Ⅳ.①R-33

　中国版本图书馆 CIP 数据核字（2022）第 130453 号

简明医学机能学实验指导（中英文双语版）

主　　编：王跃春
出版发行：北京大学医学出版社
地　　址：（100191）北京市海淀区学院路 38 号　北京大学医学部院内
电　　话：发行部 010-82802230；图书邮购 010-82802495
网　　址：http://www.pumpress.com.cn
E-mail：booksale@bjmu.edu.cn
印　　刷：中煤（北京）印务有限公司
经　　销：新华书店
责任编辑：韩忠刚　吕曼婕　　责任校对：靳新强　　责任印制：李　啸
开　　本：787 mm×1092 mm　1/16　　印张：21.5　　字数：550 千字
版　　次：2023 年 2 月第 1 版　2023 年 2 月第 1 次印刷
书　　号：ISBN 978-7-5659-2682-2
定　　价：65.00 元

前　言

在互联网＋信息化时代，迎着世界范围教育教学改革的浪潮，医学机能学实验也在大浪淘沙中接受着融合创新的洗礼。医学机能学实验教学的目的在于通过具体实验技能的训练以及科研思维的培养，使学生在加强理论知识理解和实验技能把握的基础上，初步具备进行科学研究工作的能力和素质；同时也潜移默化地培养学生的科学精神、职业道德和人文情怀。在这一过程中，一本好的教材将会起到非常重要的推动作用。

为达到培养具有创新精神的高素质医药学人才的目的，我们顺应医学机能学实验教学改革的大趋势，组织了一批在生理学、病理生理学、药理学及实验动物学教学中积累了丰富经验的一线教师和专家，联合编写了本书，以期有效地提高医学机能学实验教学质量，为医学机能学实验的教学改革和发展贡献绵薄之力。

为便于学生携带和参考，本书删繁就简，简明扼要，主要包含医学机能学实验导论、动物实验、人体实验、综合性实验、实验设计、科学研究及论文撰写与发表等内容。对学生将来从事科研工作都将有所裨益。

本书内容涵盖面大，适用范围广，不仅可用作医药院校各专业（基础医学、临床医学、预防医学、口腔、麻醉、影像、药学、检验、护理、法医等专业）本科生的医学机能学实验教材，也可作为相关专业硕士生、博士生和医务人员的参考书籍；采用中英文双语版本，扩大了本书的适用范围，尤其适合招收国际生的院校使用。

本书的出版由暨南大学教务处资助，得到了医学部和基础医学与公共卫生学院各级领导的支持和关怀；也是全体参编人员集多年教学实践经验之大成并精诚合作的结果；很多学生也在本书的编写过程中给予了很大帮助。承蒙北京大学医学出版社和成都泰盟科技有限公司大力支持，才使本书得以如期出版，在此一并致谢。

2022.8.15 于暨南园

Foreword

In the age of increasing reliance on the Internet, we are faced with an inevitable demand of pedagogical reform at the global level. The teaching of medical functional experiments also requires innovation in this wave of reform. The purpose of teaching medical functional experiments is to train medical and science students' specific experimental and analytical skills, as well as to cultivate innovative and critical thinking abilities, so that students can develop the aptitude and attribute required of an independent researcher, who should possess technical knowledge based firmly on thorough understanding of the scientific, theoretical and conceptual basis. As an added benefit, the teaching of medical functional experiments will also help students to nurture their scientific spirit, professionalism, ethical thinking and humanistic attitude. In this context, the appropriate set of educational tools for such a programme must contain a comprehensive textbook which will play a crucial role in the promotion of effective learning.

In order to achieve the goal of cultivating high-quality medical talents with innovative spirit and conformed to the general trend of teaching reform of medical functional experiments, we have invited a group of front-line teaching staff and experts, who have substantial teaching experience in physiology, pathophysiology, pharmacology and experimental animal science, to contribute to this textbook. We hope that this textbook could effectively improve the quality of teaching of medical functional experiments, and makes a small contribution to the reform and development of the teaching in this field.

In order to facilitate students to carry and read, this textbook is simplified and concise. The areas covered include the introduction to medical functional experiments, animal experiments, human experiments, comprehensive experiments, experimental design, and the publication of papers. We believe that this book will be beneficial to both the teachers and students who plan to engage in scientific research.

This textbook covers a wide range of topics and has a broad spectrum of applications. Not only it can be used as a medical functional experiments textbook for undergraduates majoring in basic medicine, clinical medicine, preventive medicine, stomatology, anesthesiology, medical image science, pharmacy, medical laboratory science, nursing, forensic science in medical colleges and universities, but also can be used as a reference book for postgraduate students and medical staff in related subjects. This textbook was written in both Chinese and English so that it is also suitable for colleges and universities that recruit international students.

The publication of this textbook has been funded by the Teaching Affair Office of Jinan University and supported by School of Basic Medicine and Public Health of Jinan University. It is also the result of the years of teaching experience and sincere cooperation. We are grateful for the enormous support of Peking University Medical Press and Chengdu Techman Software Co., Ltd. and a lot of others who made great contribution to this project so that the textbook could be published on schedule.

August 15, 2022 in Jinan Garden

目　录

第一章　医学机能学实验导论

医学机能学是医药院校的重要基础课程，主要包括生理学、病理生理学和药理学，广义上也包括细胞与分子生物学。随着现代新型医学模式的建立和发展，对上述各学科中的实验教学内容、实验方法和技术进行精选、组合、融合和创新，以适应信息时代医学教育发展的趋势，从而形成独立开设的医学机能学实验课程。

医学机能学实验主要是为医学生或医学相关专业的学生设计的，包括临床医学、药学、护理学、口腔医学、中医学、预防医学、生物医学等学科和专业。医学机能学实验的课程目标包括知识技能获取、能力素质培养和情感价值养成等方面。首先，通过基本的机能学实验训练，学生可学会实验仪器的正确使用，初步掌握基本操作技术，逐步掌握获得机能学知识的科学方法。其次，学生可从设计实验和撰写实验报告的训练中了解研究论文的写作及论文发表的过程和技巧；培养学生的科学思维方法以及问题意识，提高其提出问题、观察问题、分析问题和解决问题的科研素养；锻炼学生的团队合作能力、沟通表达能力和科学精神。最后，可在实验的过程中，培养学生对生命的敬畏之心、对动物的关爱之情、对医德的关注和追求以及服务国家和民众的意志等。总之，本课程不仅在理论和实验技能层面为后续课程的学习奠定了坚实的基础，还有助于培养具有国际视野、创新精神和岗位胜任力的新型综合型医学人才。

本实验指导由 4 个章节、37 个实验组成，包括经典动物实验、人体实验、设计性实验、整合实验和创新性实验等。实验内容的选择主要考虑以下几个方面：可以帮助学生更好地理解医学机能学的基本原理，把握医学机能学实验的基本技能（如脑脊髓损毁术、气管插管术、颈总动脉插管术、颈浅表静脉插管术、股动脉插管术、左心室插管术、输尿管插管术、灌胃术、体外肠管灌流术等）；可以对学生的科学研究能力进行基本的训练和提高；能引导学生树立正确的世界观、科学观和价值观，如在实验设计中遵循求实、创新的科学精神，在动物手术过程中注意保护福利，在人体生理学实验中体现人文关怀。

本实验指导保留了暨南大学基础医学院生理学系、病理生理学系及药理学系多年来一直开展的经典实验和核心实验，并按照生理学实验、病理生理学实验和药理学实验的顺序来编排，因此在使用时具有较大的灵活性。由于每个学期的具体实验教学内容及进度均有所不同，可根据各个专业的培养方案、教学大纲的具体要求进行组合，如护理学专业可以偏重人体实验，而临床医学专业除了保留的动物实验和人体实验之外，还要安排综合性及创新性实验；在暨南大学，我们有来自世界各地的学生，因此，在实验设计的难度以及综合性、创新性实验的比例方面也应根据生源地的不同进行调整。综合性实验主要是基于器官系统整合的理念，在一次实验中同时采用两种或两种以上实验技能，研究两个或两个以上器官系统的活动，如在研究缺氧对心血管系统活动的影响实验中，要采用气管插管术和颈动脉插管术；而在血压变化对尿生成的影响实验中，要采用气管插管术、颈动脉插管术和输尿管插管术等。创新性实验主要是指学有余力的学生在掌握了基本实验技能的基础上，在教师的指导下，结合导师的科研课题自行设计的实验，往往是形态 - 功能 - 分子生物学整合性实验。其创新性是第一位要考虑的因素，需经过开题报告论证其可行性之后再进行实验。难度比较大，因此此类实验的比例要控制在适当范围内。

本着"以学生为中心、产出为导向"的教学理念，从学生实际需要出发，结合暨南大学"侨校＋名校"的特色和现有的实验条件，我们编写了这本简明双语实验指导。本书的特点是语言简洁明了，课本便于携带，内容易把握，对后续学习和进一步科学研究也有指导性意义。

第一节 医学机能学实验的发展及分类

一、医学机能学实验的发展

人类怎样理解客观世界，又如何获取知识？实践尤为关键，科学史尤其是医学史也有力地证明了实践的重要性。从公元前 4 世纪到公元前 3 世纪，古希腊生物学奠基人亚里士多德最早开展了动物实验，他运用解剖学技术证明了各种动物的内部差异，这是第一个关于动物实验的西方文献。而在古罗马，盖伦通过对各种动物的活体解剖，进而对人体的生理功能进行了研究，这对医学的发展产生了巨大影响。在 17 世纪，英国医生威廉·哈维用验尸的方法对几种动物进行了许多实验，他首先确定了血液循环的具体途径，并指出心脏是循环系统的中心。1628 年他出版了《心与血的运动》（*De Motu Cordis*），这是第一部基于实验的生理学著作，标志着现代生理学的诞生。而血液循环的发现使生理学成为了一门学科，并逐步建立了生理学的科学研究方法，开创了实验生理学的新时代。到了 19 世纪，人们意识到只有临床观察和尸体解剖才能全面和深刻地了解疾病，于是他们开始制备带有人类疾病的动物模型，以研究疾病的原因、发生过程和条件等，并且进一步揭示各种疾病的临床表现与身体内在变化之间的联系，明确疾病发生和发展的机制，从而理解疾病的本质。1865 年，法国生理学家克劳德·伯纳德成为第一个用活体动物对各种疾病进行研究的倡导者，他提出用动物代替人类来进行实验，从而创造了"实验医学"。"实验医学"现在被称为"动物实验研究"，指用动物而不是人类来做实验。当时，动物实验等实验方法非常强大，因此开启了医学的黄金时代。

随着自然科学的发展，医学科学在过去几个世纪里取得了举世瞩目的成就，并逐渐形成了许多分支，实验科学是其中的重要分支。此外，随着医学各分支的进步，出现了许多实验技术，一般分为四类技术：形态学、功能科学、分子生物学和细胞生物学技术。然而，在医学教育和科学研究领域，绝大多数医学基础实验研究依赖于使用多种实验技术，因为在复杂的自然环境中，使用单一实验技术得到的结果往往是片面的，对事实和客观规律的认识也带有一定的偶然性。在科学技术日新月异的时代，综合应用医学实验室技术显得尤为重要，而医学机能学实验技术在医学研究中得到了广泛的应用，同时，其他实验技术也被广泛地应用于医学机能学的实验研究中。近年来，机能与形态的整合，各器官系统的贯通以及基础与临床一体化虚拟仿真实训系统的研发等已成为医学机能学实验改革发展的趋势。温州医科大学的龚永生教授提出"以实验引领医学综合创新，以机能实验引领基础医学实验整合"的观点，同时希望将医学机能学实验从课程上升为学科，并将信息技术与教育教学进行深度融合，以教学平台为依托建设科学创新平台和医学科普平台等。在国家教育教学改革的浪潮中，我们必将迎来医学机能学实验无限美好的未来。

二、医学机能学实验研究的层次和实验类型

1. 医学机能学实验研究的层次

（1）细胞水平：生命体的基本结构和功能单位是细胞，在细胞水平进行研究是了解器官的功能。细胞的生理特性取决于组成细胞的大分子物质的物理和化学特征，因而分子水平的研究是研究细胞的功能，例如肌肉细胞的收缩功能和内分泌细胞的分泌功能。

（2）器官和系统水平：器官和系统层面的研究目标是探索人体器官和系统的基本功能、活动方式及其影响因素。例如，呼吸系统的作用是什么？呼吸是怎样进行的？哪些因素可以影响呼吸活动？

（3）整体水平：整体水平研究的目的是研究器官和系统之间的相互作用，以及人体与环境之间的相互作用。人有复杂的情感活动和心理活动。这些活动可以影响许多体细胞活动和内脏活动，并导致相应的行为学表现。人类生活在不同的家庭和社会中，来自外部环境的信息会影响情绪、情感和意志等，从而对身体产生积极或消极的影响。

因此，医学机能学实验主要在分子、细胞、器官和整体水平进行，主要包括以下几种基本的实验类型。

2. 医学机能学实验的类型

（1）人体实验和动物实验：医学机能学实验的理论知识来源于以狗、猫、兔、大鼠、小鼠、青蛙等动物为实验对象的实验研究，而随着实验医学的发展，越来越多的实验可以在人体上进行。根据不同的实验对象，医学机能学实验可分为人体实验和动物实验：人体实验可包括与临床观察相关的血压和心率测定、心电图和脑电图的记录等；而动物实验则包括多种动物模型，如疾病动物模型或转基因动物模型。

（2）体内实验和体外实验：医学机能学实验的主要方法有体内研究和体外研究。在体内研究中，实验是在完整动物身上进行的，有急性和慢性实验，前者是在麻醉或脑损毁动物身上进行的，而后者则是在清醒的动物身上进行很长时间的实验。在体外研究中，实验是在细胞、组织或器官上进行的，可以进行复杂的实验以更深入地了解细胞和分子水平的

生命活动机制。与整个生物体的研究相比，体外研究显示出其简单性、物种特异性和便利性。体外研究的另一个优点是，无需从实验动物的细胞反应中"外推"，即可研究人体细胞，而且体外研究可以小型化和自动化，产生高通量筛选方法，用于检测药理学或毒理学中的分子。体外研究的主要缺点是，从体外结果推断完整生物体的生物学特性可能具有不一致性，甚至可能出现相反的结果，因此，研究者必须足够小心，以免得出对生物体和系统生物学而言错误的结论。

（3）急性实验和慢性实验：急性实验可细分为体外实验和体内实验。急性实验具有以下优点：实验条件易于控制，结果易于分析。而许多需要长期和动态地进行观察和检测的实验，属于慢性实验，具有以下优点：有可能在有意识的条件下持续观察生命活动，其结果近似于生理状态；缺点是机体的状况过于复杂，难以分析结果。

第二节　医学机能学实验室的基本规范及安全守则

鉴于医学机能学实验的重要性，每个人都应该珍惜在实验室进行实验的机会。为保证实验过程的顺利进行，确保实验结果的客观、真实、可靠，我们制定了以下实验室基本规范及安全守则，需要大家严格遵守和执行。

一、实验课要求

1. 课前要求

（1）预览教学进度表，明确要做哪个实验。

（2）仔细阅读实验指导，知道为什么做这个实验以及如何做这个实验。

（3）复习与实验相关的理论知识，预测可能的实验结果并提出问题。

2. 课中要求

（1）准时进入实验室，不能出示请假许可或提前离开实验室的同学将被认定为缺勤。

（2）进入实验室要穿白大衣，不允许穿拖鞋。

（3）上课时应把手机设置为静音模式，不要大声喧哗。

（4）在课程开始时仔细听教师讲课，尤其要关注决定实验能否成功完成的注意事项。

（5）在教师进行实验演示时，一定要认真、仔细地观察。

（6）将与实验无关用品移出工作台，保持实验区干净、整洁，以免发生错误和意外。

（7）在教师指导下正确使用各种设备和软件。如果设备出问题，应该及时告诉教师，请求处理。

（8）按照实验程序逐步进行实验，耐心观察实验现象，及时、准确地做笔记，保留所有数据的完整记录，并及时将收集的数据与教材中的相关资料进行关联。

3. 课后要求

（1）清理实验台，清洗实验器材，并按要求摆放或归还。小组成员应分工合作，各司其职。

（2）动物标本和纸巾、手套等要分开处理，标本应放入黄色塑料袋，按要求存放于指定地点。非医疗垃圾投入普通垃圾桶。

（3）班长安排一组学生清扫整个实验室，包括打扫地面和清除垃圾。

（4）整理原始数据并进行初步的统计分析，再根据实验报告的格式和要求认真书写实验报告，并按时提交。

二、实验室基本规范及安全守则

（1）进入实验室，必须穿白大衣，禁止穿拖鞋、短裤及过短的裙子，长发同学应将头发束好。

（2）进入实验室，需要熟悉实验室的消防通道出口、消防辅助套件及锐化容器位置。

（3）实验室内禁止进食和嬉戏。实验期间不得进行任何与实验无关的活动，保持实验室安静，不得喧哗。实验时若因故需要离开，应向教师请假。

（4）按实验操作规程使用实验器材和试剂，注意个人防护，小心使用剪刀、刀片、针头和其他利器，避免打碎玻璃仪器。

（5）废弃的利器和碎玻璃须放置到利器盒中。强酸、强碱具有强烈腐蚀性，用时要特别小心，切勿溅在皮肤、衣服和实验台上。

（6）所有的实验室化学品都是潜在的危险来源，要按照说明进行使用；不能用嘴接触任何化学物质或移液器；涉及化学溶液的实验必须佩戴护目镜。如果不小心将任何化学品溅到自己身上，要立即告知教师。

（7）实验室内各组的仪器和器材由各组自己使用，不得与别组调换，以免混乱。如遇仪器损坏或故障，应及时报告教师或实验准备室技术人员，以便维修或更换。

（8）禁止用接触过试剂和动物的手套触摸电脑开关、键盘、鼠标，设备开关、桌椅、门把手和窗户把手等。

（9）麻醉药品按需取用，不得私自将药品带出实验室。

（10）掌握实验动物的正确抓握方法，避免被抓咬。如被抓咬，需使用大量清水冲洗、然后用碘伏消毒，告知教师，并立即去医院就诊。

（11）爱护实验动物，严格遵循动物实验"3R"原则，人道地对待实验动物，减少实验动物不必要的浪费，减轻动物痛苦。实验动物在处置前需要进行安乐死。

（12）在人体实验中，如果您有心脏或呼吸系统疾病，请不要自愿成为受试者。如果受试者在实验中感到不适，应立即停止实验并通知教师。如果受试者服用了特殊药物或怀孕，要提前告知教师。

（13）实验结束后，清洁并归还使用过的仪器设备，金属器械要用干毛巾擦干；同时清理实验台面，将实验椅归位。值日生负责清理实验动物笼具和托盘、清洁地面、处理垃圾。

第三节　医学机能学实验常用试剂的配制

医学机能学实验最常使用的溶液主要包括：生理盐水、任氏液和台氏液，分别适用于人类、两栖动物和哺乳动物。

一、生理盐水（normal saline，NS）

生理盐水为 0.9% 的氯化钠水溶液，其渗透压与人体血浆和组织液的渗透压相等，不会引起细胞脱水或让细胞吸收过多的水分，可以维持细胞的正常形态和功能。静脉滴注 NS 常用于不能服用口服液体药物的患者。配制方法：将 9 g 氯化钠溶解到 800 mL 蒸馏水中，充分搅拌使之溶解，再加入 200 mL 蒸馏水。此时，氯化钠的浓度为 0.154 mol/L，而氯化钠分解产生的钠离子和氯离子的摩尔浓度均为 0.154 mol/L，渗透系数为 286.44。等离子体渗透压范围为 280~310 mOsm/L，如果渗透压 <280 mOsm/L 称为低渗液，>310 mOsm/L 为高渗液，NS 的渗透压接近等离子体渗透压，所以是等渗液。

二、任氏液（Ringer's solution）

任氏液中含有氯化钠、氯化钾、氯化钙、碳酸氢钠和磷酸二氢钠，称为复方氯化钠注射液，由英国生理学家林格（Ringer）发明。任氏液类似于生理盐水，有时在调节电解质和体液酸碱平衡时效果更好。由于钠、钾、钙、氯等离子在实验中能维持两栖动物身体组织和器官的生理活性，所以常用于两栖类动物的离体实验，例如离体的青蛙心脏可在任氏液中长时间跳动。按表 1-1 配制任氏液。

表 1-1　任氏液的配制

物质	浓度（g/L）	物质	浓度（g/L）
氯化钾	0.14	碳酸氢钠	0.20
氯化钠	6.50	磷酸二氢钠	0.01
氯化钙	0.12		

配制方法：
（1）将氯化钠、氯化钾、碳酸氢钠和磷酸二氢钠先溶解在 800 mL 蒸馏水中。
（2）用蒸馏水稀释至 980 mL。
（3）将氯化钙溶解在 20 mL 的蒸馏水中。
（4）将氯化钙溶液加入上述溶液中，不断搅拌以免产生不溶性钙盐沉淀。
（5）用 1 mol/L 盐酸溶液或 1 mol/L 氢氧化钠溶液将 pH 调整为 6.50。

三、台氏液（Tyrode's solution）

与任氏液相比，台氏液主要用于哺乳动物的体外实验，其成分中含有镁，并使用碳酸氢盐和磷酸盐作为缓冲液，成分中的葡萄糖作为能量来源。在兔离体小肠平滑肌实验中，要不断向台氏液中输入氧气，以保持肠道肌肉的正常生理功能。此外，台氏液也常用以清洁哺乳动物的组织。按表1-2配制台氏液。

表1-2　台氏液的配制

物质	浓度（g/L）	物质	浓度（g/L）
氯化钾	0.20	碳氢化钠	1.00
氯化钠	8.00	磷酸二氢钠	0.05
氯化镁	0.1	葡萄糖	1.00
氯化钙	0.20		

第四节　医学机能学实验报告的格式及写作要求

书写实验报告是整个实验的最后一步，但也许是最重要的一步。它描述了实验者所做的所有工作，并通过正确地呈现结果、讨论和结论，反映作者对实验的理解和思考，也是教师评价学生综合能力的重要依据之一。实验报告不同于研究论文，但基本要素相同。因此，书写实验报告有助于学生在未来成功地发表研究论文。

一、一般要求

（1）使用所需的报告纸格式（详情请参阅下文及附录1~3）。
（2）填写每个空白，并清楚地标记姓名和学生编号。
（3）遵循标准格式书写实验报告的各个部分。
（4）尽可能提供准确的图表、表格或图片。
（5）清晰手写或打字。
（6）独立完成实验报告（如果抄袭报告，双方得分都将为零）。
（7）按时提交实验报告。

二、实验报告的基本格式

在医学机能学实验中，某些实验强调操作技能或手术方法，如神经-肌肉标本的制备；有些实验注重观察和检测现象的变化，如胃肠道运动的生理特性；还有一些实验则强调结果和分析，如各因素对尿液形成的影响。但大多数实验，尤其是综合性实验，包括以上三个方面。

一般而言，典型的机能学实验报告包括以下内容：目的、原理、实验材料、实验步骤和观察项目、结果、讨论、结论和参考文献。

1. 目的
简要说明实验的目的，一般一个实验有一个或两个实验目的，即了解实验要验证的原理和掌握本实验所涉及的方法和技术等。

2. 原理

简要介绍与本次实验相关的理论知识。

3. 实验材料

简要列出实验材料，包括实验对象（动物或人体）、仪器设备或试剂耗材等。

4. 实验步骤和观察项目

详细描述实验步骤以逐步完成实验。

5. 结果

详细描述实验的结果，尽量以图或表格的形式呈现结果。

（1）图至少应包括：图、放置在图下方的标题、图中添加的刺激标记（图 1-1）。

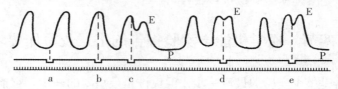

E：期前收缩　P：代偿性间隙。

图 1-1　蛙心的期前收缩和代偿性间隙

（2）表的上方应有一个标题，表的下方应添加注释（表 1-3 和表 1-4）。

（3）设计表格时，可以将观察项目放在左侧（从上到下），并将结果设置在右侧（表 1-3 和表 1-4）。

表 1-3　脊蛙屈肌反射观察

观察项目	屈肌反射（+/–）
正常的右腿	
去掉右脚的皮肤的右腿	
正常的左腿	
切断左侧坐骨神经的左腿	
刺激左侧坐骨神经外围端	
刺激左侧坐骨神经中心端	
破坏脊髓	

+代表正屈肌反射，– 代表负屈肌反射。

表 1-4　不同条件下青蛙心脏的心率（次 / 分）

观察项目	静脉窦	心房	心室
对照			
阻断 1			
阻断 2			

阻断 1：阻止从静脉窦到心房的传导；阻断 2：阻止从心房到心室的传导。

（4）对于量化数据，应确定正确的单位，如体重、速度、长度、身高、心率、血压、呼吸速率等都有对应的单位。

6. 讨论

（1）根据已知的理论知识按实验顺序对结果进行详细分析。

（2）讨论要针对本次实验的结果进行解释，不要涉及任何与本次结果无关的内容。

（3）在对结果进行评估和分析时，可以考虑以下几个方面：①将实验数据与参考书中的预期结果进行比较；②运用医学知识分析各种现象的产生原因和机制；③当产生非预期结果时，要分析可能的原因并提出合理的解释，探讨如何避免由不受控制的变量或意外因素引起的错误。

（4）为之后的实验提出建议。

7. 结论

（1）从结果和讨论中提炼出一般性的、高度概括的原理，通常用一两个句子来表达。

（2）结论不同于结果，不要用简单地列出结果来代替结论。

8. 参考文献

建议至少列一个参考文献并保持统一的格式或样式。

第五节 医学机能学实验病例讨论

机能学的三大组成学科（生理学、病理生理学和药理学）是从基础医学通向临床医学的桥梁性学科，生理学重点讨论机体如何在神经系统和内分泌系统的调控下维持内环境的稳态，一旦各器官系统的生理功能不能相互配合、相互协调，机体就会产生疾病；病理生理学的主要任务是研究疾病发生的原因和条件，疾病过程的机能、代谢的动态变化以及这些变化的发生机制，揭示疾病发生、发展和转归的规律；而药理学则是在生理学和病理生理学的基础上探讨药物对疾病的治疗作用及机制。机能学实验不仅要求学生通过实验验证前人已总结出的理论知识，更应培养学生用所学的理论知识对疾病（包括复制的动物疾病模型和临床实际病例）进行综合分析并提出药物治疗方案的临床思维能力和岗位胜任力。因此，适当地开展病例讨论不仅能将教学内容和实际病例相结合以做到"早临床、多临床"，而且能将抽象的理论知识感性化、情境化以激发学生的学习兴趣，同时在案例分析中还能培养学生的医学人文关怀能力。

一、病例讨论在教学中的实施

1. 在理论课中的实施

课中病例讨论是指每一章节在课程讲授前均附有一个典型病例，病例能够贯穿本章的主要内容，并在病例后提出相关问题，引出本次课的主要内容。在讲解基本知识和基本理论的过程中，一直以病例为中心进行启发式教学。这种以病例为中心的启发式教学，能使学生主动参与教学过程，带着疑问听课，带着兴趣思考，对所讲的内容印象加深。

2. 在理论课后的实施

课后病例讨论是指在系统讲授完某一章节相关的理论知识，学生对病因、发病机制、机体机能代谢变化、临床表现及防治原则等有了初步认识后，教师通过智慧教学工具或网络教学平台等形式把病例展示给学生，然后在实验课中以小组为单位开展病例讨论，以加深学生对该病的了解，达到对章节内容全面系统的掌握。

二、病例讨论的基本步骤

1. 精心选取典型病例

以小组为单位的病例讨论一般在系统讲授完某一章节相关的理论知识，学生对病因、发病机制、机体机能代谢变化、临床表现及防治原则等有了初步认识后开展。病例来源主要有本校附属医院或其他医院以往的病例、文献上报道的病例等。但无论病例来源于何种形式，都必须包括病人的一般情况、病史、体格检查及其他辅助检查的真实描述。通过病例讨论，可以加深学生对该病的系统性了解，达到对本章内容全面系统的掌握，使理论知识活学活用。

2. 布置病例讨论内容

教师提前 1 周通过班级微信群或在线学习平台将经典病例发送给学生。学生将根据病例提供的资料来查阅教科书及相关资料，讨论并制作 PPT，分析导致相关症状与体征的直接和间接原因。

3. 课堂开展病例讨论

上课时，由小组选派代表总结本组的讨论结果，提出不能解决的或新发现的问题，其他学生可以补充，意见不一致时还可以全班展开辩论，讨论过程中指导教师给予适当的引导。

课堂病例讨论的要点：
①疾病的诊断结果及诊断标准
②疾病的病程演变过程及发生原理
③患者主要症状产生的机制
④临床药物治疗的最佳方案及机制

4. 教师进行总结

对于相对简单、学生意见统一的问题，简要总结；对于相对复杂、学生分歧比较大、需要综合分析的问题要进行详细讲解，以加深学生的理解。

三、病例讨论的要点

1. 导向性

在讨论中，作为主导的教师必须对讨论进行有效控制和正确导向。教师可以采用各种办法，积极引导学生围绕主题展开讨论，在学生各抒己见、集思广益、互相启发的基础上，灵活点拨，引导思考，适时讲解，帮助学生解决问题，达成对知识点的共识。

2. 启发性

在讨论中，教师要利用一些有助于引发学生深度思考并转变思维方式的教学策略，努力使学生开阔视野，活跃思路，学会思考，多侧面、多角度、全方位地认识问题，要提出一些带有启发性的问题，循循善诱，使学生在讨论中找到重点和要害，得出正确的结论。

3. 双向性

讨论是师生双方共同的思维活动，因此，教师在讨论中的谈话、讲述、讲解要有助于师生间信息的传递和沟通。这样，教师才能在讨论中及时发现问题，并通过有针对性的讲解，及时帮助学生解决讨论中的难点，使讨论达到预定目标。切忌教师包揽一切，信息单向传递，使"讨论式"变为"讲授式"。

四、病例讨论示例

1. 简单病例讨论

病史和主诉：患者女，25 岁，被汽车撞伤后左季肋部疼痛并伴有头晕、无力，撞伤后半小时被送往医院急诊科就诊。患者主诉左季肋部疼痛、头晕、无力。

体格检查：患者面色苍白、四肢冰冷、痛苦面容。体温 35℃，心率 115 次 / 分，血压 70/45 mmHg。全腹轻度压痛及腹胀、肌紧张，以左上腹明显。移动性浊音（＋），肠鸣音减弱，其他查体未见异常。

辅助检查：腹腔穿刺抽出不凝血。

问题：

（1）病人的初步诊断是什么？有何依据？

（2）病情的演变过程有哪些？

（3）病人的紧急处理原则有哪些？

2. 复杂病例讨论

病史和主诉：患者男，38 岁，半年前出现劳累后心悸、气短，1 个月前频发胸闷、气短、憋气，不能平卧，双下肢水肿，近 1 周发展至全身水肿。患者主诉咳喘、胸闷、端坐呼吸 3 日。无手术及输血史，无心肌梗死和心绞痛病史。

体格检查：患者端坐呼吸，气促，不能平卧，颈静脉怒张。血压 130/86 mmHg，心率 110 次 / 分。心界向左右两侧扩大，心尖区可闻及收缩期吹风样杂音，两肺遍布中小水泡音。腹部膨隆，移动性浊音阳性。肝大，锁骨中线肋下 6 cm，肝区叩痛。患者乳房以下身体不同程度凹陷性水肿。

心电图检查：窦性心动过速，心率 110~130 次 / 分，偶发室性期前收缩二联律。

超声检查：发现胸腔积液和腹水。各心腔均明显扩大，室壁弥漫性运动减弱，可见二尖瓣和三尖瓣瓣膜关闭不全。左心室舒张期末内径 77 mm（正常值 49 ± 4 mm），左心室收缩期末内径 67 mm（正常值 30 ± 5 mm），左心室射血分数 28%（正常值 50%~70%）。

诊断：慢性心力衰竭，室性期前收缩二联律。

治疗经过：入院后首先给予去乙酰毛花苷注射液 0.4 mg + 呋塞米 20 mg 静脉滴注，并针对心力衰竭和液体潴留采取了以下口服治疗措施。（qd，每天一次；tid，每天三次；bid，每天两次）

（1）控制液体潴留：　　　　　氢氯噻嗪　　　　50 mg qd

　　　　　　　　　　　　　　　呋塞米　　　　　20 mg qd

　　　　　　　　　　　　　　　螺内酯　　　　　40 mg tid

（2）强心：　　　　　　　　　地高辛　　　　　0.125 mg qd

（3）抗心室重塑：　　　　　　依那普利　　　　2.5 mg bid

问题：

（1）该患者的病程是如何演变的？病人为什么出现心脏扩张？

（2）患者心尖区为什么能听到收缩期吹风样杂音？其产生的机制如何？

（3）本病例治疗中应防止哪些水、电解质代谢紊乱发生？应采取哪些措施？

（4）哪些治疗措施可使扩张的心脏缩小？实施这些措施时应注意什么问题？

第二章　医学机能学实验中的动物实验

第一节　实验动物的分类及选择

一、实验动物的分类

实验动物是经人工培育、遗传背景清楚、对其微生物和寄生虫实行控制，用于科研、教学、生产、检测、鉴定及其他科学实验的动物。按遗传学特征分类，实验动物可分为近交系、封闭群和杂交群；按微生物、寄生虫控制程度分类，可分为普通动物、清洁级动物、无特定病原体动物和无菌动物。

1. 按遗传学特征分类

（1）近交系（inbred strain）：在一个动物群体中，任何个体基因组中99%以上的等位位点为纯合时定义为近交系。经典近交系是经至少连续20代的全同胞兄妹或亲子交配培育而成的品系，品系内所有个体都可以追溯到起源于第20代或以后代数的一对共同祖先。该品系动物在基因位点纯合性、遗传组成的同源性、独特性、遗传特征的可辨性、表型均一性和长期遗传的稳定性上均高度一致。但由于"近交衰退"现象，个体敏感，生活力、繁殖力等较差。常见的有 BALB/c 小鼠、C57BL/6J 小鼠、F344 大鼠、Lewis 大鼠等。

（2）封闭群（closed colony）：以非近亲交配方式进行繁殖生产的一个实验动物种群，在不从外部引入新个体的条件下，至少连续繁殖4代以上的群体。该群体动物在遗传组成杂合性、遗传特征的稳定性、繁殖率、抗病力上均有较好表现，同时存在许多有价值的突变基因。常用于药物筛选、毒理实验和教学使用等，常见的有昆明（KM）小鼠、ICR 小鼠、NIH 小鼠、Wistar 大鼠和新西兰兔等。

（3）杂交群（hybrid）：指由两个不同近交系杂交产生的后代群体，子一代动物简称F1。该群体的动物虽然基因不是纯合子，但其个体同样具有相同的基因型，在遗传和表型上的均质性高，同时克服了"近交衰退"现象，具有杂交优势，适应性和抗病力强，广泛地应用于营养、药物、病原和激素的生物评估等。

2. 按微生物学特征分类

（1）普通级动物（conventional animal）：指不携带所规定的人畜共患病病原体和动物烈性传染病原的动物。此类动物饲养于开放系统，主要有豚鼠、地鼠、实验猫、实验兔、实验犬和灵长类等。2003 年我国已经取消普通级的小鼠和大鼠。

（2）清洁级动物（clean animal）：指除普通级动物应排除的病原外，不携带对动物危害大和对科学研究干扰大的病原的实验动物，饲养于屏障环境中。该等级动物是我国特殊国情下的产物，随着国力提高，市场上已基本没有清洁级动物，部分省市地方标准中也已取消清洁级动物级别。

（3）无特定病原体级动物（specific pathogen free animal）：指除清洁动物应排除的病原外，不携带主要潜在感染或条件致病和对科学实验干扰大的病原的实验动物，简称SPF动物。此类动物饲养于屏障环境或隔离系统中，广泛应用于科学研究中，主要有大鼠、小鼠、豚鼠等。

（4）无菌动物（germ-free animal）：指不携带可检出的一切生命体的实验动物。在无菌动物体内人为植入一种或数种已知的微生物的动物，称为悉生动物（gnotobiotic animal）。无菌动物和悉生动物都必须饲养于隔离环境中，所接触的物品均须严格灭菌，广泛应用于微生态与各种疾病的关系研究、营养与代谢和抗肿瘤研究等。

二、实验动物的选择

医学机能学实验（medical functional experiment）是在人工控制的特定条件下，对生命现象进行客观的观察和分析，以获取生理学、病理生理学以及药理学知识。医学机能学的研究离不开实验动物，实验动物的选择是动物实验研究工作的重要环节，不同实验的研究目的不同、要求不同，选择的动物也各不相同，主要考虑的因素如下。

1. 选择质量合格的标准化实验动物

实验动物的质量包括遗传学质量和微生物学质量。实验动物都需要有明确的遗传背景，根据实验选择不同遗传学质量的近交系、封闭群或杂交群。实验动物的微生物学质量也是多样的，异常的病原微生物感染对动物实验结果正确与否有直接的影响。选用经遗传学、微生物学、营养学、环境卫生学的控制而培育的标准化实验动物，才能排除因实验动物带细菌、带病毒、带寄生虫和潜在疾病对实验结果的影响；也才能排除因实验动物遗传上不均一，导致的个体差异和反应不一致；便于把所获得的实验研究成果在国际间进行学术交流。

2. 选择符合实验目的和要求的实验动物

不同种属的动物具有各自不同的解剖、生理特点，熟悉并掌握这些种属的差异，选择合适的实验动物，能为动物实验提供很多便利条件，减少实验准备方面的麻烦，降低操作的难度，使实验容易成功，有助于获得理想的动物实验结果。如大鼠无胆囊，可用来做胆管插管，收集胆汁，进行消化功能方面的研究；兔的体型适中，性情比较温顺，耳朵较大，血管清晰，便于静脉反复注射，因此广泛应用于各系统生理学实验的研究，如血压、呼吸等急性实验；离体的蛙心能维持较长时间的活动，常用来进行心脏生理功能的研究；兔颈部的交感神经、迷走神经和降压神经都是独立走行、单独存在的，所以，可用以观察降压神经对心血管活动的影响，如果错选用犬或鸡，从大体解剖上很难找出降压神经，使实验无法进行。

3. 选择易获得、易饲养的实验动物

生理学实验研究用动物的种类虽然相当广泛，但在具体选择实验用动物时必须考虑所选择的实验动物是否容易得到，是否经济，是否易于饲养和管理。一般来说，兔、大鼠、小鼠和蟾蜍等数量多，来源广，又易于管理，是医学生理学研究最常用的实验动物。

4. 选择合适的动物个体

在选择实验动物时，动物的年龄、性别、体重也应考虑在内。一般实验选用成年动物，如内分泌腺体实验最好选择成年动物中较年轻的。若选用幼龄动物，由于幼龄时期机体的大部分内分泌腺体尚在发育，未达到标准状况或成熟阶段，其获得的结果不具有典型意义。此外，不同性别的动物对药物的敏感性不同，如用戊巴比妥钠对大鼠进行麻醉，雌性的敏感性是雄性的 2.5~3.8 倍；食盐急性毒性实验中，雌性小鼠较敏感，而雄性小鼠对慢性毒性较敏感。因此，在实验研究中，为了避免人为因素干扰，如无特别需要，选用实验动物时应雌雄个体数量大致相等，个体大小适中。

三、机能学实验常用的实验动物

1. 两栖类动物

（1）青蛙（frog）

①遗传背景：青蛙属于脊索动物门，脊椎动物亚门，属两栖纲，滑体亚纲，无尾目，蛙科，侧褶蛙属，黑斑侧褶蛙种的两栖类动物。

②生物学特性：青蛙颈部不明显，无肋骨。前肢的尺骨与桡骨合并，后肢的胫骨与腓骨合并，因此爪不能灵活转动，但四肢肌肉发达。蛙类的生殖特点是雌雄异体、水中受精，孵化成蝌蚪，用鳃呼吸，经过变异，成体主要用肺呼吸，兼用皮肤呼吸，属于卵生。心脏在离体以后，仍能较持久地节律性搏动。

（2）蟾蜍（toad）

①遗传背景：蟾蜍属于脊索动物门，脊椎动物亚门，属两栖纲，滑体亚纲，无尾目，蟾蜍科，蟾蜍属，蟾蜍蛙种的两栖类动物，体表有许多疙瘩，内有毒腺，俗称癞蛤蟆。在我国分为中华大蟾蜍和黑眶蟾蜍两种。成体蟾蜍是医学实验中常用的一种实验动物。

②生物学特性：蟾蜍身体宽短粗壮，全身皮肤极粗糙，体背布满大小不等的瘰疣，可分泌蟾蜍素。腹面不光滑、乳黄色，有棕色或黑色的细花斑，背面肤色随季节变化，且雌、雄不同，在繁殖季节时，雌性蟾蜍体表颜色较淡，雄性蟾蜍体表为黑绿色。

2. 啮齿类动物

（1）小鼠（mouse）

①遗传背景：小鼠属于脊索动物门，脊椎动物亚门，哺乳纲，啮齿目，鼠科，小鼠属，小鼠种，含20对染色体，是目前世界上用量最大、用途最广、品种（系）最多、研究最充分的一种实验动物。

②生物学特征：小鼠尾长约与体长相等，成年鼠尾长不大于 15.5 cm，尾部被有短毛

和环状角质鳞片。食管缺乏黏液分泌腺体，内壁有一层厚的角质化鳞状上皮，有利于灌胃操作；胃容量小（1.0~1.5 mL），功能较差，不耐饥饿；肠道较短，盲肠不发达；胆囊、胰脏分散在十二指肠、胃底及脾门处，色淡红，不规则，似脂肪组织；淋巴系统很发达，没有腭或咽扁桃体，外界刺激可使淋巴系统增生，易患淋巴系统疾病；无汗腺，尾有四条明显血管，背腹面各有一条动脉，两侧各有一条静脉。小鼠的基本生理参数：小鼠体温38（37~39）℃，心率600（328~780）次/分，呼吸频率163（84~230）次/分，收缩压113（95~125）mmHg，舒张压81（67~90）mmHg，血容量占体重的8.4%。

（2）大鼠（rat）

①遗传背景：大鼠属于脊索动物门，脊椎动物亚门，哺乳纲，啮齿目，鼠科，大鼠属，大鼠种，含21对染色体。实验大鼠为野生褐色鼠的后代，起源于亚洲，于14~18世纪传至欧洲，18世纪中期野生大鼠和白化变种鼠首次用于实验。

②生物学特征：外貌与小鼠相似，成年体重是小鼠的10倍多，大鼠汗腺极不发达，尾巴是散热器官，覆有短毛和环状角质鳞片。大鼠不能呕吐，因此不能用于做催吐实验。其肠道较短，盲肠较大，功能不发达；不耐饥饿，肠内不能合成维生素C；胰腺分散，位于十二指肠和胃弯曲处；无胆囊，胆汁通过胆总管直接进入十二指肠；胆总管括约肌松弛，不具有浓缩胆汁和贮存胆汁的功能。大鼠基本生理参数：大鼠的体温39（38.5~39.5）℃，心率475（370~580）次/分，呼吸频率85.5（66~114）次/分，麻醉时收缩压116（88~138）mmHg，舒张压91（58~145）mmHg，血容量占体重的7.4%。

（3）豚鼠（guinea pig）

①遗传背景：豚鼠属于脊索动物门，脊椎动物亚门，哺乳纲，啮齿目，豚鼠科，豚鼠种，染色体共32对。1780年，Laviser首次用豚鼠做热原试验。由于豚鼠具有易于在实验室内饲养、易于实验操作以及适用于医学、生物学研究的多种特性，在19世纪和20世纪初，豚鼠逐渐在科学研究用动物中占有了突出的地位。

②生物学特性：豚鼠耳蜗管发达，听觉灵敏，听域远大于人，常用于听力实验；其消化系统有典型的草食性动物特征，咀嚼肌发达，胃壁很薄，黏膜呈皱襞状，胃容量约为20~30 mL；肠管较长，约为体长的10倍，盲肠发达，约占腹腔容积的1/3，充满时，大约占体重15%；食量大，对粗纤维消化能力强，消化率达到38.2%。豚鼠体内缺乏左旋葡萄糖内酯氧化酶，自身不能合成维生素C；对抗生素处理敏感，尤其是青霉素，还有杆菌肽、红霉素、金霉素等，轻则发生肠炎，重则造成死亡；对组胺等物质极其敏感，常用于哮喘模型的制作和抗过敏实验。

3. 哺乳类动物

（1）兔（rabbit）

①遗传背景：兔属于脊索动物门，脊椎动物亚门，哺乳纲，兔形目，兔科，真兔属，含22对染色体。生物医学研究应用的家兔是由野生穴兔经过驯化而育成，多为欧洲兔的后代。

②生物学特征：家兔耳廓大，血管清晰，便于血管注射和采血。兔眼球大，适于眼科

研究。家兔为单胃，胃底特别大，小肠和大肠的总长度为体长的 10 倍。盲肠发达，占腹腔的 1/3。在回盲处有特有的圆小囊，囊壁富有淋巴滤泡，其黏膜不断外泌碱性液体，可以中和盲肠中微生物分解纤维素所产生的各种有机酸，有利于消化吸收。颈神经血管束中降压神经易于分离，其末梢分布在主动脉弓血管内，属于传入性神经。

（2）犬（dog）

①遗传背景：犬属于脊索动物门，脊椎动物亚门，哺乳纲，食肉目，犬科，犬属，犬种动物，含 39 对染色体，常用于动物实验的品种是比格犬。

②生物学特征：犬是红绿色盲，故不能用红绿色作条件刺激进行条件反射实验。犬具有发达的血液循环和神经系统，内脏与人相似，比例也近似；胸廓大，心脏较大；肠道短，约为体长的 5 倍；肝较大，胰腺分左右两叶，胰岛小，数量多；皮肤汗腺极不发达，趾垫有少许汗腺。雄犬无精囊和尿道球腺，有一块阴茎骨。雌犬有乳头 4~5 对。

第二节　医学机能学动物实验的基本操作

掌握正确的动物实验操作技巧可以有效防止实验者被动物咬伤抓伤或被锐器扎伤，同时也能最大限度地减少实验动物应激、维持动物正常生理状态，保证实验动物福利和实验的顺利进行。

一、两栖类动物实验基本操作技能

1. 抓取与固定

蛙类一般不伤人，固定比较容易。用左手握持动物，以左手食指和中指夹住左前肢，用左拇指按住右前肢，拉直后肢，再用无名指和小指夹住即可，右手进行给药等操作。对蛙和蟾蜍进行毁髓等复杂操作或手术时，可选择将其背部向上固定，拇指压住其背部，用食指压住其头部前端，使头向前俯，中指抵住其胸部，使得其头部与脊柱相连处凸起（图 2-1A）。当进行解剖或其他生理学实验时，也可根据需要选择解剖台或固定板，按照实验需要体位，用钉或针将四肢固定于板上。由于蟾蜍两耳部突起的毒腺可喷射毒性较强的毒汁，所以在捉拿固定时，切勿挤按其局部，以避免毒汁射进眼中。

2. 毁髓操作

根据图 2-1A 方法固定后找到枕骨大孔，右手将探针经枕骨大孔垂直刺入，再向其头部方向推进刺入颅腔，并左右摆动探针捣毁脑组织。退回探针，针尖转向其后肢方向与脊柱平行插入椎管，一边深入一边旋转破坏脊髓（图 2-1B~D）。

3. 给药（淋巴囊注射）

由于蛙的皮肤弹性差，针头刺破后皮肤不易闭合使得药液外溢，故注射时针头须通过一层隔膜再进入皮下淋巴囊。腹淋巴囊给药时，针头自大腿上端刺入，经过大腿肌层入腹壁肌层，再进入腹壁皮下淋巴囊。注射量为每只 0.25~1 mL。

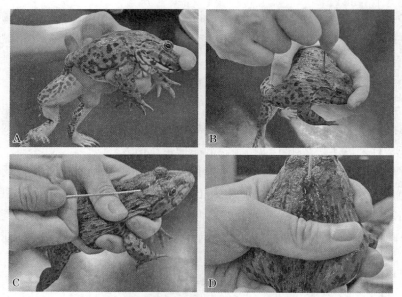

图 2-1　两栖类动物的抓取、固定与毁髓操作

二、啮齿类动物实验基本操作技能

1. 抓取与固定

（1）小鼠的抓取与固定：有双手抓取法、单手抓取法和固定器固定法三种方法。

双手抓取法（图 2-2A~C）：用一只手抓取鼠尾根部提起，置于鼠笼或粗糙台面上，向后轻拉鼠尾。当小鼠向前爬行时，用另一只手的拇指和食指抓住小鼠的两耳及颈部皮肤。翻转手掌，掌心向上，将鼠体置于手掌心中，拉直后肢，使鼠体呈一条直线，用无名指按住鼠尾，小指按住后肢即可。注意捏住的皮肤要适量，太多太紧会导致小鼠窒息，太少太松小鼠会回头咬伤实验操作者。

单手抓取法（图 2-2D~F）：抓取时，用一只手（一般是左手）的拇指与食指捏住鼠尾后端，无名指和小指将鼠尾根部按压在手心的后部，然后松开拇指和食指，再用拇指和食指抓住小鼠两耳及颈部的皮肤，固定后翻转过来即可。本方法适用于操作熟练的实验人员，或一只手已持器械、药品或避免污染等情况。

固定器固定法（图 2-2G~I）：需要进行尾静脉注射或采血等操作时，可将小鼠装入塑料、有机玻璃、金属等材料制成的小鼠固定器中。抓取小鼠尾部，使小鼠接近固定器，待其钻入后固定好位置或盒盖，使尾巴留在外面供操作。

（2）大鼠的抓取与固定：抓取及固定固定方法基本与小鼠相同。大鼠较安静时右手捏住鼠尾根部提起。不能抓尾尖，也不能悬空时间过长。对于体重比较大的大鼠，应该用另一只手托住大鼠的前半部躯体。在大鼠向前爬行时，用另一只手拇指和食指抓住大鼠两耳及颈部皮肤，其他 3 个手指抓住大鼠背部皮肤，翻转手掌使大鼠呈仰卧位，使大鼠身体呈一条直线，右手固定后肢和尾部（图 2-3A~C）。给药时，用左手的拇指和食指抓住大鼠颈

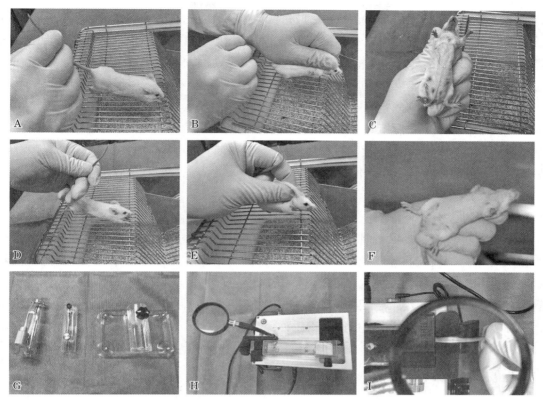

图 2-2　小鼠的抓取与固定

（参见彩插）

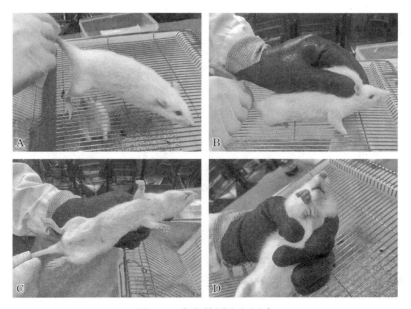

图 2-3　大鼠的抓取与固定

背部皮肤，其余3指抓住背部，固定后肢；或者拇指和食指扣住大鼠颈部，使其头部不得随意转动，其前肢固定或形成十字交叉，其余3指将躯干部固定于手掌，即可进行一般的操作（图2-3D）。在进行一些特殊需求操作时，也可使用大鼠固定器进行固定。大鼠在惊恐或被激怒时易将实验操作者咬伤，故抓取时应注意安全，初学者应佩戴帆布防咬手套。

（3）豚鼠的抓取与固定：豚鼠性情非常温顺，一般不会咬人。抓取幼小豚鼠时，可以双手捧起来。抓取成熟豚鼠时，先用一只手掌迅速扣住鼠背，抓住其肩胛上方，以拇指和食指环握颈部，中指和无名指轻轻扣住胸廓；或像抓取大鼠一样抓住双耳及颈背部皮肤，另一只手托住臀部。体重小者可用一只手抓取，体重大者抓取时宜用双手。

2. 给药

（1）灌胃：用量准确，适用于急性毒性实验。

小鼠灌胃法（图2-4A）：将针尖圆滑的灌胃针接在注射器上，吸入药液，一只手抓住小鼠双耳及颈部皮肤将动物抓取固定，体位为头高尾低（头高位），另一只手持注射器，将灌胃针从动物嘴部侧面插入动物口中，再轻轻摆正并沿口腔顶壁和咽后壁缓慢插入食管。针插入时应无阻力，若感到阻力或动物挣扎时，应立即停止进针或将针拔出，以免损伤或穿破食管或误入气管。注射完药液后，轻轻退出胃管，动作宜轻柔，以免损伤食管及膈肌。当灌胃针插入3~4 cm，见有胃液回流时，即可将药物注入。灌胃量应不超过体重的1%，小鼠单次灌胃量0.2~1 mL。

大鼠灌胃法（图2-4B）：与小鼠基本相同，灌胃针进入深度约为4~6 cm左右。为防止插入气管，可先回抽注射器针栓，若无空气抽出说明不在气管内，即可注药。大鼠单次灌药量1~4 mL。

豚鼠灌胃法与大鼠和小鼠基本相同，单次灌药量1~5 mL。

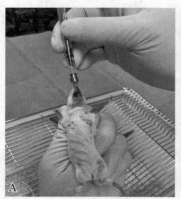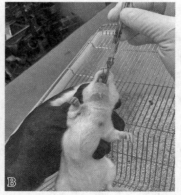

图2-4　大、小鼠的灌胃

（2）注射

①皮下注射：是将药物推进皮下结缔组织，经毛细血管、淋巴管吸收进入血液的循环过程。小鼠通常在背部进行皮下注射，具体操作为局部消毒后，左手拇指、食指捏起皮肤，使其呈三角窝，右手持注射器垂直于皮下凹窝，迅速刺入皮肤，刺入后放开左手，抽

动针栓若无回血，即可注射（图2-5）。大鼠皮下注射部位可在背部或后肢外侧皮下，操作时轻轻提起注射部位皮肤，将注射针头刺入皮下，推注药液。豚鼠皮下注射部位可选两肢内侧、背部、肩部等皮下脂肪少的部位。通常选择大腿内侧，注射针头与皮肤呈45°刺入皮下，确定针头在皮下推入药液，拔出针头后，拇指轻压注药部位。针头拔出后，以左手在针刺部位轻轻捏住皮肤片刻，以防药液流出。正确刺入皮下时，针头可自由摆动。如若给药剂量大，可分点注射。

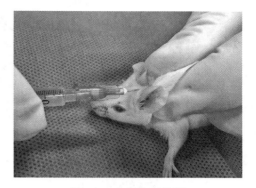

图2-5　小鼠皮下注射

②皮内注射：是将药液注入皮肤的表皮与真皮之间，多用于接种或过敏试验。注射时，先对注射部位进行脱毛处理，后以左手将皮肤捏成皱襞，右手持注射器使针头与皮肤呈30°刺入皮肤内，注射完成后注射部位应呈现小丘疹状隆起。皮内注射若推入阻力小，表明注于皮下，应重新进针。注射完成后不要用力压迫，以免药液流出。

③腹腔注射：吸收能力很强，注射剂量可以大些。小鼠做腹腔注射时，以左手抓取动物，使腹部向上，呈头低尾高位，并逆毛消毒；右手持注射器将针头刺入左（或右）下腹部皮下，使针头向前推0.5 cm，再以45°斜穿过腹肌，此时有抵抗力消失的落空感，固定针头，回抽无液体，即可缓慢注入药液（图2-6）。一次可注射量为0.1~0.2 mL/10 g体重。腹腔注射时切勿使针头向上注射，以防刺伤内脏。大鼠、豚鼠的腹腔注射可参照小鼠腹腔注射法。

④肌肉注射：小鼠肌肉注射，可将动物固定后，一手拉直动物一侧后肢，另一手持注射器刺入后肢大腿外侧肌肉内注液（图2-7）。小鼠一次注射量每只不超过0.1 mL。

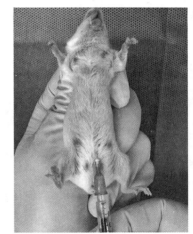

图2-6　小鼠腹腔注射

大鼠、豚鼠的肌肉注射具体操作方法与小鼠基本一致，大鼠和豚鼠一次注射量每只不超过0.5 mL。

⑤静脉注射：小鼠多采用尾静脉注射，一般选择左右侧边的两条静脉，并从尾远端（距尾尖1/3处）皮肤薄处开始注射，容易刺入。先将小鼠固定于固定器内，将尾巴留在外面。注射前以右手食指轻弹尾部，或先将鼠尾浸入40~50℃温水中，或用酒精擦拭使血管扩张，并软化表皮角质；再用手指夹住尾巴根部，阻断尾静脉血流，使之充盈；而后从下托起尾巴，手持注射器平行于尾巴呈一定角度（15°~30°）刺入静脉（图2-8A）。刺入后先回抽看是否有回血，若有回血且推注药液无阻力、沿静脉血管可见一条白线说明针头正确刺入血管内。一次注射量为0.05~0.1 mL/10 g体重。黑色小鼠尾部血管不易被看见，可采用带有灯光的尾静脉注射仪帮助确认血管（图2-8B），提高成功率。月龄较小或体形较小

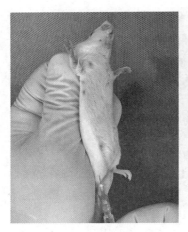

图 2-7　小鼠肌肉注射

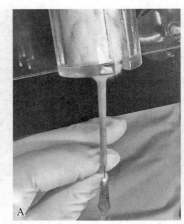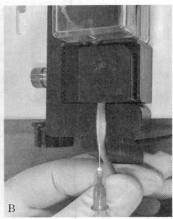

图 2-8　小鼠尾静脉注射

（参见彩插）

的小鼠，可选用胰岛素注射器进行注射。大鼠的静脉注射操作方法与小鼠基本一致，但大鼠的尾部皮肤表面有较厚的鳞片，穿刺比较困难，可选择在距离尾侧 1/4~1/3 处进针。

3. 采血

大、小鼠的采血方法基本通用，可根据采血量、采血频率、血型及检测目的选择合适的采血方式。

（1）剪尾采血：这种方法适用于采血量少的实验，如血细胞计数。采血前宜先使鼠尾充血，可用 50℃水浸泡，擦干并消毒尾部后，剪去尾尖 1~2 mm 采血，自尾根部向尾尖按摩，血即自尾尖流出。采血完成后用棉球压迫止血并用 6% 液体火棉胶涂在伤口处止血。每次采血量最多 0.1 mL。

（2）割尾采血：使用锋利的刀片在尾巴上割破一段静脉，血由切口流出，可以交替切割并从尾尖部开始。采血完成后可用棉球按压止血。

（3）眼眶后静脉丛采血：本方法适用于短期重复采血，小鼠一次可采血 0.2~0.3 mL，大鼠一次可采血 0.5~1.0 mL。首先准备好玻璃毛细管，临用前折断成 1~1.5 cm 长，根据需要浸入抗凝剂中，取出干燥。采血前动物需要麻醉，采血时左手拇指和食指抓住鼠双耳及颈背部皮肤，使头部固定，轻轻压迫颈部两侧，阻碍静脉回流，使眼球充分外凸、眼眶静脉丛充血；右手持毛细管尖端刺入内眼角与眼球之间，轻轻向眼底部方向移动，并旋转毛细管以切开静脉丛，保持毛细管水平位，小鼠刺入 2~3 mm，大鼠刺入 4~5 mm，当感觉有阻力时即停止刺入，血液即流出（图 2-9）。采血完成后立即拔出毛细管，放松左手并用棉球按压即可止血。小鼠、大鼠、豚鼠均可采用此法采血。

（4）心脏采血：动物麻醉后背卧固定，心前区被毛消毒，右手持注射器，在左侧 3~4 肋间心尖冲动最明显处垂直进针刺入，抽出血液（图 2-10A）。也可从上腹部进针穿过横膈膜刺入心室采血，动作宜轻柔（图 2-10B）。大、小鼠均可用此法采血。

（5）摘眼球采血：小鼠麻醉后，左手抓住小鼠双耳及颈背部皮肤使眼球突出，并

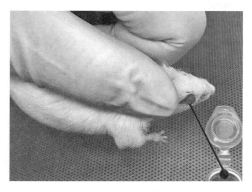

图 2-9　小鼠眼眶后静脉丛采血

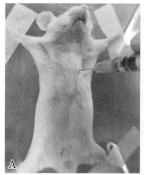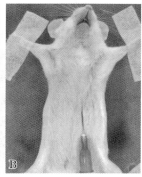

图 2-10　小鼠心脏采血

将小鼠侧卧位放置，右手持眼科弯镊夹取眼球根部迅速摘除眼球，血液即从眼眶流出（图2-11）。一般可取得相当于动物体重4%~5%的血液量。采血完成动物即死亡，只适用于一次性采血。

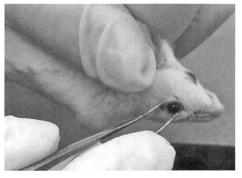

图 2-11　小鼠摘眼球采血

三、哺乳类动物实验基本操作技能

1. 抓取与固定

（1）徒手固定法：连同耳部抓取兔颈背部皮肤一起提起，后用另一只手托住其臀部使兔体重主要落在这只手上（图2-12A）。兔一般不咬人，但其爪锐利，当其被捉拿挣扎时，极易引起操作人员被抓伤，应防避其四肢的活动。另外不能只提拿兔双耳、双后腿、腰或背部皮肤以避免造成兔耳、肾、颈椎的损伤或皮下出血。

（2）固定器固定法：麻醉后兔的固定一般采用盒式固定架或台式固定架（图2-12B）。适用于耳缘静脉采血、注射、血压测定等外科手术性实验。

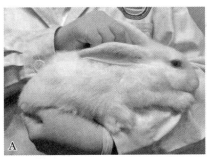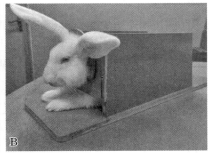

图 2-12　兔的抓取与固定

2. 给药

（1）灌胃法：适用于急性毒性实验，用量准确。

给兔、犬等动物灌胃时，应使用开口器，避开动物臼齿和犬齿，以免咬坏灌胃管。用兔固定器将兔固定，操作者将开口器横放于兔口中，将兔舌压在开口器下面，将胃管经开口器中央小孔插入，慢慢沿兔口腔顶壁插入食管约 15~18 cm。插管完成后将胃管的外口端放入水杯中，如有气泡从胃管逸出，说明不在食管内而是在气管内，应拔出来重插；如无气泡逸出，则可将药推入，每次灌入液量可达 80~120 mL。灌胃完毕，可用少量清水冲洗胃管，然后拔出。拔出胃管时，应捏住胃管的开口端，慢慢抽出；接近咽喉部时，动作应加快，迅速通过，以防残留液体进入咽喉、气管。

（2）口服法：适用于慢性实验和固体剂型药物。

口服法是把药物混入饲料或饮水中让动物自由摄取。此方法优点是简单方便，缺点是不能准确定量，且动物个体间差异较大。大动物给药时，如药物为固体剂型时，可直接将药物用镊子或手指放入实验动物口中，设法使其口服咽下。

（3）注射给药

①耳缘静脉注射：兔耳部血管分布清晰，耳中央是一条动脉，外缘是静脉。因内缘静脉较深且不易固定，故较少使用，而外缘静脉较浅且容易固定，故较常用。耳缘静脉沿耳背后缘行走，剪除其表面皮肤上的毛并用酒精湿润局部后血管即显现。注射前可先轻弹或揉擦耳尖部并轻压耳根部，使耳缘静脉充血。尽可能从远心端进针，用左手食指和中指夹住静脉近心端，无名指和小指垫在耳下，先刺破皮肤再刺入静脉，后顺着血管平行方向深入 0.5~1 cm，松开食指和中指，左手拇指和食指移至针头刺入部位压住，将针头与兔耳固定后推入液体（图 2-13）。若注射时阻力较大或出现局部肿胀，说明针头没有刺入静脉，应立即拔出针头，在原注射点的近心端重新刺入。注射完拔出针头，用碘酒棉球压在针孔上止血。若实验过程中需多次静脉给药，可用头皮针注射并用动脉夹将针头与兔耳固定以备用。

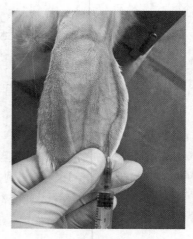

图 2-13　兔耳缘静脉注射

②腹腔注射：兔腹腔注射时，需将兔仰卧位固定，使其腹部朝上，并剪去下腹部注射部位的被毛。注射位置位于下腹部近腹白线两侧 1 cm 处，呈 45° 刺入，当针头穿过腹肌有落空感时，说明针头已经进入腹腔；固定针头，如回抽无液体，即可进行注射。

③皮下注射：兔皮下注射方法参照小鼠皮下注射法，选择组织疏松部位的皮下进行注射，多为颈部和肩部（图 2-14）。

④肌肉注射：通常在后腿肌肉处进行注射，将兔固定后，酒精消毒被毛，左手手指将注射部位的皮肤绷紧，右手持注射器与皮肤呈 60°，迅速刺入肌肉，回抽无回血，即可进行注射（图 2-15）。一次注射量不超过 2 mL。

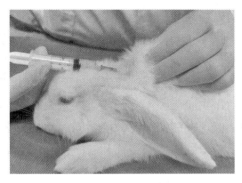
图 2-14　兔皮下注射

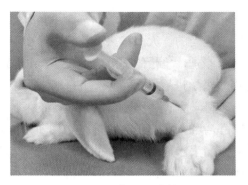
图 2-15　兔肌肉注射

⑤皮内注射：首先，剪去皮内注射区域的被毛，然后用脱毛剂进行脱毛，间隔 1 天后才可进行皮内注射，注射方法与大、小鼠相同，一次性注射量约为 0.1 mL。

3. 采血

（1）耳缘静脉采血：操作方法与耳缘静脉注射给药方法相同（图 2-13）。局部去毛使血管扩张，注射器穿刺成功后即可抽血；也可只用针头不连接注射器，让血液直接滴在有抗凝剂的容器内；还可以用刀片割破耳缘静脉，让血液自然流出滴入有抗凝剂的容器内。采血完成后，用纱布或棉球压迫止血，采血量每次 5~10 mL。

（2）耳中央动脉采血：兔耳中央有一根较粗，颜色鲜红的中央动脉。采血方法与兔耳缘静脉采血方法类似。将兔用固定器固定后，左手固定兔耳，右手持注射器在中央动脉的远心端沿着与动脉平行的向心方向刺入动脉，穿刺成功即可见动脉血进入针管。由于兔耳中央动脉容易发生痉挛，故抽血前必须让兔耳充分充血，且动作要轻柔。采血用针头过细或室内温度较低均不利于采血。

（3）心脏采血：兔麻醉后仰卧固定，并对进针区域剪毛、消毒。在左侧第 3~4 肋间处，或以左手食指触摸到心脏搏动最明显处为进针点，将采血针垂直刺入胸腔，进针深度约 3 cm，当有落空感时，可感觉到针尖随心脏有节律搏动，此时说明已插入心脏，即有血液进入注射器内。如此时还无血液流入注射器，可边退针（或进针）边抽吸，一旦抽到血液，立即固定针头。针头只能上、下垂直进退针，不可在胸腔内左右摆动，以免刺破心脏。

第三节　实验动物福利与动物实验伦理

一、概述

动物在科学中的使用可以追溯到公元前 3 世纪的埃里斯特拉图斯和赫拉菲勒斯以及公元 2 世纪的盖伦。人类从自身利益出发对动物的使用会造成某些道德困境。一些人认为动物有权利，使用它们是错误的，无论是食用、研究用、役用还是作为宠物饲养，甚至包括把它们当作害虫杀死。另一个群体认为，人类以任何我们认为合适的方式使用动物都是可以被接受的。大多数人介于这两个极端之间。几十年来，关于动物实验的争论此起彼伏，从未停止，争论的部分内容与一个世纪前基本相同。一个重要论点是，动物实验是否对重要的医学进展不可或缺。许多反对团体认为，动物实验从来没有带来任何医学进步，它误导了科学家，并且随着替代技术的发展，活动物实验已经没有必要了。毫无疑问，在现代麻醉药和止痛药出现之前，它确实是残酷的。但现在的情况已大不相同：动物医学的进步使无痛手术成为可能，并且动物使用者都强烈意识到维护动物福利的必要性。不论在过去还是将来，动物实验在医学进步中都发挥着重要作用。

二、实验动物福利

世界动物保护协会（World Animal Protection）2000 年世界大会上，提出了针对动物福利立法的五大自由：享有不受饥渴的自由，即保证充足清洁的饮用水和食物；享有生活舒适的自由，即提供适当的生活栖息场所；享有不受痛苦伤害的自由，即保证动物不受额外的痛苦，并得到充分适当的医疗待遇；享有生活无恐惧和悲伤的自由，即避免各种使动物遭受精神创伤的状况；享有表达天性的自由，即提供适当的条件，使动物天性不受外来条件的影响而被压抑。实验动物的福利不是片面地保护动物，而是在兼顾对动物利用的同时，考虑动物的福利状况，并反对使用那些极端手段和方式。哈斯汀斯中心（The Hastings Center）关于动物研究伦理的报告指出，"动物福利与确保对动物的人道待遇有关：包括保持良好的健康，最大限度地减少痛苦等负面状态，增强积极状态，并让动物自由地表达自然天性"。良好的动物福利还需要疾病预防和兽医治疗，为其提供适当的庇护所、管理、营养、人道处理和人道屠宰。

三、动物实验的"3R"原则

1959 年，英国动物学家 W.M.S.Russel 和微生物学家 R.L.Burch 共同提出了以动物实验和实验动物减少、替代和优化为核心的动物实验替代方法理论。随着人们理解的不断加深，"3R"（减少、替代和优化）原则已经成为实验动物福利的核心价值观。

减少（reduction）是指如果某一研究方案中必须使用实验动物，同时又没有可行的替代方法，则应把使用动物的数量降低到实现科研目的所需的最小量。替代（replacement）是指使用低知觉或没有知觉的实验材料代替活体动物，或使用低等动物替代高等动物进行实验，并获得相同实验效果的科学方法。优化（refinement）是指通过为动物提供适宜的生活条件，改善和完善实验程序，避免、减少或减轻实验给动物造成的疼痛和不安，保证动物实验结果的可靠性、精确性和代表性，提高实验动物福利的科学方法。

1993 年，美国芝加哥"伦理化研究国际基金会"在"3R"的基础上，增加了"责任"（responsibility）作为第 4 个原则。在动物实验中增强伦理观念，呼吁实验者对人类和动物都要有责任感。提倡动物福利并不等于不能利用动物和进行动物实验，而是如何合理、人道地利用动物，实现科研需要和善待动物福利的平衡。

四、动物实验的伦理审查

为了使动物实验符合伦理要求，研究人员应该分析实验的动机：进行动物实验是否有充分的理由？是否有其他替代实验方法？因此，在开展动物实验之前甚至在动物实验过程中，必须应用"3R"原则来评估动物实验，考虑如何减少动物遭受的痛苦。

伦理审查的原则包括必要性原则、保护原则、福利原则、伦理原则、利益平衡性原则、公正性原则、合法性原则以及符合国情原则。审查内容包括实验的目的、必要性、意义和实验设计，拟使用动物的信息（包括选择实验动物种类和数量的原因），对动物造成的可预期的伤害及防控措施（包括麻醉、镇痛、仁慈终点和安乐死等），动物替代、减少动物用量、降低动物痛苦伤害的主要措施及利害分析等。

动物实验的伦理审查在科研项目的申请、实施等阶段越来越受科技工作者和科研管理单位的重视，各省及各使用单位均设立了严格审查机制；而教学用实验动物的伦理审查一直不受重视，教学实验动物的使用者均是未来科学研究的从业人员，其伦理审查更应该引起重视。暨南大学教学实验动物伦理申请于每学期伊始向大学实验动物伦理委员会提出实验伦理审核申请，不断优化实验方案及操作手段。

第四节　BL-420 生物数据采集和分析系统简介

一、BL-420 系统概述

BL-420 生物数据采集和分析系统（简称 BL-420 系统）是配置在计算机上的 4 通道生物信号采集、放大、显示、记录和处理系统，可应用于生理、药理、毒理和病理等实验，是研究生物机能活动的主要设备和手段之一。它由计算机、BL-420 系统硬件和 BL-420F 生物信号显示与处理软件（简称 BL-420F 软件）三个主要部分构成，如图 2-16 所示。

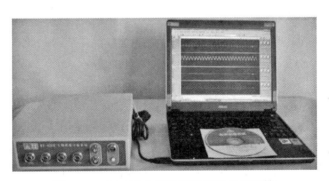

图 2-16　BL-420 生物数据采集和分析系统

二、BL-420 系统原理

在生物电信号或通过传感器引入的生物非电信号的检测中，往往会因为信号非常微弱（比如降压神经放电，其信号为微伏级信号），或生物信号中夹杂的幅度比生物电信号本身的强度还要大的众多声、光、电等干扰信号（比如电网的 50/60 Hz 信号），导致有用的生物机能信号无法被观察到。BL-420 系统的工作原理（图 2-17）是首先将原始的生物机能信号进行放大、滤波等处理，然后对处理的信号通过模数转换进行数字化并将数字化后的生物机能信号传输到计算机内部，计算机则通过专用的生物机能实验系统软件（BL-420F 软件）接收从生物机能信号放大、采集卡传入的数字信号，然后对这些收到的信号进行实时处理，进行生物机能波形的显示及生物机能信号的存贮，并根据使用者的命令对数据进行处理和分析，如平滑滤波、微积分和频谱分析。

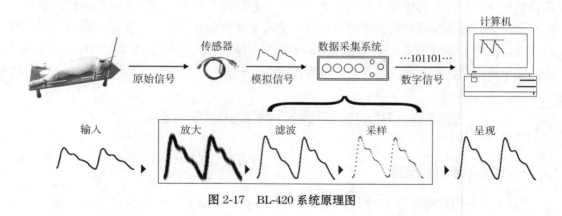

图 2-17　BL-420 系统原理图

三、BL-420F 软件工具条介绍

BL-420F 软件的整个工具条参见图 2-18。

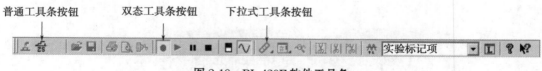

图 2-18　BL-420F 软件工具条

工具条是一组命令的集合，它把一些常用的命令以方便、直观（图形形式）的方式呈现在使用者面前。工具条上的每一个图形按钮称为工具条按钮，当工具条按钮以雕刻效果（灰色）显示时，表明该工具条按钮当前不可用，不会响应用户输入。

BL-420F 软件的主工具条上共有 23 个工具条按钮和一个特殊实验标记编辑选择组框，其中有两个工具条按钮是下拉式工具条按钮。

下面对工具条按钮命令做详细的介绍。

1. 系统复位

系统复位命令用于对 BL-420 系统的所有硬件及软件参数进行复位，即将这些参数设置为默认值。这个命令在系统处于非实时实验及反演状态时起作用。

2. 零速采样

零速采样命令与暂停命令相似，在实时状态下执行该命令会导致波形停止移动，并且停止任何数据的存盘记录，但波形的变化会在屏幕的新数据出现端显示，测量的最新点数据值也在硬件参数调节区的右上角显示。这个命令主要用于观察极慢速信号的变化，比如，1 h 后才会发生变化的信号可使用这个功能进行观察。这个命令在系统处于实时采样状态时起作用。

3. 打开

该命令用于打开一个以前记录的数据文件（.tme 类型文件）。BL-420F 软件对记录原始数据波形数据的文件默认采用"temp.tme"的命名方法。

4. 另存为

选择此命令，将弹出"另存为"对话框，如图 2-19 所示。"另存为"命令只在数据反演时起作用，该功能可以将正在反演的数据文件另外起一个名字进行存贮，或将该文件存贮到其他目录下。

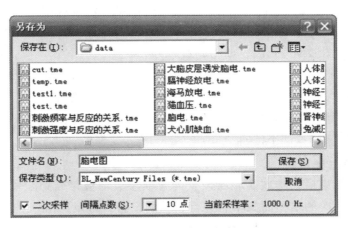

图 2-19 "另存为"对话框

5. 打印

该命令为打印当前屏幕显示波形。选择该命令，首先会弹出"定制打印对话框"，如图 2-20 所示。

设置"打印整个文件"参数，将把反演的整个数据文件打印出来。一般情况下，不要轻易设置这个参数，因为一个文件的数据包含很多无效数据，通常需要打印几十页打印纸。较好的做法是用数据剪辑功能将有用数据剪辑在一起组成一个较小的数据文件，再使用打印整个文件功能。

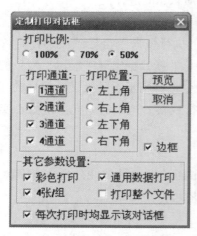

图 2-20　定制打印对话框

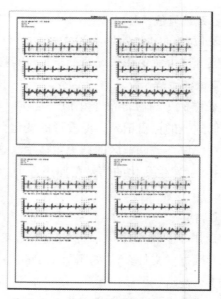

图 2-21　打印预览图形（4 张／组）

6. 打印预览

选择该命令，首先会弹出"定制打印对话框"，如图 2-20 所示。根据该对话框选择好打印参数之后，按下"预览"命令按钮可以进入到打印预览状态，打印预览显示的波形与从打印机打印出的图形是一致的，如图 2-21 所示。

注意：打印和打印预览功能与通道显示窗口相联系。当进行数据反演或实时实验时，如想使用打印或打印预览功能，需要将通道显示窗口设置为激活状态，否则这两个功能按钮为灰色，不能使用。如果在打印时这两个按钮为灰色，只需在任何一个通道显示窗口中单击鼠标左键即可激活这两个按钮。

7. 上一次实验配置

当一次实验结束后，本次实验所设置的各项参数均被存贮到配置文件 config.las 中，如果想要重复上一次的实验而又不想进行繁琐的设置，可以点击"上一次实验配置"命令，计算机将自动把实验参数设置成与上一次实验时完全相同。

8. 数据记录

"数据记录"命令是一个双态命令，即每执行一次命令，其所代表的状态就改变一次。当记录命令按钮的红色实心圆标记处于按下状态时说明系统正处于记录状态，否则系统仅处于观察状态而不进行观察数据的记录。

9. 开始

选择该命令，将启动数据采集，并将采集到的实验数据显示在计算机屏幕上；如果数据采集处于暂停状态，选择该命令，将继续启动波形显示；反演时，该命令用于启动波形的自动播放。

10. ▮▮ 暂停

选择该命令，将暂停数据采集与波形动态显示；反演时，该命令用于暂停波形的自动播放。

11. ▮ 停止

选择该命令，将结束当前实验，同时发出"系统复位"命令，使整个系统处于开机时的默认状态，但该命令不复位已设置的屏幕参数，如通道背景颜色，基线显示开关等；反演时，该命令用于停止反演。

12. ▮ 切换背景颜色

选择该命令，显示通道的背景颜色将在黑色和白色这两种颜色中进行切换。不管以前设置的通道背景颜色是什么，该命令无条件将背景设置为黑色或白色。

13. ∿ 格线显示

这是一个双态命令，用于显示或隐藏背景标尺格线。

14. ✎ 测量

测量按钮是一个下拉式工具按钮，在这个按钮上按住鼠标左键不放将弹出一个下拉式子工具条，如图 2-22 所示。这个子工具条上包括 4 个与测量相关的命令："区间测量""两点测量""频率测量""心功能参数测量"。

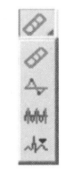

图 2-22　测量子工具条

（1）✎ 区间测量：该命令用于测量任意通道波形中选择波形段的时间差、频率、最大值、最小值、平均值、峰-峰值、面积、最大上升速度及最大下降速度等参数，测量的结果显示在通用信息显示区中。如果测量过程中 Excel 电子表格被打开，那么测量的数据将同时被写入到 Excel 电子表格中。

区间测量步骤：

①单击"区间测量"命令按钮，此时将暂停波形扫描；

②将鼠标移动到需要进行区间测量的波形段（任意通道中）的起点位置，单击鼠标左键进行确定，此时将出现一条垂直直线，代表选择的区间测量起点；

③移动鼠标，另一条垂直直线出现并随鼠标左右移动而移动，在通道显示窗的右上角将动态地显示两条垂直直线之间的时间差，单击鼠标左键确定终点；

④此时，在两条垂直直线区间内将出现一条水平直线（图 2-23），该直线用来确定频率计数的基线（对心电信号进行区间测量时，心率分析采用模板分析法，故水平基线不作

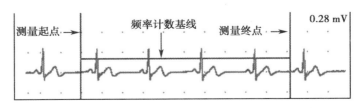

图 2-23　区间测量示意图

为频率计数线）。水平基线会随鼠标的上下移动而移动，其所在位置的值将显示在通道的右上角，按下鼠标左键确定该基线的位置，完成本次区间测量；

⑤重复步骤②～④，对不同通道内的不同波形段进行区间测量；

⑥在任何通道中单击鼠标右键都将结束本次区间测量。

（2）　两点测量：该命令用于测量任意通道中，某段波形的最大值、最小值、平均值、峰-峰值、两点之间的时间差、信号的变化速率及变化率，这些信息均显示在通用信息显示区中。其中，信号的变化速率指相对于时间的变化量，即第二点的值减去第一点的值然后再除以两点间的时间差得到，单位为 mV/ms；信号的变化率指相对于第一点值的变化量，即第二点的值减去第一点的值然后再除以第一点的值得到，单位为 %。

两点测量步骤：

①单击"两点测量"命令按钮，此时将暂停波形扫描；

②在要测量的波形段的起点位置单击鼠标左键确定第一点位置。此时，会出现一根红色的直线，一端固定在确定的第一点上，另一端随着鼠标的移动而移动，用于确定第二点；

③确定第二点后，单击鼠标左键，红色直线固定，完成本次两点测量（图 2-24）；

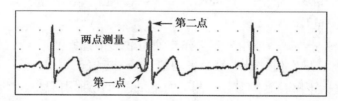

图 2-24　两点测量示意图
（参见彩插）

④重复步骤②③，对不同通道内的不同波段进行两点测量；

⑤在任何通道内按下鼠标右键都将结束本次两点测量。

（3）　频率测量：该命令用于手动测量某种波形的频率。

由于 BL-420F 系统记录的波形曲线多样，如胃肠道电活动极慢，降压神经电活动又极快；心脏电活动很有规律，而脑电活动规律性较差。虽然显示的波形有所不同，但它们的真正差异并没有被计算机反映出来，因为计算机总是使用一些有限的频率算法来计算波频。因此，在波形变异较大或主次波混杂的情况下，计算机可能无法辨识，从而得不到正确的波形频率。此时需要采用手动测量的方法。

频率测量步骤：

①单击"频率测量"命令按钮；

②选择第一个主波位置按下鼠标左键；

③选择第二个主波位置按下鼠标左键；

④选择第三个主波位置按下鼠标左键，完成一次测量（图 2-25）；

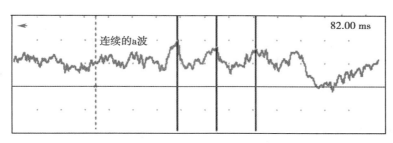

图 2-25　频率测量示意图

⑤重复步骤②～④，对不同通道内的不同波段进行频率测量；

⑥在任何通道中按下鼠标右键都将结束本次频率测量。

（4）　心功能参数测量：该命令用于手动测量一个心电波形上的各种参数，包括心率、R 波幅度、ST 时段等 13 个参数。这是一个开关命令，仅可在命令打开状态下测量。

心功能参数测量方法有两种：整体测量和局部测量。整体测量可一次测量出所选择心电波形的全部参数（13 个），局部测量则每次测量 1 个参数。如果在测量过程中已经通过工具条上的"打开 Excel"命令按钮打开了 Excel 电子表格，那么测量的数据将直接被写入到 Excel 电子表格。

整体测量方法：使用区域选择功能选择一个完整的心电波形。注意，因为整体测量使用选择波形段的时间宽度计算心率，所以应尽量选择一个完整周期的心电波形，否则测量的心率不准确。选择完成后单击鼠标右键弹出心功能参数测量快捷菜单，选择"整体测量"命令完成整体测量，如图 2-26 和图 2-27 所示。

局部测量方法：一次测量一个数据。由于测量的数据要么是一个时间差值，要么是一个幅度差值，所以必须配合 Mark 标记来完成测量。以测量 PR 间期为例，首先确定测量的起点和终点，使用 Mark 标记确定一个点，用移动光标确定另一个点，然后单击鼠标右键弹出快捷菜单，选择"PR 间期"命令完成测量，如图 2-26 和图 2-27 所示。

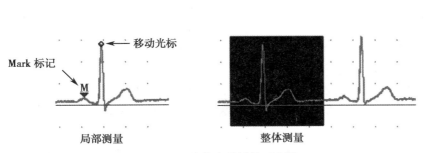

图 2-26　心功能参数测量示意图

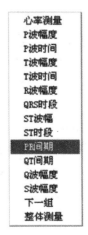

图 2-27　心功能参数测量快捷菜单

33

15. 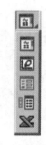 图形剪辑窗口

图形剪辑窗口按钮是一个下拉式工具按钮，单击这个下拉式工具按钮会弹出与窗口相关的子工具条，如图2-28所示。子工具条上包含5个命令："图形剪辑窗口""X-Y输入窗口""参数设置窗口""区间测量数据显示窗口""打开Excel"。

（1）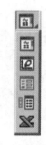 图形剪辑窗口："图形剪辑窗口"分为图形剪辑页和图形剪辑工具条两部分（图2-29）。

"图形剪辑页"在图形剪辑窗口的左边，占图形剪辑窗口的大部分空间，用于拼接和修改从原始数据通道剪辑的波形图。剪辑的图形只能在剪辑页的白色区域内移动。

图2-28　图形剪辑窗口子工具条

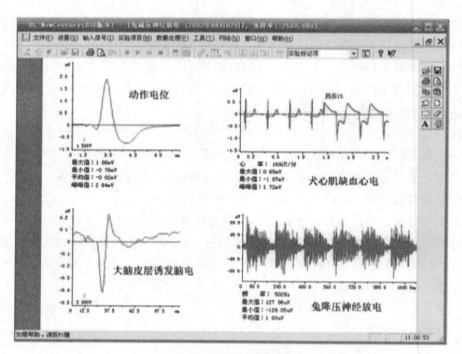

图2-29　图形剪辑窗口

"图形剪辑工具条"占据图形剪辑窗口的右边，包含12个与图形剪辑相关的命令按钮："打开""存贮""打印""打印预览""复制""粘贴""撤销""刷新""选择""擦除""写字""退出"。

（2） X-Y输入窗口：点击该命令，出现"X-Y向量图"对话框，如图2-30所示。

"X-Y向量图"对话框中的"类型选择"参数可以设定所描绘的X-Y向量图的类型："心电向量环（X-Y向量）""压力-变化率环（p-dp/dt）""压力-速度环（p-dp/dt/p）"。后两种类型为分析血压与血压变化速率关系的X-Y曲线，其使用须事先对某一通道的实验数据进行了微分处理。

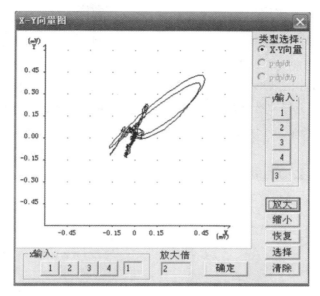

图 2-30　"X-Y 向量图"对话框

"x 输入"指的是 X-Y 向量图中 X 轴方向所选择的输入通道，可为 1、2、3 或 4 通道中的任意一个；"y 输入"代表 Y 轴方向的输入通道。

"X-Y 向量图"对话框中有 5 个功能按钮："放大""缩小""恢复""选择""清除"。"放大"按钮将 X-Y 向量图在原来基础上放大 1 倍；"缩小"按钮的功能与"放大"按钮功能相反；"恢复"按钮将放大或缩小的图形恢复到 1 倍大小；"选择"按钮用于在 X 轴的输入通道上选择一段波形完成 X-Y 向量图，选择波形段的方法与区间测量选择波形段的方法相同；"清除"按钮用于清除不需要的 X-Y 向量图形。

（3）▦参数设置窗口：该命令可以在实验过程中改变某些有自选参数设置的实验模块的初始参数设置。针对选定的实验模块，弹出对应的对话框。

（4）▦区间测量数据显示窗口：BL-420F 软件具有双视显示系统，两套显示系统的测量数据都显示在通用信息显示区中。实时实验时，实时测量是从右视中取得原始数据进行计算，且自动刷新通用显示区内的测量结果，如果想分析左视内数据，则无法显示测量结果。

选择"区间测量数据显示窗口"命令可以打开区间测量数据显示窗口（图 2-31），用于显示左视的区间测量结果。其也可用于显示右视的区间测量结果。

（5）✖打开 Excel：该命令用于打开 Excel 电子表格应用程序。如需将 BL-420F 软件中的测量结果，如区间测量结果、血流动力学测量结果或心功能参数测量结果直接写入 Excel 中，必须打开 Excel 电子表格，在 BL-420 软件和 Excel 电子表格程序间建

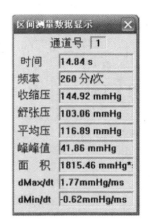

图 2-31　区间测量数据
显示窗口

立一种写入关系。该命令在整个 BL-420F 软件运行期间只能执行一次。故在 BL-420F 软件未退出之前，不能关闭 Excel 电子表格，否则将不能再将数据写入 Excel 中。

16. 选择波形放大

这个功能能将很小的波形细节放大，便于观察和分析。在使用区域选择功能选择了一段波形细节后，即可选择"选择波形放大"命令，将弹出"波形放大窗口"，如图 2-32 所示。在该窗口中还可对波形进一步放大或缩小。

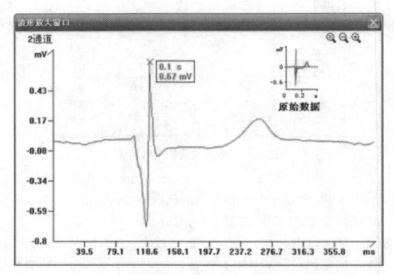

图 2-32　波形放大窗口

17. 图形剪辑

"图形剪辑"指从通道显示窗口中选择的一段波形连同这段波形中测出的数据一起以图形的方式发送到 Windows 操作系统的一个公共数据区内，便于以后将图形粘贴到 BL-420F 软件剪辑窗口或任何可以显示图形的 Windows 应用软件如 Word、Excel 或画图中，方法是选择这些软件"编辑"菜单中的"粘贴"命令即可。

"图形剪辑"的操作步骤如下：

①在实时实验过程或数据反演中，按下"暂停"按钮使实验处于暂停状态，此时，工具条上的"图形剪辑"按钮处于激活状态，按下该按钮系统将处于图形剪辑状态；

②使用区域选择功能，选择一个通道或同时选择多个通道的一段波形，如图 2-33 和图 2-34 所示。

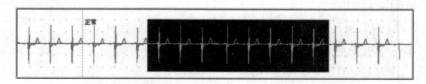

图 2-33　在一个通道显示窗口中进行区域选择

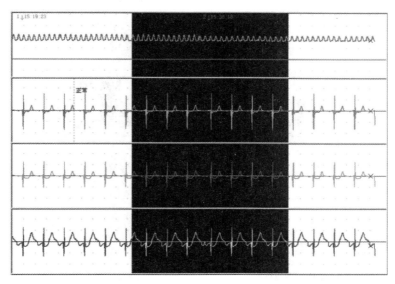

图 2-34　对多个通道显示窗口中相同时间段的区域进行区域选择

③进行区域选择后，"图形剪辑窗口"将出现，上一次选择的图形将自动粘贴进入"图形剪辑窗口"中；

④选择"图形剪辑窗口"右边工具条上的退出按钮退出"图形剪辑窗口"；

⑤重复步骤①～④，剪辑其他波形段的图形，然后拼成一幅整体图形，便于打印、存盘或复制到 Word、Excel 等应用程序中。

18. 数据剪辑

"数据剪辑"是将选择的一段或多段反演实验波形的原始采样数据按 BL-420F 软件的数据格式提取出来，并存入指定名字的 BL-420F 软件格式文件中。该格式文件可以被 BL-420F 软件读取并继续进行分析和数据提取等操作。该命令须对某个通道的数据进行区域选择后才起作用。

数据剪辑的操作步骤如下。

①在整个反演数据中查找需要剪辑的实验波形；

②将需要剪辑的实验波形进行区域选择，可同时选择多个数据；

③按下工具条上的数据剪辑命令按钮，完成一段波形的数据剪辑；剪辑的数据段以灰色显示，如图 2-35 所示；

④重复步骤①～③，对不同波形段进行数据剪辑；

⑤停止反演时，一个以"cut.tme"命名的数据剪辑文件将自动生成，可根据需要重命名剪辑文件，但命名的文件不能与打开的反演文件重名。数据剪辑的文件存贮在"\data"子目录下，扩展名为 tme。

19. 数据删除

"数据删除"可将原始数据中的无用数据删除掉，剩下的有用数据构成一个新的文件。

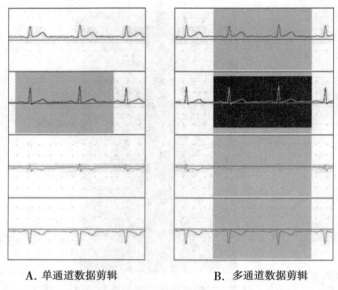

A. 单通道数据剪辑　　　　B. 多通道数据剪辑

图 2-35　数据剪辑

该功能仅对只有少量数据是无效数据的文件有用。

需要注意的是，"数据剪辑"和"数据删除"不能同时使用，如果一个文件先使用了"数据剪辑"，"数据删除"功能则变得无效，反之亦然。

20. 　通用标记

实时实验过程中，单击该命令，在波形显示窗口的顶部将添加一个通用实验标记，形状为向下的箭头，箭头前面是该标记的数值编号，编号从 1 开始顺序进行，如"20↓"，箭头后面则显示添加该标记的时间。一次实验中，最多能添加 200 个这样的通用实验标记。

21. 垂体后叶激素 　特殊实验标记编辑选择组框

特殊实验标记编辑选择组框实际上并不是一个工具条按钮，放在工具条上是为了方便操作。

BL-420F 软件的部分实验模块有预先设置的相关特殊实验标记组。当有预设特殊实验标记组的实验模块被选择时，该组框就会列出这个实验模块中所有预先设定的特殊实验标记，如图 2-36 所示。在编辑框中编辑，按"Enter"按钮确认后可以添加新的实验标记。这样，编辑的实验标记可以直接添加到实时实验的波形上，同时被自动存盘到相应的实验标记组中。

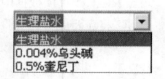

图 2-36　特殊实验标记列表

对于没有预先设定特殊实验标记组的实验，也可以在编辑组框中输入新的实验标记，输入完成后，新的实验标记可以直接加到实时显示的波形上，但不被存盘。如需新增实验标记组需要使用特殊实验标记编辑对话框。

实时实验中，从特殊实验标记编辑选择组框中选择或编辑一个特殊实验标记，然后在波形需要添加特殊标记的位置单击鼠标左键即可，如图 2-37 所示。注意，选择的标记只能被添加一次，如需再次添加同样的标记，需从组框中再选一次该标记。添加完标记后，还可移动（重定位）、编辑或删除添加的特殊实验标记。用鼠标指向特殊实验标记的名称，按下鼠标左键不放移动鼠标即可移动标记。

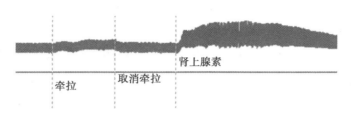

图 2-37　添加特殊实验标记

数据反演时，在显示的特殊实验标记附近单击鼠标右键，在弹出的窗口快捷菜单中选择"编辑特殊标记"命令，将弹出"特殊标记编辑对话框"，如图 2-38。在该对话框的编辑框中修改原有的特殊实验标记内容，按下"确认"按钮，编辑后的结果生效；如果按下"取消"按钮，此次编辑无效。应注意，要添加的标签不得超过 30 个汉字或 60 个英文字母。

22. **L** 打开特殊实验标记对话框
单击该命令，可以打开"实验标记编辑对话框"，如图 2-39 所示。

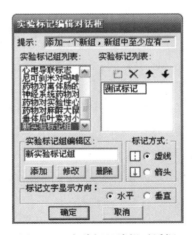

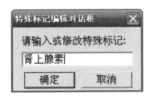

图 2-38　特殊标记编辑对话框　　　图 2-39　实验标记编辑对话框

在"实验标记编辑对话框"中，选择一个已经编辑好的特殊实验标记组，或新建一个特殊实验标记组，按"确定"按钮选择该组特殊标记。

（1）添加：按下"添加"按钮，在实验标记组列表的最下方将出现一个"新实验标记组"选项，同时在"实验标记列表"中自动为该实验标记组添加一个名为"新实验标记组"的新标记。此时，在"实验标记组编辑区"中也显示"新实验标记组"，该名称可以修改并按"修改"按钮生效,如图 2-39 所示。

(2)修改:使修改后的特殊实验标记组的组名修改生效。

(3)删除:删除选择的整个特殊实验标记组,包括它内部的所有特殊实验标记。

(4)编辑实验标记列表:实验标记列表框不仅具有普通列表框的列举数据功能,还具有在列表框中加入新列表数据、修改和删除列表数据等功能。其顶部有 4 个功能按钮:"添加""删除""上移""下移"。

添加按钮将添加一个组内特殊标记,选择该按钮,在实验标记列表框最后一行将出现一个空白的编辑框,并且出现一个闪动的文本编辑光标,表示现在可以编辑这个新添加的特殊实验标记。

删除按钮将删除当前选择的特殊实验标记。

上移按钮将当前选择的特殊实验标记上移一个位置。

下移按钮将当前选择的特殊实验标记下移一个位置。

(5)标记方式:特殊实验标记在标记处除了有文字说明外,还有一个标记点指示,可选择以虚线或箭头方式进行标记,如图 2-40 所示。

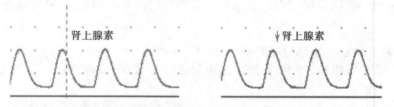

图 2-40 特殊实验标记的标记方式

(6)标记文字显示方向:特殊实验标记的文字根据需要可水平显示也可垂直显示。

23. 关于

该命令包含 BL-420F 软件的版本、版权信息及本台计算机的一些配置信息。

24. 帮助

该命令能实现上下文相关的及时帮助功能。选择该命令后,鼠标指示将变成一个带问号的箭头,此时用鼠标指向屏幕的不同部分,按下鼠标左键,将弹出关于指定部分的帮助信息。

第五节 医学机能学经典动物实验

实验一 坐骨神经 - 腓肠肌标本制备

1. 目的

(1)掌握损毁蟾蜍或青蛙脑和脊椎的方法。

(2)掌握坐骨神经 - 腓肠肌标本的制备方法。

2. 原理

两栖类动物组织的生理特性与恒温动物相似，但它们生存的环境较简单，离体组织容易维持生理活性。因此，蟾蜍或青蛙坐骨神经 - 腓肠肌标本常在医学机能学实验室被用于研究兴奋性、兴奋性过程以及刺激引起骨骼肌收缩的一般规律和特点。

坐骨神经在大腿各大肌群之间（即半膜肌与股外侧肌和股内侧肌之间）向下延伸，腓神经位于两个小腿肌肉之间，即腓骨肌和腓肠肌之间的深部。

3. 实验材料

（1）实验动物：青蛙。

（2）实验器材：青蛙解剖装置（蛙板、玻璃分针、骨剪、组织剪、眼科剪、图钉、滴管、培养皿、锌铜弓）、探针、BL-420 系统。

（3）实验试剂：任氏液。

4. 实验步骤和观察项目

（1）破坏脑和脊髓

①操作者用左手抓住青蛙使其背面朝上，且头部远离操作者（图 2-41A）。

②用探针沿青蛙头骨正中线找到颅骨表面的凹陷处，此为枕骨大孔的位置（图 2-41B）。

③将探针从枕骨大孔处垂直插入并向其头部方向刺入颅腔，左右旋转以损毁大脑（图 2-41B）。

④在上述同一位置再次插入探针，向其后肢方向刺入椎管，前后提插以破坏脊髓（图 2-41C）。

脑和脊髓被破坏的表现：角膜反射消失；下肢突然伸直，随后因肌张力下降而变得松软。

（2）切除躯干和内脏

①找到骶髂关节（图 2-41D），在骶髂关节上方 1~2 cm 处切断青蛙脊柱，此处是坐骨神经沿脊髓出现的部位（图 2-41E）。

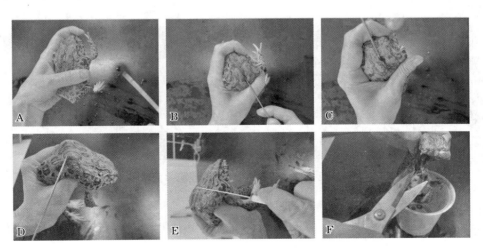

图 2-41 脑脊髓破坏及躯干和内脏去除步骤

②剪断并丢弃头部、上肢及内脏，保留脊柱和腿部（图 2-41F）。

（3）去皮

①撕掉皮肤，将标本放置在含有任氏液的培养皿中。

②青蛙去皮后，要清洁双手及使用过的器具。

（4）标本的分割

①用骨剪沿中线将脊柱剪成两半（图 2-42A）。

②在耻骨联合中心做一个切口，将两条腿分开（图 2-42B），将两只腿放在装有任氏液的培养皿中。

（5）坐骨神经 - 腓肠肌标本的准备

①用图钉将其中一个标本固定在蛙板上，背侧（将蛙翻过来）向上放置（图 2-42C）。

②用一根玻璃分针沿着脊柱将坐骨神经分离至髋关节（图 2-42D）。

③分离跟腱并在跟腱下穿一根线，然后在肌腱处结扎，留适当长度的线以便后续实验（图 2-42E）。

④将坐骨神经向下游离至膝关节（图 2-42F）。

⑤将坐骨神经的脊柱段和大腿段相连接，坐骨神经上部与一小块脊柱相连（图 2-42G）。

⑥剪断腓肠肌肌腱，向上分离到膝关节处，剪断胫骨和腓骨（图 2-42H）。

⑦剪去膝关节周围的肌肉，剪断股骨（图 2-42I）。

⑧修剪与脊柱相连的坐骨神经，完成坐骨神经腓肠肌标本（图 2-42J）。

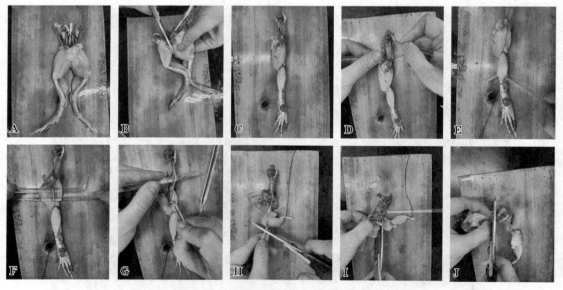

图 2-42　制作坐骨神经 - 腓肠肌标本的步骤

（参见彩插）

（6）测试标本的兴奋性

①完成的坐骨神经腓肠肌标本由一小块脊柱、坐骨神经及腓肠肌组成（图 2-43A）。

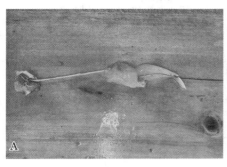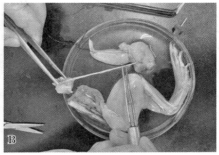

图 2-43　坐骨神经 - 腓肠肌标本的组成及其兴奋性检测

（参见彩插）

②用锌铜弓刺激神经，观察肌肉收缩情况以测试标本的兴奋性（图 2-43B）。

5. 注意事项

（1）不要过度牵拉神经。

（2）不要用尖锐的物品或手触碰标本。

（3）在实验过程中，始终用任氏液保持标本湿润。

（4）通过切断与神经伴行的周围组织以分离坐骨神经。

6. 相关问题

（1）刺激神经引起肌肉收缩的条件和过程是什么？

（2）用锌铜弓测试组织兴奋性的原理是什么？

（3）如何正确使用锌铜弓？

实验二　刺激强度对肌肉收缩的影响

1. 目的

观察刺激强度与骨骼肌收缩强度之间的关系。

2. 原理

在神经科学中，阈电位是刺激引起膜电位去极化并启动动作电位的临界膜电位水平，它决定着刺激的强度是否足以产生动作电位（action potential，AP）。能引起动作电位的最小刺激为阈刺激，其对应的强度为阈强度，而阈下刺激是指强度小于阈强度的刺激，阈下刺激可以产生局部电位，而局部电位是可叠加的，一旦局部电位的总和达到了阈值，AP即可爆发。阈电位的值可以随许多因素变化，如钠离子或钾离子电导的变化可引起阈值发生变化。同时，样本兴奋性的降低可能会使其对刺激难以作出反应。

对一个骨骼肌细胞而言，阈刺激是能引起肌细胞收缩的最小的刺激。肌细胞的兴奋性可以通过阈刺激来评估，引起肌细胞收缩的阈强度越低，该肌细胞的兴奋性越高。一块骨骼肌是由许多兴奋性不同的肌细胞组成的，阈下刺激不能引起其中任何骨骼肌细胞收缩，阈刺激只会引起兴奋性最高的骨骼肌细胞收缩，而阈上刺激能使骨骼肌中较多的肌细胞发生收缩。在一块骨骼肌组织中，每个骨骼肌细胞都有自己确定的阈刺激，因而，一块骨骼肌的收缩强度取决于参与收缩的、兴奋的骨骼肌细胞的数量，如果持续增加刺激的强度，当骨骼肌中所有的肌细胞都已经兴奋和收缩后，再增加刺激强度，骨骼肌收缩的幅度也不会继续增加。因此，引起一块肌肉中所有肌细胞收缩的最小刺激强度，就称为其最大刺激或最适刺激，它可以引起肌肉产生最大的反应。刺激强度与肌肉收缩的关系如图2-44所示。

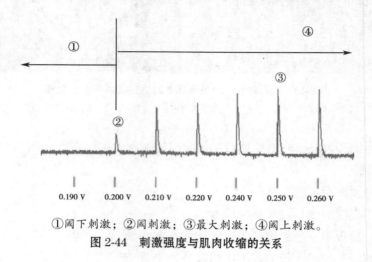

①阈下刺激；②阈刺激；③最大刺激；④阈上刺激。

图2-44　刺激强度与肌肉收缩的关系

3．实验材料

（1）实验动物：青蛙。

（2）实验器材：青蛙解剖装置、电子刺激器、万能支架、探针、机械 - 电换能器、BL-420系统。

（3）实验试剂：任氏液。

4．实验步骤和观察项目

（1）参考实验—制备坐骨神经 - 腓肠肌标本。

（2）用机械 - 电换能器将标本与BL-420系统的输入孔相连。

（3）调整刺激电极，使其与坐骨神经密切接触。

（4）用BL-420系统的电输出对坐骨神经进行电刺激，记录骨骼肌收缩曲线。

①用最弱的刺激电流来刺激标本，此时肌肉无收缩，刺激均为阈下刺激。

②逐渐增大刺激的强度，直到肌肉首次出现轻微收缩，这时的刺激为阈刺激，对应的强度为阈强度。

③继续增加刺激强度，肌肉收缩幅度会随着刺激强度的增加而相应增加，但是会达到一个"饱和点"，此时再增加刺激强度，收缩幅度不再进一步增加，此饱和点对应的刺激为最大刺激或最适刺激。

5．注意事项

（1）不要过度拉伸神经。

（2）在实验过程中，始终用任氏液保持标本湿润。

（3）不要用尖锐的物品或手触摸标本。

（4）在两个刺激之间应该有 30 s 的停顿。

（5）在记录曲线的过程中，要保持实验条件的稳定，不要触碰标本或相关设备。

6. 相关问题

（1）什么是"全或无"原理？是谁第一个提出了"全或无"原理？

（2）当我们讨论阈下刺激、阈刺激和阈上刺激的概念时，对单一神经纤维和一束神经纤维是同一回事吗？

（3）在阈刺激和最适刺激之间，肌肉收缩随着刺激强度的增加而相应增加，如何解释这一现象？

实验三　刺激频率对肌肉收缩的影响

1. 目的

观察刺激频率与肌肉收缩方式之间的关系。

2. 原理

当 AP 沿着运动神经传到肌细胞时，它会引起肌细胞膜发生去极化并产生 AP，AP 沿着肌细胞膜传到三联管，可使肌浆网释放钙离子，启动肌肉收缩过程，而钙离子泵通过主动转运恢复胞浆中的钙离子水平，此时肌肉收缩停止，转为舒张。

肌肉单收缩是指一次刺激引起一次收缩，包括潜伏期、缩短期和舒张期。在较低频率的刺激下，单收缩相继发生，不发生重合；随着刺激频率的增加，新的收缩将在前一次收缩结束之前发生，导致第二次收缩被部分地加到第一次收缩上，因此肌肉收缩强度随着刺激频率的增加而增加，在较高频率的刺激下，连续的收缩融合在一起，但可以区别开来，收缩曲线呈锯齿形，称为不完全强直收缩；当频率继续上升到某一临界水平时，肌肉的连续收缩将融合在一起，收缩曲线看上去是完全平滑和连续的，称为完全强直收缩。因此，有效刺激的频率决定了肌肉收缩的形式（图 2-45），且刺激频率越高，肌肉收缩的幅度也越大。

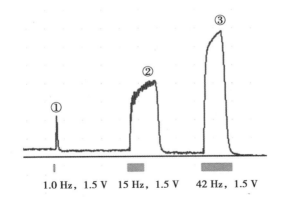

　　1.0 Hz，1.5 V　　15 Hz，1.5 V　　42 Hz，1.5 V

①单收缩；②不完全强直收缩；③完全强直收缩。

图 2-45　肌肉收缩随刺激频率变化模式

3. 实验材料

（1）实验动物：青蛙。

（2）实验器材：青蛙解剖装置、电子刺激器、万能支架、机械 - 电换能器、BL-420 系统。

（3）实验试剂：任氏液。

4. 实验步骤和观察

（1）参考实验一制备坐骨神经 - 腓肠肌标本。

（2）用机械 - 电换能器将标本与 BL-420 系统的输入孔相连。

（3）把刺激电极放在坐骨神经或肌肉上，并使其密切接触。

（4）用 BL-420 系统的电输出对坐骨神经进行电刺激，调整刺激频率，记录骨骼肌收缩曲线。

5. 注意事项

（1）不要过度牵拉神经。

（2）在实验过程中，始终用任氏液保持标本湿润。

（3）不要用尖锐的物品或手触碰标本。

（4）在两次串刺激之间应该有 30~60 s 的停顿。

（5）在记录曲线的过程中，要保持实验条件的稳定，不要触碰标本或相关设备。

6. 相关问题

（1）肌肉收缩可以叠加，引起肌肉收缩的 AP 是否也可以叠加呢？为什么？

（2）刺激频率是如何决定肌肉收缩形式的？

（3）比较单收缩、不完全强直收缩和完全强直收缩，并且分析三者差异的生理意义。

实验四　神经干动作电位的引导

1. 目的

（1）学习坐骨神经标本的制备。

（2）记录坐骨神经复合动作电位的双相 AP 和单相 AP。

（3）观察刺激强度与神经干复合动作电位幅值的关系。

2. 原理

在一条神经干中有成千上万根神经纤维，它们的直径、大小各不相同，因此，在神经干表面记录到的是复合动作电位（compound action potential，CAP）。CAP 是所有神经纤维所产生的动作电位的代数和。细胞外记录法可以用来记录 CAP。

在本实验中，我们用一个屏蔽的神经盒来记录神经干动作电位（后文简称为神经干 AP），如图 2-46 所示。神经屏蔽盒内与神经标本接触的电极包括：刺激电极、接地

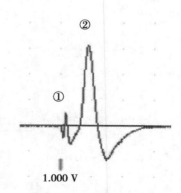

1.000 V

①刺激伪迹；②神经干 AP。

图 2-46　刺激伪迹和神经干 AP

电极和记录电极。神经屏蔽盒的防护罩起到隔离外部环境干扰的作用。在神经干表面放置记录电极，可以记录细胞外去极化区和静息区的电位差。在记录到 CAP 之前，我们可以观察到刺激伪迹（stimulus artifact），如图 2-46 所示，刺激伪迹是刺激开始的标志，其大小随刺激强度的增加而增大，过大的刺激伪迹会影响 AP 的波形。

每个神经纤维都有自己的阈刺激。因此，神经干 AP 的振幅取决于其中兴奋性神经纤维的数目。兴奋的神经纤维越多，神经干 AP 的幅值越大。当所有的神经纤维受到刺激兴奋时，CAP 的振幅将达到最大。阈强度可以通过逐渐增加刺激强度直到触发 AP 来确定，这种精细的控制和记录可以通过计算机软件来实现。

当神经受到刺激时，其膜外电位低于刺激部分的静息电位（resting potential，RP）。随着神经冲动的传导，该处膜外电位恢复为 RP，神经干表面两点之间膜电位的变化称为神经干 AP。在正常神经干表面放置两个导电极，当一个刺激连续穿过两个电极时，会产生两个反向的电位偏转，称之为双相 AP（图 2-47）。如果两个记录电极之间的神经组织受到损伤，则刺激只穿过第一个记录电极，而不能通过第二个记录电极，在这种情况下，会记录到一个单向的电位偏转，称为单相 AP（图 2-47）。

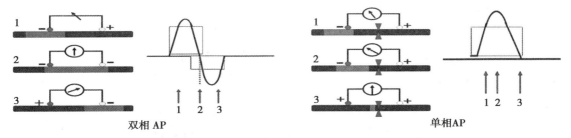

双相 AP　　　　　　　　　　　　单相 AP

图 2-47　神经干的双相 AP 和单相 AP

3. 实验材料

（1）实验动物：青蛙。

（2）实验器材：青蛙解剖装置、电子刺激器、神经标本屏蔽盒、万能支架、BL-420系统。

（3）实验试剂：任氏液。

4. 实验步骤和观察项目

（1）参考实验一的实验步骤（1）~（4）。

（2）制备坐骨神经标本

①用图钉将标本背部向上固定在蛙板上，沿坐骨神经沟小心地解剖和分离坐骨神经的脊柱段和大腿段。

②将坐骨神经向上分离至髋关节，向下分离至膝关节，可观察到延伸至膝关节的坐骨神经被分成了两部分，切断此处覆盖神经的肌腱（图 2-48A）。

③将小腿的肌肉分开，找到腓神经和胫神经，将神经向下游离到脚踝处（图 2-48B和图 2-48C）。

④切断与神经并行的周围组织，使坐骨神经脱离周围组织，小心不要切断神经。

⑤用一根棉线在脚踝处结扎腓神经和胫神经，在打结处的外端剪断，留下一段 4~5 cm 长的棉线用于移动标本（图 2-48D）。

⑥从脊柱发出的地方用一根棉线结扎坐骨神经，切断线结与脊柱之间的神经，留下一段 4~5 cm 长的棉线用来移动神经。

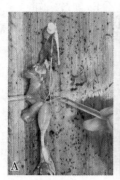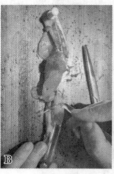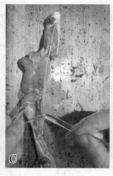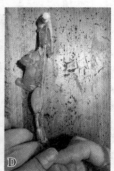

图 2-48　坐骨神经的分离
（参见彩插）

（3）标本放置：将神经干置于神经屏蔽盒内的刺激电极和记录电极上，确保刺激电极与神经干的近端（粗）密切接触，而记录电极与神经干远端（细）密切接触（图 2-49）。

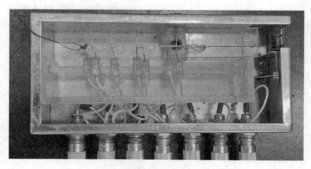

图 2-49　神经屏蔽盒内神经干的放置

（4）CAP 波形观察：将神经屏蔽盒的电极连接到 BL-420 系统（图 2-50），用足够强度的电刺激来刺激神经干，记录 CAP。所记录的波形包括一个在刺激后立即出现的刺激伪迹，随后出现的双相成分是真正的神经干 AP。

①从弱刺激开始，逐步增大刺激，确定 CAP 的阈刺激强度；改变刺激强度，观察 CAP 是否有变化，观察刺激强度与 CAP 波幅的关系，并找出引起最大 CAP 的最小刺激强度。

②先用镊子或止血钳将两个记录电极中间的神经夹伤，然后给予同等强度的刺激，这时引导出单相 AP；将其与损伤前的双相 AP 进行比较。

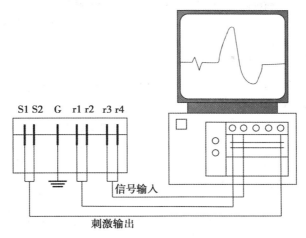

图 2-50 神经屏蔽盒与 BL-420 系统的连接

5. 注意事项

（1）分离时不要损伤神经，以免影响实验结果。

（2）坐骨神经标本应尽可能长，以 8 cm 以上为最佳。

（3）经常用任氏液湿润标本以保持其良好的兴奋性。

（4）保持神经干与电极密切接触，记录电极与记录电极之间的距离应尽可能长。

（5）避免在神经上滴加过多的任氏液。

（6）避免强电流刺激损伤神经。

6. 相关问题

（1）过大的刺激伪迹会造成 AP 波形的改变，我们可以通过什么方式减少刺激伪迹？

（2）CAP 具有"全或无"的特性吗？

（3）为什么 AP 的正相波振幅小于 AP 的负相波振幅？

实验五 蛙心起搏点观察

1. 目的

（1）确定和观察青蛙心脏起搏点及传导途径。

（2）观察记录青蛙心脏不同部位自律性的高低。

2. 原理

心脏的特殊传导系统具有自动节律性，但各部分的自律性高低不同，两栖类动物以静脉窦的自律性最高。正常心脏每次兴奋都从自律性最高的部位开始，依次传到心房、心室，相继引起心房、心室收缩，把自律性最高的部位称为心脏的起搏点。当正常的自律性受到影响而发生改变时，心房、心室的活动也发生相应变化；如果起搏点下传的冲动受阻，心脏下部的活动会暂时停止，甚至表现出自己的自律性。

两栖动物的正常起搏点位于静脉窦，是腔静脉和右心房之间稍膨大的区域。青蛙心脏的每个部位都有其内在的跳动速率，例如静脉窦大约是 72 次 / 分，心房大约是 60 次 / 分，心室大约是 25 次 / 分。去极化速度最快的细胞能控制所有其他细胞的收缩速度，因此它们充当心脏的起搏器。当速率较快的起搏器的下传信息被阻断时，才有可能观察到起搏速率较慢区域的潜在自律性。

青蛙的心脏有三个腔室，一个心室两个心房，这在解剖学上与哺乳动物不同（图 2-51 和图 2-52）。青蛙的心脏在室温下功能良好，即使从胸腔中暴露出来，也会继续跳动一段时间。因此，本实验以青蛙为实验对象。

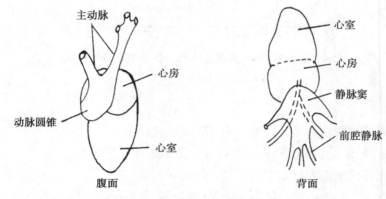

图 2-51　青蛙心脏的结构

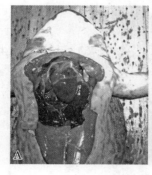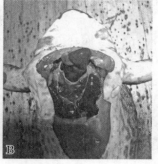

A 腹侧；B 背侧。

图 2-52　青蛙的心脏

（参见彩插）

3. 实验材料

（1）实验动物：青蛙。

（2）实验器材：青蛙解剖装置、计时器、棉线。

（3）实验试剂：任氏液。

4. 实验步骤和观察项目

（1）取青蛙一只，破坏脑和脊髓，将其固定于蛙板。

（2）打开胸腔，剪开心包，暴露心脏。

（3）在窦房沟、房室沟处各预置一段手术用的丝线。

（4）观察静脉窦、心房和心室的跳动的次序，并记录各部位在单位时间内的跳动次数。

（5）找到静脉窦和心房交界的半月形白线（窦房沟）处，用棉线结扎以阻断静脉窦和心房之间的传导，观察心房、静脉窦的跳动是否停止及其跳动频率有何变化。

（6）用预先穿过的棉线在房室沟处结扎（斯氏第二结扎），阻断房室之间的传导，观察心室是否停止跳动及心房和心室的跳动情况，分别记录各部位在单位时间内的跳动次数。

（7）松开结扎线，使心房、心室恢复跳动，记录各部位在单位时间内的跳动次数并观察其跳动节律是否一致。

（8）将实验结果填入表 2-1 中。

表 2-1　心脏跳动频率（次/分）

观察项目	静脉窦	心房	心室
对照			
结扎窦房沟			
结扎房室沟			

5. 注意事项

（1）用任氏液经常湿润标本。

（2）不要用尖锐的物品或手去触摸标本。

（3）在静脉窦和心房之间进行结扎时，注意尽量靠近心房进行结扎。

6. 相关问题

（1）正常起搏点是如何控制整个心脏的跳动频率的？

（2）临床上使用的心脏起搏器的工作原理是什么？使用时要注意些什么呢？

实验六　期前收缩和代偿间隙

1. 目的

观察青蛙心脏的期前收缩和代偿间隙现象。

2. 原理

心室肌细胞有很长的不应期，从收缩期一直延续到舒张的早期（图 2-53）。任

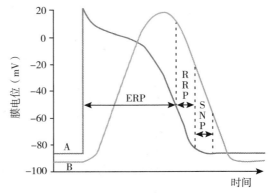

A. 动作电位；B. 收缩曲线；

ERP. 有效不应期；RRP. 相对不应期；SNP. 超常期。

图 2-53　AP 期间兴奋性与心室肌肉收缩的关系

何刺激都不能在有效不应期内引发新的收缩；随着肌肉的舒张，其兴奋性逐渐恢复，虽然此时兴奋性仍低于正常水平，但给予额外更强的刺激，肌肉仍可以产生收缩；在不应期之后和正常起搏点的正常冲动到达心肌之前，额外有效刺激可以诱发心肌产生额外的收缩，称为额外收缩或期前收缩（extrasystole），如图 2-54 所示。心肌额外收缩也有其自身的绝对不应期，如果正常窦房结产生的冲动刚好落在期前收缩的绝对不应期中，则不能引起心肌收缩，因此会导致较长时间的心脏舒张，称为代偿性间隙（compensatory pause），如图 2-54 所示。

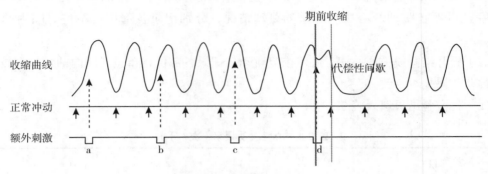

图 2-54　蛙心期前收缩和代偿性间歇

3. 实验材料

（1）实验动物：青蛙。

（2）实验器材：青蛙解剖装置、电子刺激器、万能支架、蛙心夹、BL-420 系统。

（3）实验试剂：任氏液。

4. 实验步骤和观察项目

（1）破坏青蛙的脑与脊髓。

（2）在心脏舒张期用蛙心夹夹住心尖 2 mm 左右。

（3）将蛙心与仪器连接好，如图 2-55A 所示。

（4）调整刺激电极的两极，使其在收缩期和舒张期均与心室密切接触，如图 2-55B 所示。

（5）记录心脏收缩曲线，辨认收缩期和舒张期。

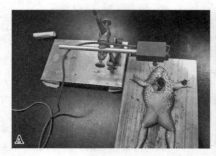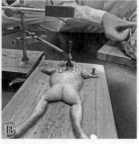

图 2-55　青蛙心脏与仪器连接

（6）分别在心脏的收缩期与舒张期用中等强度的单脉冲刺激心室，观察心脏对刺激的不同反应。

5. 注意事项

（1）不要过度牵拉心脏。

（2）经常用任氏液润湿标本。

（3）电极的两极在收缩期和舒张期都要与心肌接触。

（4）每两次刺激间隔 30 s。

（5）在记录曲线的过程中保持实验条件稳定，不要触碰标本或相关设备。

6. 相关问题

（1）蛙心会出现强直性收缩吗？

（2）额外收缩是否一定会伴随着代偿性间歇？为什么？

实验七 呼吸运动的调节

1. 目的

（1）掌握气管插管的基本技术。

（2）观察各种因素对呼吸运动的影响。

2. 原理

肺的主要功能是从外部环境中获取氧气，为细胞供氧，并排出体内细胞代谢产生的二氧化碳。呼吸运动在中枢神经系统的控制下进行，呼吸控制系统对人体内部环境的变化非常敏感，PCO_2、pH 和 PO_2 等的变化会通过呼吸调节反射改变肺泡通气量，最终将这些变量恢复为正常值。化学感受器有两种类型：外周化学感受器（peripheral chemoreceptor，PCRs）和中枢化学感受器（central chemoreceptor，CCRs）。PCRs 位于颈动脉和主动脉弓，主要对 PO_2 敏感，但也对 CO_2 和 pH 变化有反应，它们在受到刺激时会迅速增加呼吸运动，因此被称为低氧感受器。CCRs 位于延髓，它们对细胞外液和脑脊液（cerebrospinal fluid，CSF）中的 CO_2 和 pH 变化敏感，缺氧对 CCRs 无兴奋作用。虽然因为存在血脑屏障（blood brain barrier，BBB）等原因，CCRs 往往反应较慢，但其对呼吸的影响更大。

除了化学因素的影响外，肺牵张反射也可以影响呼吸。肺牵张反射有两种类型：肺扩张反射和肺缩小反射。前者是由于肺部过度充气而导致肺牵张感受器被激活，该感受器通过迷走途径将刺激信息发送至呼吸中枢，从而使吸气受到抑制，及时转为呼气。而肺缩小反射是因为肺缩小导致肺壁（胸膜）中的感受器被激活，并通过迷走途径将刺激信息发送至呼吸中枢，从而抑制呼气，及时转为吸气。当迷走神经的一侧被切断时，因为肺牵张反射的效率降低了一半，呼吸会变得较深较慢；而切除两侧迷走神经后，由于肺牵张反射已完全不起作用，所以呼吸变得更深更慢。

3. 实验材料

（1）实验动物：家兔，2.0~2.5 kg。

（2）实验器材：哺乳动物手术器械（皮钳、组织剪、止血钳、组织镊、手术刀片、手术刀柄、眼科剪、眼科镊、缝合线、缝合针、持针器）、兔台、机械 - 电换能器、电子刺激器、气管插管、注射器、长度为 50 cm 的橡胶导管、充满 CO_2 的气囊、充满 N_2 的气囊、棉线、纱布、万能支架、BL-420 系统。

（3）实验试剂：25% 氨基甲酸乙酯（乌拉坦）溶液、3% 的乳酸溶液。

4. 实验步骤和观察项目

（1）麻醉和固定

①麻醉：经耳缘静脉注射 25% 乌拉坦溶液 4 mL/kg。麻醉成功的主要体征是：角膜反射消失，疼觉减弱或消失，四肢松软。

②固定：将麻醉的兔子仰卧位固定在手术台上。

（2）清除喉头及颈部前的毛发。

（3）在甲状腺软骨的下缘沿着正中线做一长约 5~7 cm 的切口。

（4）游离两侧的迷走神经，如图 2-56 所示。

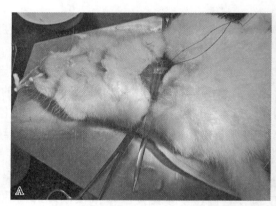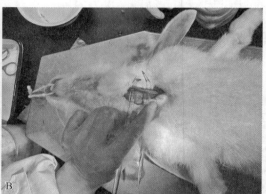

图 2-56　迷走神经的分离

（参见彩插）

（5）用止血钳分离气管两侧及气管与食管之间的结缔组织，分离覆盖气管的肌肉，暴露并分离气管，并在气管下放置一根棉线。

（6）气管插管术

①在喉头下方约 2~3 cm 的位置，用手术刀在两个软骨环之间的前壁做一个横切口，再在横切口中间向头部做一纵向切口，形成了一个反向的"T"形切口，见图 2-57A。

②用棉球清理伤口的分泌物和血液。

③一手拉住气管下的棉线，将适当直径的气管插管插入气管，见图 2-57B。

④用置于气管下的棉线固定气管插管。

（7）观察记录

①记录正常的呼吸运动曲线，确认吸气和呼气对应的部分，检查其节律和频率。

②二氧化碳的作用：将充满 CO_2 的气囊连接管靠近气管插管（不连接），观察呼吸运

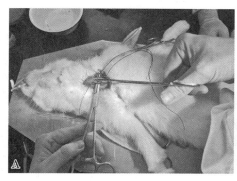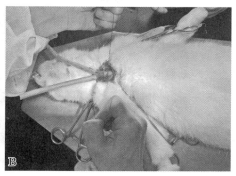

图 2-57　气管插管
（参见彩插）

动的变化；取走气囊，再观察呼吸运动的恢复情况。

③缺氧的影响：夹闭气管插管的一个分支，将一个充满 N_2 的气囊连接到气管插管的另一个分支，观察呼吸运动的变化；再取走气囊，观察呼吸运动的恢复情况。

④无效腔的影响：将一根 50 cm 长的橡胶导管与气管插管的另一分支相连，观察呼吸运动的变化。

⑤血液 pH 值的影响：将 2 mL 3% 的乳酸溶液通过耳缘静脉注入，观察呼吸运动的变化。

⑥迷走神经的影响：切断一侧迷走神经，观察呼吸运动的变化；再切断另一侧迷走神经，观察呼吸运动的变化。

5. 注意事项

（1）使用麻醉剂的注意事项

①根据家兔体重计算准确的麻醉剂用量。

②从耳缘静脉远心端开始注射。

③注射前一半剂量的麻醉剂时可以较快，越后越慢。

④仔细观察动物的反应，切忌麻醉时过量、过快。

⑤补充注射麻醉剂时注意要小于原剂量的 1/5。

（2）分离神经与血管的注意事项

①不应使用齿状镊分离，以免造成神经与血管结构或功能上的损坏。

②用玻璃分针分离神经和血管的细支，以保留正常的结构。

③当分离多根神经或血管时，在其下面置放浸泡过生理盐水的不同颜色的线进行识别。

④用湿纱布覆盖切口。

6. 相关问题

（1）缺氧和血液中二氧化碳过多对呼吸运动的影响有何不同？请比较其作用机制。

（2）迷走神经在节律性呼吸运动中的功能是什么？

（3）谁发现了 PCRs？他是如何设计实验来确定 PCRs 的位置和功能的？

实验八　心血管系统活动的调节

1. 目的

（1）掌握动脉插管的基本技术。

（2）观察神经和激素等因素对心脏和血管活动的影响。

2. 原理

心血管活动主要由神经系统和体液因素控制和调节。本实验以血压为心血管活动的指标，验证各种药物和迷走神经对心血管系统的影响。

（1）压力感受器的作用：在主动脉弓和左右颈内动脉的颈动脉窦中均有压力感受器。它们可以感受血压的变化，通过压力感受性反射维持正常的动脉血压，使组织获得适量的血液。压力感受器的敏感刺激是其所在的血管壁所受到的牵拉，搏动性牵拉越大，它们产生 AP 的频率就越高。压力感受器对维持稳定血压的反应非常快，但它们只对短期变化作出反应。

（2）迷走神经的作用：心脏的副交感神经支配是由迷走神经介导的。迷走神经支配窦房结（sinoatrial node，SN），并使心脏易于发生房室传导阻滞。迷走神经分泌乙酰胆碱，与心脏 M 受体结合产生作用。乙酰胆碱增加窦房结细胞第 4 期 K^+ 的外流，减少 Ca^{2+} 的内流。因此，迷走神经的激活会引起心率减慢和血压降低。

（3）肾上腺素的作用：肾上腺素在短期应激反应中起着至关重要的作用。它是由肾上腺髓质分泌的。当注射肾上腺素到血液中时，肾上腺素可与骨骼肌小动脉中平滑肌的 α、β1 和 β2 受体结合。肾上腺素与 α 受体结合导致血管收缩，与 β1 受体结合导致心脏活动增加，与 β2 受体结合导致血管舒张。肾上腺素增加心率和搏出量，而搏出量的增加会导致血压的升高。

（4）去甲肾上腺素的作用：去甲肾上腺素作为一种激素由肾上腺髓质释放到血液中，但它也是神经系统中的一种神经递质，在突触传递过程中从去甲肾上腺素能神经元中释放出来。当注射到血液中时，去甲肾上腺素与骨骼肌小动脉平滑肌的 α 和 β2 受体结合。与 α 受体结合导致血管收缩，与 β2 受体结合导致血管舒张，但去甲肾上腺素对 α 受体的亲和力远高于对 β2 受体的亲和力。因此，去甲肾上腺素最终会引起血管收缩，而不是血管舒张。故激活交感神经系统会直接增加心率和血压。

（5）乙酰胆碱的作用：乙酰胆碱是第一个被确认的神经递质，是所有自主神经节的神经递质。当乙酰胆碱与心脏 M 受体结合时，会导致窦房结细胞在第 4 期增加 K^+ 的外流，减少 Ca^{2+} 的内流。因此，注射乙酰胆碱可减弱心肌纤维的收缩，导致心率减慢和血压下降。心脏的副交感神经支配是由迷走神经介导的，迷走神经支配窦房结，使心脏易受房室传导阻滞的影响。

3. 实验材料

（1）实验动物：家兔，2.0~2.5 kg。

（2）实验器材：哺乳动物手术器械、兔台、机械 - 电换能器、电子刺激器、保护电极、聚乙烯管、注射器、三通管、棉绳、棉线、纱布、万能支架、动脉夹。

（3）实验试剂：液状石蜡、肝素溶液（1：1000 单位/毫升）、25% 氨基甲酸乙酯（乌拉坦）溶液、3% 乳酸溶液、生理盐水、0.01% 肾上腺素溶液、0.01% 去甲肾上腺素溶液、0.01% 乙酰胆碱溶液。

4. 实验步骤和观察项目

（1）麻醉：经耳缘静脉注射 25% 乌拉坦溶液 4 mL/kg。麻醉成功的主要体征是：角膜反射消失，疼觉减弱或消失，四肢松软。

（2）固定：将麻醉后的家兔仰卧位固定于解剖台上。

①四肢固定：用棉绳打活结套在前腿肘关节上方和后腿脚踝上方，先固定后肢，再固定前肢，均与手术台两侧的铁棒进行固定。

②头部固定：用一根棉绳通过动物的两上门齿与手术台前端的铁棒进行固定。

（3）分离血管神经：分离双侧颈总动脉和迷走神经。

①在甲状软骨下缘沿着颈部的正中线做一约 5~7 cm 的切口，钝性分离皮下组织和肌肉。

②找到气管，左侧和右侧颈总动脉就位于气管两侧。与颈总动脉平行的神经分别是迷走神经（最粗的一条）、交感神经和降主动脉神经（细如头发）。

③分离颈总动脉和迷走神经约 2~3 cm 长（图 2-58A），用不同颜色的棉线放在神经和血管下方以便识别。在左侧颈总动脉下面放置两根棉线以便固定。

（4）颈动脉插管：一般对左侧颈总动脉进行插管。

①用棉线结扎左颈总动脉远心端，用动脉夹夹闭动脉近心端，在结扎线和动脉夹之间留 3 cm 长的血管，如图 2-58B 所示。

②在结扎线下方的动脉管壁上与动脉长轴呈 45° 用眼科剪做一个"V"形切口，如图 2-58B 所示。

③向心脏方向插入已经充满了肝素溶液的动脉导管，如图 2-58C 所示。

④用动脉下的棉线进行结扎，使动脉导管固定在动脉内，如图 2-58D 所示。

⑤检查三通管的封闭性，然后放开动脉夹，使血液通过动脉导管与机械-电换能器相通。

（5）记录血压曲线

①记录正常血压曲线，观察收缩期和舒张期的变化。

②夹闭右侧颈总动脉 15 s 左右，观察血压和心率的变化。

③用一对保护电极勾住迷走神经，用中等强度进行刺激，观察血压和心率的变化。

④对右侧迷走神经进行双重结扎，从结扎线中间切断，然后用保护电极分别刺激外周端和中枢端，观察血压和心率的变化。

⑤从耳缘静脉注射 0.3 mL 的 0.01% 的肾上腺素溶液，观察血压和心率的变化。

⑥从耳缘静脉注射 0.3 mL 的 0.01% 的去甲肾上腺素溶液，观察血压和心率的变化。

⑦从耳缘静脉注射 0.3 mL 的 0.01% 的乙酰胆碱溶液，观察血压和心率的变化。

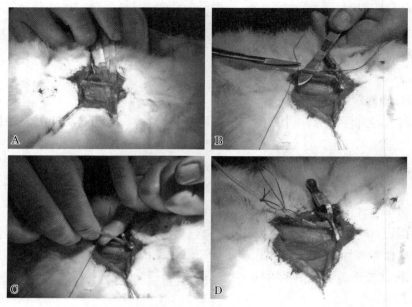

图 2-58　动脉插管

（参见彩插）

5. 注意事项

同实验七。

6. 相关问题

（1）去甲肾上腺素和肾上腺素对心脏和血管的作用有何不同？谈谈两者在临床上的应用。

（2）第一个发现乙酰胆碱的科学家是谁？他是如何发现乙酰胆碱的，其意义是什么？

（3）缺氧和过量的 CO_2 均可增加心血管活动，其作用机制是什么？

（4）去甲肾上腺素是如何被发现的，其意义是什么？

实验九　消化道平滑肌的生理特性

1. 目的

（1）学习肠道平滑肌的体外灌注法。

（2）通过观察某些化学物质对消化道平滑肌运动的影响，研究消化道平滑肌的生理特性。

2. 原理

肠神经系统（enteric nervous system，ENS）是存在位于肠道壁中的独立神经系统，该系统控制胃肠道的运动和分泌。尽管 ENS 可以独立于周围神经起作用，但副交感神经系统和交感神经系统可以增强或抑制胃肠道功能。自主神经纤维末梢的囊泡主要含有乙酰胆碱和去甲肾上腺素，偶尔还有其他神经递质。

平滑肌具有高度可收缩性，平滑肌膜上有许多钠通道或钙通道。当受到神经或其他化学因素的刺激时，钠或钙内流启动 AP，从而诱导肌浆网释放钙离子，或使细胞外钙离子进入细胞。钙离子可激活钙调蛋白，之后引起横桥磷酸化，从而活化横桥，导致横桥与肌动蛋白结合，启动肌丝滑行引起肌肉收缩。因此，平滑肌的收缩在很大程度上依赖于细胞内钙离子的浓度。

平滑肌具有不同程度的紧张性和自律性。在静息膜电位的基础上，自动去极化和复极化会产生慢波，其振幅（大约 10~15 mV）和频率（持续几秒钟）较小。当慢波达到一定水平（大于 –40 mV）时，可以启动 AP 和平滑肌收缩。食物的机械牵拉、温度和化学物质都是胃肠道平滑肌的敏感刺激。

3. 实验材料

（1）实验标本：2~3 cm 长的小肠段（家兔）。

（2）实验器械：恒温水浴锅、恒温浴槽、弯针、棉线、机械 - 电换能器、BL-420系统。

（3）实验试剂：台氏液、25% 氨基甲酸乙酯（乌拉坦）溶液、0.01% 肾上腺素溶液、0.01% 乙酰胆碱溶液、0.01% 硫酸阿托品、1 mol/L HCl 溶液、1 mol/L NaOH 溶液。

4. 实验步骤和观察项目

（1）仪器及标本准备

①准备恒温浴槽，向其中加入台氏液，预热至 38℃。

②动物麻醉：经耳缘静脉注射 25% 乌拉坦溶液 4 mL/kg。

③打开腹腔，在胃与十二指肠连接处，迅速分离一段小肠管并将其取出体外。

④在台氏液中清洗后，将取出的肠管剪成长度为 2~3 cm 的肠段，供各组使用。

⑤用棉线扎住肠段的两端，将一端固定到恒温浴槽中的 L 型钩上，另一端通过棉线固定到换能器上。

⑥通过机械 - 电换能器记录小肠的收缩情况，见图 2-59。

（2）观察记录小肠的收缩曲线

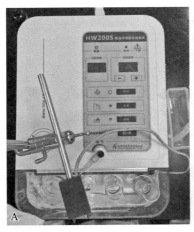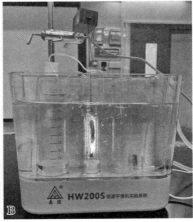

图 2-59　实验仪器及标本连接

①记录正常的小肠收缩曲线。

②在浴槽中加入 1~2 滴 0.01%肾上腺素溶液，观察到变化之后，用台氏液冲洗 3 次，进行下一项。

③在浴槽中加入 1~2 滴 0.01%乙酰胆碱溶液，观察到变化之后，用台氏液冲洗 3 次，进行下一项。

④在浴槽中加入 1~2 滴 0.01%硫酸阿托品溶液，观察变化，不用台氏液冲洗，直接进入下一步。

⑤在浴槽中加入 1~2 滴 0.01%乙酰胆碱溶液，观察到变化之后，用台氏液冲洗 3 次，进行下一项。

⑥在浴槽中加入 1~2 滴 1 mol/L HCl 溶液，观察到变化之后，用台氏液冲洗 3 次，进行下一项。

⑦向浴槽中加入 1~2 滴 1 mol/L NaOH 溶液，观察到变化后，用台氏液冲洗 3 次，进行下一项。

⑧将浴槽中 38℃台氏液换成室温下的台氏液，观察小肠运动的变化。

5. 注意事项

（1）在切断肠管前，结扎肠系膜血管。

（2）每次在进行下一项操作之前，先用 38℃的台氏液洗涤 3 次，使前一次试剂的作用效果消失。

（3）经常检查台氏液温度和恒温浴槽中的氧气流量，并尽快做完全部实验。

6. 相关问题

（1）加入 1 mol/L HCl 溶液与加入 1 mol/L NaOH 溶液对肠道收缩的影响有无可能是一致的？为什么？

（2）0.01%硫酸阿托品溶液在乙酰胆碱之前或之后加入浴槽，肠收缩情况会有怎样的变化？

（3）如何证明钙离子对小肠平滑肌收缩具有重要作用？

实验十 影响尿生成的因素

1. 目的

（1）练习腹部手术操作。

（2）学习输尿管插管的基本技术。

（3）观察各因素对尿生成的影响。

2. 原理

肾脏是泌尿系统的重要器官，在调节内环境稳态方面起着重要的作用。肾脏发挥作用的一种最常见的方法是清除体内代谢产生的废物，包括尿素、肌酐、尿酸等。肾脏还能排除体内产生或摄入的大多数毒素和其他外来物质，如农药、药物和食品添加剂。肾脏的第二个功能是调节水和电解质平衡。为了维持内环境稳态，水和电解质的排泄与摄入必须精确地相适应，从而稳定体液渗透压和电解质浓度，调节酸碱平衡，进而通过控制总血容量来稳定动脉血压。肾脏的这种调节功能维持了细胞进行各种活动所必需的稳定内环境。

肾脏通过生成尿液来执行其主要的排泄功能，尿的形成包括肾小球滤过、肾小管再吸收和分泌。任何作用于这些过程的因素都会导致尿液的质量和数量发生改变。

3. 实验材料

（1）实验动物：家兔，2.0~2.5 kg。

（2）实验器材：哺乳动物解剖设备、兔台、棉线、计滴器、保护电极、聚乙烯管、三通管、纱布、注射器、葡萄糖试纸、BL-420 系统。

（3）实验试剂：25% 氨基甲酸乙酯（乌拉坦）溶液、生理盐水、20% 葡萄糖溶液、0.01% 去甲肾上腺素溶液、呋塞米、抗利尿激素。

4. 实验步骤和观察项目

（1）麻醉：经家兔耳缘静脉注射 25% 乌拉坦溶液 4 mL/kg。

（2）固定：将麻醉后的家兔仰卧位固定于手术台。

（3）分离右侧迷走神经，穿线，备用。

（4）分离颈浅静脉，并在其下方穿线，结扎远心端，做一个"V"形切口，插入一个充满生理盐水的聚乙烯管，用线将插管固定在静脉中，且该管的另一端与三通管连接以便注射药物。

（5）输尿管插管术（图 2-60）

①清除下腹部皮肤处的毛发，在耻骨上方 2 cm 处作长度为 5~7 cm 的正中切口。

②沿腹白线剪开腹部肌肉，剪开腹膜，打开腹腔。

③找到膀胱和两侧输尿管，钝性分离输尿管。

④在一侧输尿管下方穿线，在膀胱附近结扎。

⑤在输尿管管壁上做一个"V"形切口，将充满生理盐水的聚乙烯管插入输尿管，并将其固定。

⑥将导尿管与计滴器相连，通过 BL-420 系统记录尿液滴数。

⑦上述操作结束后，用一块蘸有生理盐水的温纱布覆盖在家兔的腹部。

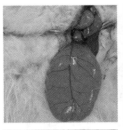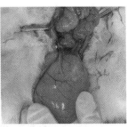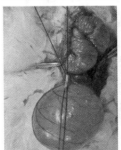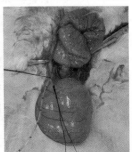

图 2-60　输尿管插管
（参见彩插）

（6）观察项目

①记录正常尿量作为对比。

②静脉注射 20 mL 38℃的生理盐水，观察记录尿量的变化，尿量恢复后进行下一项实验。

③静脉注射 0.5 mL 0.01% 去甲肾上腺素溶液，观察记录尿量的变化，尿量恢复后进行下一项实验。

④静脉注射 5 mL 38℃的 20% 葡萄糖溶液。在注射前对尿糖进行定性检测，并在注射后尿量增加的高峰期重复检测。

⑤刺激迷走神经外周端，观察记录尿量的变化，尿量恢复后进行下一项实验。

⑥静脉注射 5 mg/kg 的呋塞米，观察记录尿量的变化，尿量恢复后进行下一项实验。

⑦静脉注射 2 U 的抗利尿激素，观察记录尿量的变化。

⑧将上述实验结果填入表 2-2，也可以自行设计表格来记录结果。

表 2-2　各因素对尿量和尿糖的影响

观察项目	尿量（滴 / 分）	尿糖（+/−）
对照组		
生理盐水		
0.01% 去甲肾上腺素溶液		
20% 葡萄糖溶液		
刺激右迷走神经		
呋塞米		
抗利尿激素		

5. 注意事项

（1）应记录实验项目给药前后的尿量以作对比（每个实验项目给药前的尿量可用对照组的尿量表示）。

（2）只有当上一个实验的因素的影响减弱或消失时，才进行下一个项目。

（3）多次注射时应注意保护耳缘静脉。应先从远端开始注射，然后逐渐向根部靠近。

（4）在对颈动脉进行手术操作前，应先进行腹部手术，以免腹部手术引起家兔挣扎使动脉导管脱落或折断，从而引起失血甚至死亡。

6. 相关问题

（1）如何避免血凝块堵塞聚乙烯管道从而影响尿液收集？

（2）注射高渗葡萄糖后尿量会明显增加吗？其原理是什么？

（3）呋塞米利尿的分子机制是什么？临床上用于哪些情况？

实验十一　反射弧分析

1. 目的

通过分析反射弧的组成，证实反射弧的完整性及反射弧与反射活动之间的关系。

2. 原理

机体大多数的活动是由感受器受到的刺激所引发的，每种类型的感受器只对某一类的刺激高度敏感，这种类型的刺激被称为适宜刺激。来自体表和一些深部组织的感受器首先将感觉信息传输到中枢神经系统，然后传到大脑中的多个感觉区域，经过大脑的信息整合，一方面产生特定感觉，另一方面发出传出冲动使机体对刺激作出反应。神经系统对机体的调节是通过反射活动完成的，神经调节的基本模式是反射。反射的结构基础是反射弧，它由感受器、传入神经元、中枢神经系统、传出神经元和效应器五个部分组成，其结构和功能的完整性是实现反射作用的前提条件。

当有害的刺激作用到皮肤的感受器上，受刺激的部位产生肢体屈肌的收缩，此过程称为屈肌反射。这种反射可由脊动物来实现。脊动物是指除了脊髓外，中枢神经系统的其他部分被实验者破坏的动物。本次实验通过破坏反射弧的各个组成部分来证实反射弧完整性是实现反射的基础。

3. 实验材料

（1）实验动物：青蛙。

（2）实验器材：青蛙解剖装置、探针、万能支架、试管夹、纱布、瓷盘、烧杯。

（3）实验试剂：任氏液、0.5%硫酸溶液。

4. 实验步骤和观察项目

（1）制备脊蛙：破坏脑髓并保持脊柱的完整，用试管夹夹住青蛙下颌使其悬挂在铁架台上。

（2）在培养皿中加入适量的0.5%硫酸溶液。

（3）将青蛙左后肢的脚趾放到0.5%硫酸溶液中（图2-61A），观察屈肌反射是否产生。用烧杯中的自来水清洗残留在青蛙皮肤上的硫酸并擦干皮肤。

（4）彻底去除左脚上的皮肤。重复步骤（3），用硫酸刺激该脚脚趾（图2-61B），查看是否出现屈肌反射。

（5）将青蛙右后肢的脚趾放到0.5%硫酸溶液中，观察屈肌反射是否产生，用烧杯中的自来水清洗残留在青蛙皮肤上的硫酸并擦干皮肤。

（6）找出右侧的坐骨神经并在神经上进行双重结扎，在两个结扎点中间切断神经（图2-61C）。

（7）将青蛙右后肢的脚趾放到0.5%硫酸溶液中（图2-61D），观察屈肌反射是否产生。

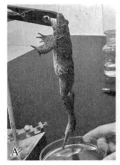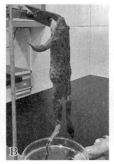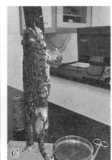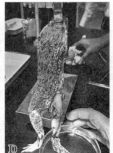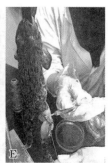

图2-61　青蛙屈肌反射的反射弧分析

（8）分别刺激神经的中枢和外周端，观察各有什么现象发生（图 2-61E）。

（9）取另外一只青蛙，破坏脑和脊髓，重复步骤（3）或（5），观察屈肌反射是否产生。

5. 注意事项

每次使用硫酸后，要使用自来水清洗皮肤受刺激的部分，并用纱布擦干，以免稀释硫酸溶液。

6. 相关问题

（1）谁是第一个提出脊动物概念的人？为什么本实验需要制备脊动物？

（2）如果增加硫酸的浓度，在屈肌反射的基础上我们还可以观察到什么反射？

（3）屈肌反射的生理意义是什么？在完整机体中诱导的屈肌反射还会有什么表现？

实验十二　缺氧模型制备与观察

1. 目的

（1）复制小鼠低张性缺氧和血液性缺氧模型。

（2）比较不同类型缺氧模型动物的呼吸变化、血液颜色和发病机制的异同。

2. 原理

大气中的氧通过呼吸进入肺泡后弥散入血并与血红蛋白结合，再由血液循环输送到全身被组织、细胞利用。组织氧供减少或不能充分利用氧，导致组织代谢、功能和形态结构异常变化的病理过程称为缺氧（hypoxia）。根据引起缺氧的原因和血氧变化的特点，缺氧分为低张性缺氧、血液性缺氧、循环性缺氧、组织性缺氧四种类型，本实验主要复制低张性缺氧和血液性缺氧两种实验模型。

（1）低张性缺氧（hypotonic hypoxia）：是以动脉血氧分压降低、血氧含量减少为基本特征的缺氧，又称乏氧性缺氧（hypoxic hypoxia）。引起低张性缺氧的原因有吸入气氧分压降低、外呼吸功能障碍、静脉血分流入动脉等，其共同特征是动脉血氧分压、氧含量、血氧饱和度均降低。本实验将小鼠放入盛有钠石灰（$NaOH \cdot CaO$）的密闭缺氧瓶内，由于瓶内氧气逐渐被小鼠利用，而呼出的 CO_2 被钠石灰吸收，因此缺氧瓶内空气的氧分压逐渐降低而不伴有 CO_2 浓度的增加，所以此种类型的缺氧为低张性缺氧。

（2）血液性缺氧（hemic hypoxia）：是由于血红蛋白含量减少或血红蛋白性质改变，使血液携氧能力降低或与血红蛋白结合氧不易释放所引起的缺氧。本实验详细介绍一氧化碳中毒和亚硝酸盐中毒所引起的血液性缺氧。

① 一氧化碳（CO）中毒：CO 可与血红蛋白（hemoglobin，Hb）结合形成碳氧血红蛋白（carboxyhemoglobin，HbCO）而失去携氧能力。CO 与 Hb 的亲和力是氧的 210 倍，而当 CO 与 Hb 分子中的某个血红素结合后，将增加其余 3 个血红素对氧的亲和力，使与 Hb 结合的氧不易被释放，氧解离曲线左移，导致缺氧。

② 亚硝酸盐中毒：Hb 中的二价铁（Fe^{2+}）可在氧化剂如亚硝酸钠（$NaNO_2$）的作用下被氧化成高铁血红蛋白（methemoglobin，$Hb-Fe^{3+}OH$），高铁血红蛋白中 Fe^{3+} 因与羟基结合牢固而失去结合氧的能力。当血红蛋白分子中的 4 个 Fe^{2+} 中有一部分被氧化成 Fe^{3+} 后，

剩下的 Fe^{2+} 虽能与氧结合但不易解离，导致氧解离曲线左移，组织缺氧。

$$Hb\text{-}Fe^{2+} \xrightarrow{\quad NaNO_2 \quad} Hb\text{-}Fe^{3+}$$

当体内存在还原剂时，被氧化的 Fe^{3+} 可还原为 Fe^{2+}，恢复血液携氧能力。本实验将 5% 亚硝酸钠溶液注入小鼠腹腔内，复制血液性缺氧模型，同时取另一只小鼠，用 1% 亚甲蓝（methylene blue）注入小鼠体内对抗 $NaNO_2$ 的作用，使被氧化的 Fe^{3+} 还原为 Fe^{2+}，恢复血液携氧能力，从而探讨 $NaNO_2$ 中毒的解救原理。

$$Hb\text{-}Fe^{3+} \xrightarrow{\quad 亚甲蓝 \quad} Hb\text{-}Fe^{2+}$$

3. 实验材料

（1）实验动物：小鼠，22~25 g，雌雄不限。

（2）实验器材：小鼠缺氧装置（图 2-62）、CO 发生装置（图 2-62）、剪刀、镊子、1 mL 注射器、1 mL 移液器。

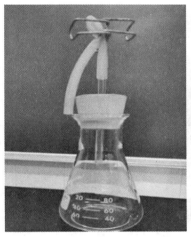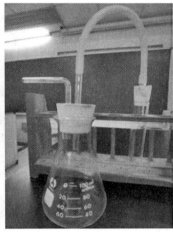

图 2-62　小鼠缺氧装置（左）和 CO 发生装置（右）

（3）实验试剂：钠石灰（NaOH·CaO）、甲酸、浓硫酸（H_2SO_4）、生理盐水、5% 亚硝酸钠（$NaNO_2$）、1% 亚甲蓝。

4. 实验步骤和观察项目

（1）低张性缺氧（A 鼠）：取 1 只小鼠放入盛有钠石灰（5 g）的缺氧瓶中，塞紧瓶塞、夹闭橡胶管并用水密封缺氧瓶，观察小鼠一般状况、呼吸频率和皮肤与黏膜颜色直至死亡。

（2）血液性缺氧

①一氧化碳中毒（B 鼠）：取 1 只小鼠放入缺氧瓶中，用 1 mL 移液器分别取 4 mL 甲酸和 2 mL 浓硫酸加入试管内并塞紧瓶塞，将已盛有小鼠的缺氧瓶（不放钠石灰）与一氧化碳发生装置相连接（原理见附录 4），观察小鼠一般状况、呼吸频率和皮肤与黏膜颜色直至死亡。

②亚硝酸盐中毒：取体重相近的 2 只小鼠（C 鼠和 D 鼠）分别作如下处理。

C 鼠：小鼠腹腔注射 5% 亚硝酸钠 0.3 mL 后立即再注入生理盐水 0.3 mL，观察小鼠一般状况、呼吸频率和皮肤与黏膜颜色直至死亡。

D 鼠：小鼠腹腔注射 5% 亚硝酸钠 0.3 mL 后立即再注入 1% 亚甲蓝溶液 0.3 mL，观察小鼠一般状况、呼吸频率和皮肤与黏膜颜色直至死亡。

（3）正常对照组（E 鼠）：取 1 只正常小鼠作为对照鼠，观察其一般状况、呼吸频率和皮肤与黏膜颜色，在其他模型全部复制完成后脱臼处死。

（4）用剪刀和镊子分别剖开 A、B、C、D、E 小鼠的下腹部，暴露肝脏并比较 5 只小鼠的肝脏颜色。

（5）根据观察和测量结果，填写表 2-3。

表 2-3　实验结果

小鼠编号	缺氧模型	一般活动	呼吸频率 （加快 / 减慢）	皮肤与黏膜颜色	肝脏颜色
A	低张性缺氧				
B	血液性缺氧 （CO 中毒）				
C	血液性缺氧 （$NaNO_2$ 中毒）				
D	亚甲蓝救治组				
E	正常对照组				

5. 注意事项

（1）缺氧瓶一定要密封，可将水加在瓶与瓶塞之间、瓶塞与玻璃管之间的缝隙中，以增加缺氧瓶的密封程度。

（2）为排除年龄因素的影响，各组小鼠的体重最好相等或接近。

（3）小鼠腹腔注射应在左下腹进行，勿损伤肝脏，也应避免将药液注入肠腔或膀胱。

（4）CO 中毒实验应注意先加甲酸再加浓硫酸，操作时注意防护，避免发生伤害事故。实验后应将废酸集中回收。

（5）一氧化碳产生后应立即与已盛有小鼠的缺氧瓶相连，否则一氧化碳挥发将影响实验效果。切勿将与大气相通的玻璃管封闭，以免产生危险。

6. 相关问题

（1）各类型缺氧时，动物血液颜色变化有何不同，为什么？

（2）各类型缺氧时，动物的呼吸变化有何不同，为什么？

（3）各类型缺氧时，动物的血气变化有何特点？其发生机制是怎样的？

实验十三　影响缺氧耐受性的因素

1. 目的

（1）复制小鼠低张性缺氧模型。

（2）观察外界环境温度、机体神经系统活动、代谢状态对小鼠缺氧耐受性的影响。

2. 原理

机体对缺氧的耐受性除受缺氧程度和发生速度影响以外，还与其他许多因素有关。代谢耗氧率是影响机体对缺氧耐受性的重要因素。当机体基础代谢率提高时，如外界环境温度升高、甲状腺功能亢进、神经及机体活动增强，代谢耗氧率增高，机体对缺氧的耐受性降低；当机体基础代谢率降低时，如外界环境温度降低、神经系统受抑制时则代谢耗氧率降低，机体对缺氧的耐受性增高。本实验通过改变小鼠所处的外界环境温度、腹腔注射中枢兴奋剂（异丙肾上腺素 + 尼可刹米）和抑制剂（戊巴比妥钠），观察外界环境温度和中枢神经系统功能状况对小鼠代谢耗氧量和存活时间的影响并计算代谢耗氧率，探讨外界环境温度和中枢神经系统功能状况对小鼠缺氧耐受性的影响。

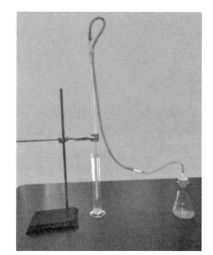

图 2-63　耗氧量测量装置

3. 实验材料

（1）实验动物：小鼠，22~25 g，雌雄不限。

（2）实验器材：小鼠缺氧装置（图 2-62）、电子天平、注射器、耗氧量测量装置（图 2-63）、恒温水浴锅。

（3）实验试剂：钠石灰、生理盐水、0.5% 戊巴比妥钠、4 mg/100 mL 异丙肾上腺素 +1 g/100 mL 尼可刹米混合液。

4. 实验步骤和观察项目

（1）外界环境温度对小鼠缺氧耐受性的影响

①取 3 个缺氧瓶，各放入 5 g 钠石灰。

②取 3 只体重相近的小鼠，称重后分别放入缺氧瓶中，编号后作如下处理。A 瓶：置于室温下；B 瓶：浸入冰水混合物中；C 瓶：浸入 42℃的水浴锅中。不盖瓶塞，将小鼠分别放入 A、B、C 瓶中适应 5 min 之后塞紧瓶塞，用弹簧夹夹闭胶管并用水密封缺氧瓶后开始计时。

③观察小鼠在瓶中的活动情况、呼吸运动和皮肤颜色，直至死亡，记录小鼠存活时间。将 B、C 瓶放回实验台面静置 15 min，待恢复室温后，用耗氧量测定装置分别测定 A、B、C 瓶内的总耗氧量（测定方法见附录 5）。

④根据小鼠体重（W）、存活时间（T）、总耗氧量（A），计算小鼠耗氧率（R）。将测得的数据填入表 2-4。

$$R\left[\mathrm{mL}/\left(\mathrm{g}\cdot\mathrm{min}\right)\right]=\frac{A\left(\mathrm{mL}\right)}{W\left(\mathrm{g}\right)\cdot T\left(\mathrm{min}\right)} \qquad (2\text{-}1)$$

（2）不同机体代谢状态对缺氧耐受性的影响

①取 3 个小鼠缺氧瓶，各放入 5 g 钠石灰。

②取 3 只体重相近的小鼠，称重后分别放入缺氧瓶中，编号后作如下处理。D 瓶：腹腔注

射生理盐水（0.1 mL/10 g 体重）；E 瓶：腹腔注射 0.5 % 戊巴比妥钠（0.1 mL/10 g 体重）；F 瓶：腹腔注射浓度为 4 mg/100 mL 异丙肾上腺素 +1 g/100 mL 尼可刹米混合液（0.1 mL/10 g 体重）。

③注射药物 5 min 后塞紧瓶塞、弹簧夹夹闭胶管并用水密封缺氧瓶后开始计时。

④观察小鼠在瓶中的活动情况、呼吸运动和皮肤颜色，直至死亡，记录存活时间。用耗氧量测定装置分别测定各瓶内的总耗氧量。

⑤按式（2-1）计算 D、E、F 小鼠的耗氧率（R）。将测得的数据填入表 2-4。

表 2-4　实验结果

动物编号	处理因素	体重 W（g）	存活时间 T（min）	耗氧量 A（mL）	耗氧率 R [mL/（g·min）]
A	室温				
B	冰水（0℃）				
C	42℃水浴				
D	生理盐水				
E	戊巴比妥钠				
F	异丙肾上腺素 + 尼可刹米				

5. 注意事项

（1）缺氧瓶一定要保证密闭（可在瓶与瓶塞、瓶塞与玻璃管的缝隙间注入少量清水，以加强缺氧瓶的密闭效果）。

（2）小鼠腹腔注射应稍靠近左下腹，勿损伤肝脏，也应避免将药液注入肠腔或膀胱。

（3）测耗氧量时，要记录耗氧量测定装置外管（量筒）液面下降的高度。

6. 相关问题

（1）本实验中引起小鼠死亡的原因各是什么？

（2）陈述影响机体缺氧耐受性的因素有哪些，并解释它们是如何起作用的？

实验十四　高钾血症及其解救

1. 目的

（1）学习高钾血症动物模型的复制方法。

（2）观察高血钾对心脏的毒性作用，掌握高血钾时心电图改变的特征。

（3）了解高钾血症治疗的基本原则。

2. 原理

正常人的血清钾浓度是 3.5~5.5 mmol/L，当血清钾浓度高于 5.5 mmol/L 时称为高钾血症（hyperkalemia）。高钾血症的常见原因有钾摄入过多、排出减少、细胞内钾转移到细胞外等。高钾血症对心肌的毒性作用极强，高钾血症患者可发生致命性心室纤颤和心脏骤停，主要表现为心肌电生理特性的改变及引发的心电图变化和心脏功能损害。高钾血症时，心肌细胞的兴奋性呈双向性改变：轻度高钾血症时心肌细胞的兴奋性增加，重度高钾血症时兴奋性降低；心肌的自律性和传导性降低、收缩性减弱，心电图主要表现为 T 波狭窄高耸，P 波压低、增宽或消失，QRS 波群振幅降低和增宽，P-R 间期延长。本实验通过耳缘静脉向家兔体内输入 1%KCl，人为造成家兔血钾浓度急剧升高（血清钾 >5.5 mmol/L），同时观察家兔注射氯化钾溶液前后的心电图的变化来研究高钾血症对心脏的毒性作用，并初步了解高钾血症的治疗原则。

3. 实验材料

（1）实验动物：家兔，2.0~2.5 kg，雌雄不限。

（2）实验器材：哺乳动物手术器械、兔台、心电图机、离心机、Na^+-K^+ 分析仪、静脉输液装置、注射器、头皮针、5 mL 抗凝管。

（3）实验试剂：25% 氨基甲酸乙酯（乌拉坦）溶液、0.3% 肝素溶液、1% 氯化钾（KCl）溶液、4% 碳酸氢钠溶液、10% 氯化钙溶液、50% 葡萄糖溶液、胰岛素。

4. 实验步骤和观察项目

（1）术前准备：取 1 只家兔，称重，耳缘静脉注射 25% 乌拉坦溶液（4 mL/kg）麻醉，将麻醉后的家兔仰卧位固定在兔台上。清除颈前部毛发。

（2）颈总动脉插管（附录 6）：沿颈部正中做一 4~5 cm 的纵形切口，逐层分离皮下组织和肌肉，暴露气管。在气管的背外侧找到颈总动脉鞘，小心地分离一侧颈总动脉（长约 3 cm），远心端用线结扎，近心端用动脉夹夹闭。用充满肝素的动脉导管剪口插管或者用 22 G 静脉留置针插管并结扎固定。

（3）采血并制备血清：由颈动脉插管放血 1 mL 至抗凝管中，上下颠倒混匀，1000 g 离心 15 min 后取上清测定实验前的血钾浓度。

（4）将心电图针形电极分别插入家兔四肢踝部皮下。导联线按右前肢（红）、左前肢（黄）、右后肢（黑）、左后肢（绿）的顺序连接。

（5）打开心电图机，选择 II 导联或 avF 导联记录一段正常心电图作为对照。

（6）将头皮针与静脉输液装置相连，排气后穿刺耳缘静脉，用胶布将头皮针固定在耳廓上。根据家兔的状况，调节 1%KCl 输液速度为 60~80 滴 / 分左右。

（7）每隔 2 min 记录一次心电图。当心电图出现 P 波低平增宽、QRS 波群压低变宽和 T 波高尖后停止滴注 KCl 溶液，按照步骤（3）中的方法再次采集和制备血清标本，测定血钾浓度。

（8）抢救：当观察到典型高钾血症的心电图改变后，分组采用下列其中一种抢救方法，观察心电图是否恢复正常，再次由颈总动脉采血 1 mL，测定抢救后的血钾浓度。

A 组：自耳缘静脉缓慢注入 4% 碳酸氢钠 6~10 mL。

B 组：自耳缘静脉缓慢注入 10% 氯化钙 1~2 mL。

C 组：自耳缘静脉缓慢注入 50% 葡萄糖 20 mL+ 胰岛素 4 U。

（9）继续维持原有输液速度滴注 1%KCl 溶液，观察心电图波形变化直至出现室颤或心跳停止为止。

（10）开胸观察心室颤动或心跳停止的状态（注意观察心脏停止在收缩期还是舒

张期）。

（11）将测得的数据填入表 2-5。

表2-5　实验结果

实验项目	心电图改变	血清钾浓度（mmol/L）
实验前		
1% KCl 滴注后		
4% 碳酸氢钠		
10% 氯化钙		
50% 葡萄糖 + 胰岛素		

5. 注意事项

（1）缓慢注射乌拉坦溶液，快速注射可能会导致动物呼吸抑制和猝死。如果动物在实验过程中仍有疼痛反应，则静脉注射小剂量乌拉坦或 1% 普鲁卡因作局部浸润麻醉。

（2）由于对高钾血症的耐受性不同，一些动物可能需要比其他动物更高剂量的 KCl 来诱发心电图的异常变化。

（3）心电图机应接入地线避免周围电磁干扰。

（4）严格控制静脉滴注氯化钾溶液的速度，以防动物因滴注过快而出现心搏骤停。推注氯化钙抢救高钾血症时速度要慢，否则易导致高血钙引起动物死亡。

6. 相关问题

（1）高钾血症对心肌有什么毒性作用？

（2）高钾血症时心电图有什么变化？解释其可能的机制。

（3）心搏骤停时处于舒张还是收缩状态？

（4）高钾血症抢救的原则是什么？

实验十五　肠缺血再灌注损伤

1. 目的

（1）复制肠缺血再灌注损伤动物模型。

（2）观察肠缺血再灌注损伤时血压的改变、小肠肠系膜微循环变化及局部小肠壁形态学改变，并探讨其可能的发病机制。

2. 原理

在缺血基础上恢复血流后，不仅不能使组织器官功能恢复，反而加重组织、器官的功能障碍和结构损伤，甚至发生不可逆损伤的现象称为缺血再灌注损伤（ischemia reperfusion injury，IRI）。缺血再灌注损伤的发生机制尚未彻底阐明，目前认为自由基作用、细胞内钙超载和白细胞的激活是缺血再灌注损伤的重要发病环节。本实验通过钳夹肠系膜上动脉一定时间造成家兔急性肠缺血，使肠黏膜损伤和屏障功能障碍，表现为广泛的上皮与绒毛分离、上皮坏死、大量中性粒细胞浸润、固有层破坏、出血及溃疡形成。当放开钳夹的肠系膜上动脉恢复血流灌注后，肠黏膜损伤和肠壁毛细血管通透性更高，并出现再灌注性低血压。

3. 实验材料

（1）实验动物：家兔，2.0~ 2.5 kg，雌雄不限。

（2）实验器材：哺乳动物手术器械、兔台、BL-420 系统、微循环灌流装置、动态微循环图像分析系统、压力换能器、动脉夹、注射器、100 mL 烧杯、动脉导管、三通管、纱布。

（3）实验试剂：25% 氨基甲酸乙酯（乌拉坦）溶液、1% 普鲁卡因溶液、生理盐水、0.3% 肝素溶液。

4. 实验步骤和观察项目

（1）术前准备：取一只家兔，称重后耳缘静脉注射 25% 乌拉坦溶液（4 mL/kg）麻醉，将麻醉后的家兔仰卧位固定在台上。清除颈部和下腹部毛发。

（2）肠系膜上动脉分离术：从胸骨剑突下 5 cm 起向下沿正中线做长约 5~10 cm 的腹部正中切口，再沿腹白线剪开腹肌，打开腹腔，用蘸有生理盐水的纱布将内脏轻轻扒向左侧，暴露右肾、脊柱和腹膜后组织。以右肾为标志，将从腹主动脉略低于右肾门处发出的肠系膜上动脉分离出来，穿线备用。

（3）肠系膜微循环观察：在腹腔右下方找到回盲交界处，移出与阑尾通过筋膜相连的一段回肠，此处肠系膜长、脂肪少，便于观察。将肠系膜平铺于含有灌流液的灌流盒中的载物台上，用解剖显微镜选定最佳观察部位和血管（同一视野中有动、静脉，动 - 静脉吻合支和毛细血管），通过电脑显示屏的放大，观察正常肠系膜微循环情况（流态、流速和口径）。

流态：按照微血管内血液流动的形态区分。

0 级：线（袋）状——能看到血液在流动，但看不清楚血细胞的形态。

Ⅰ级：粒（絮）状——能清楚地看到血细胞的形态。

Ⅱ级：瘀滞——血细胞停止不动或来回摆动。

流速：可根据所使用的软件读取流速数值。

口径：选择血管边缘清晰、管径大小合适的部位，用软件提供的测距功能测量管径粗细。

（4）经耳缘静脉注射 0.3% 肝素溶液 1ml 进行全身抗凝。

（5）颈总动脉插管（附录 6）：沿颈部正中做一 4~5 cm 的纵形切口，逐层分离皮下组织和肌肉，暴露气管。在气管的背外侧找到颈总动脉鞘，小心地分离一侧颈总动脉（长约 3 cm），远心端用线结扎，近心端用动脉夹夹闭。用充满肝素的动脉导管（或者用 22G 静脉留置针）剪口插管，结扎固定后通过压力换能器与 BL-420 系统连接，记录正常动脉血压曲线（收缩压、舒张压、平均动脉压和心率）。

（6）肠缺血再灌注模型复制：用动脉夹夹闭肠系膜上动脉 30~60 min，回纳肠管入腹腔并用两把止血钳夹闭肠壁使肠腔闭合，用蘸有生理盐水的纱布覆盖腹部切口。观察肠系膜上动脉夹闭期间的动脉血压、肠系膜微循环状况。然后松开动脉夹，用手指在肠系膜上动脉远心端触摸，感觉到有动脉搏动时，说明小肠血流恢复。记录松开结扎后 0 min、5 min、15 min、30 min 时动脉血压和肠系膜微循环状况。

（7）动物安乐死：实验结束后，静脉注射两倍剂量的乌拉坦，对动物实施安乐死。

5. 注意事项

（1）缓慢注射乌拉坦，快速注射可能导致呼吸抑制和动物猝死。手术过程中如动物仍有疼痛反应，可用少量的 1% 普鲁卡因作局部浸润麻醉。

（2）翻动肠子动作要轻柔，避免过度牵拉肠管引起低血压。

（3）不要使用锐利器械分离肠系膜上动脉，以免损伤大血管而造成大出血。

（4）用动脉夹夹闭肠系膜上动脉必须牢固可靠。动脉夹松开后，可用手指轻轻搓揉动脉夹闭处血管，以防动脉壁粘贴不能恢复血流灌注。

6. 相关问题

（1）实验中平均动脉压有何变化？试述其形成机制。

（2）再灌注前后肠系膜微循环有何变化？试述其变化的原因和机制。

实验十六　失血性休克

1. 目的

（1）复制失血性休克动物模型。

（2）观察失血前后及休克治疗前后平均动脉压、微循环等主要体征及血流动力学的改变，探讨失血性休克的发病机制、病理生理过程及治疗原则。

2. 原理

休克是机体在严重失血失液、感染、创伤等强烈致病因素的作用下，有效循环血量急剧减少，组织灌流严重不足，引起组织细胞缺血、缺氧、各重要器官功能及代谢障碍、结构损伤的病理过程。当大量液体丢失或者血管通透性增高时，可导致血容量急剧减少、静脉回流不足、心排血量减少和血压下降，组织灌注不足，引起失血性休克。休克是否发生取决于失血量和失血速度：一般 15~20 min 内失血少于全身总血量的 10%~15% 时，机体可通过代偿使血压和组织灌流量基本保持在正常范围内；若在 15 min 内快速大量失血超过总血量的 20%，则超出了机体的代偿能力，即可引起心排血量和平均动脉压下降，从而发生失血性休克。本实验通过股动脉放血的方法使家兔血压较长时间维持在正常血压的 40%，从而复制失血性休克模型。通过输液、补充血容量、使用不同血管活性药物，比较其疗效，分析它们在失血性休克治疗中的作用。

3. 实验材料

（1）实验动物：家兔，2.0~2.5 kg，雌雄不限。

（2）实验器材：哺乳动物手术器械、兔台、BL-420 系统、压力换能器、动脉夹、动脉导管、注射器、头皮针、三通管。

（3）实验试剂：25% 氨基甲酸乙酯（乌拉坦）溶液、1% 普鲁卡因溶液、0.3% 肝素溶液、去甲肾上腺素、山莨菪碱（654-2）。

4. 实验步骤和观察项目

（1）术前准备：取 1 只家兔，称重后耳缘静脉注射 25% 乌拉坦溶液（4 mL/kg）麻醉，将麻醉后的家兔仰卧位固定在兔台上。清除颈部、腹部、腹股沟处毛发。

（2）颈总动脉、股动脉插管（附录6）：在颈部、腹股沟部分离颈总动脉和股动脉，穿线备用。用动脉导管（或24G静脉留置针）行股动脉插管术，通过三通管连接注射器用于放血（注射器中含有20 mL 0.3%肝素溶液）。用动脉导管（或22G静脉留置针）刺入颈动脉进行插管固定，连接压力换能器，记录并保存正常血压曲线（收缩压、舒张压、平均动脉压）。

（3）肠系膜微循环观察：在腹腔右下方找到回盲交界处，移出与阑尾通过筋膜相连的一段回肠，此处肠系膜长、脂肪少，便于观察。将肠系膜平铺于灌流盒中的载物台上，用解剖显微镜选定最佳观察部位和血管（同一视野中有动、静脉，动-静脉吻合支和毛细血管），通过电脑显示屏的放大，观察正常肠系膜微循环情况（流态、流速和口径）。

流态：按照微血管内血液流动的形态区分。

0级：线（袋）状——能看到血液在流动，但看不清楚血细胞的形态。

Ⅰ级：粒（絮）状——能清楚地看到血细胞的形态。

Ⅱ级：瘀滞——血细胞停止不动或来回摆动。

流速：可根据所使用的软件读取流速数值。

口径：选择血管边缘清晰、管径大小合适的部位，用软件提供的测距功能测量管径粗细。

（4）休克模型复制：待家兔平均动脉压稳定后，用含有20 mL 0.3%肝素溶液的注射器经股动脉放血至3/4正常血压值，维持血压稳定10 min，观察机体代偿性反应和血压变化。继续经股动脉放血至正常血压值的40%，维持该血压值30 min。观察休克状态下肠系膜微循环情况（流态、流速和口径）。

（5）实验性治疗：分为2组进行实验性治疗，选用①或者②治疗方案，观察治疗后血压和肠系膜微循环情况（流态、流速和口径）。

①血液回输：经股动脉回输全部放出的动脉血，观察血压的变化至平稳（如输血未达到效果可补充生理盐水）。在血液回输前后分别经耳缘静脉注射山莨菪碱（654-2）（每只10 mL），观察血压的变化。

②使用血管活性药物：经耳缘静脉注射去甲肾上腺素2 mL（浓度为75 μg/mL）。当血压回降至注射前血压值时，行第二次注射。当血压回降至注射前血压值时，行第三次注射。比较三次注射时的血压变化。

（6）动物安乐死：实验结束后，采用2倍剂量麻醉剂静脉注射，对动物实施安乐死。

5. 注意事项

（1）注射乌拉坦的速度要慢，过快会导致动物呼吸抑制死亡。如手术操作过程中动物仍有疼痛反应，可用少量的1%普鲁卡因作局部浸润麻醉。

（2）动脉插管时注意区分动静脉，动脉较细，颜色淡红或者鲜红，有搏动。

（3）动脉导管或者留置针插管前要充满0.3%肝素溶液；50 mL注射器使用前需经0.3%肝素溶液灌洗并预留20 mL肝素溶液于注射器内，防止凝血。

（4）肠系膜微循环观察时应取肠系膜较长、脂肪较少的回盲部肠袢，以免系膜牵拉肠袢引起反射性低血压，同时做好肠袢保温。

6. 相关问题

（1）如何判断休克的发生？有哪些体征可帮助诊断？

（2）实验过程中所记录的动脉平均血压变化呈何形态？试述其形成的病理生理机制。

（3）实验中失血前后及治疗后肠系膜微循环有何变化？试述其发生的病理生理机制。

（4）实验动物发生休克后，单纯注射去甲肾上腺素为什么不能维持稳定的血压？动物对三次注射去甲肾上腺素的反应有何不同？为什么？

（5）本实验两次注射山莨菪碱的血压反应有何不同？舒张血管药物应在什么情况下使用？

实验十七　急性右心衰竭

1. 目的

（1）复制急性右心衰竭动物模型。观察急性右心衰竭时血流动力学的主要变化。

（2）探讨急性右心衰竭的病因和发病机制。

2. 原理

心力衰竭是指在各种致病因素的作用下，心脏的收缩和（或）舒张功能发生障碍，使心排血量绝对或相对下降，以致不能满足机体代谢需要的病理生理过程。原发性心肌舒缩功能障碍和心脏前后负荷过重是心力衰竭的两大病因。前负荷指心脏舒张的容量负荷，后负荷指心脏收缩所承受的压力负荷。本实验通过增加右心室的后负荷（静脉注射液状石蜡栓塞肺小动脉）和前负荷（大量快速输液）的方法，监测动脉血压和中心静脉压来观察急性右心衰竭时血流动力学的改变，从而加深对心力衰竭发病机制的理解。

3. 实验材料

（1）实验动物：家兔，2.0~2.5 kg，雌雄不限。

（2）实验器材：注射器、哺乳动物手术器械、兔台、BL-420系统、压力换能器、动脉夹、注射器、头皮针、三通管、动脉导管或22 G静脉留置针、输液装置、中心静脉压测量装置（图2-64）。

（3）实验试剂：25%氨基甲酸乙酯（乌拉坦）溶液、1%普鲁卡因溶液、肝素钠注射液、0.3%肝素溶液、生理盐水、液状石蜡。

4. 实验步骤和观察项目

（1）术前准备：取1只家兔，称重后耳缘静脉注射25%乌拉坦溶液（4 mL/kg）麻醉，将麻醉后的家兔仰卧位固定在兔台上，清除颈部毛发。

（2）颈总动脉和颈静脉分离：沿颈部正中做一4~5 cm的纵形切口，逐层分离皮下组织和肌肉，暴露气管。分离一侧颈动脉和两侧颈静脉。

（3）经耳缘静脉注射肝素钠注射液1 mL进行全身

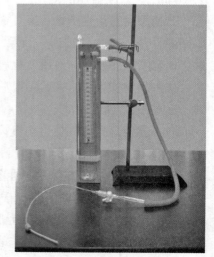

图2-64　中心静脉压测量装置

肝素化抗凝。

（4）颈总动脉插管（附录6）：颈总动脉远心端用线结扎，近心端用动脉夹夹闭。用充满肝素溶液的动脉导管（或者用22 G静脉留置针）剪口插管，结扎固定后通过压力换能器与BL-420系统连接，记录正常动脉血压曲线（收缩压、舒张压、平均动脉压和心率）。

（5）颈静脉插管（附录6）：调节中心静脉压测量装置使其"0"位和家兔腋中线处于同一平面，经右侧颈静脉插入中心静脉压插管。插管过程可见中心静脉压测量装置液面不断降低，插入约5~6 cm时液面停止下降且随呼吸波动，该高度即为中心静脉压值。固定插管，记录中心静脉压值（CVP）。经左侧颈静脉插管连接输液装置，以小于10滴/分的速度输液维持管道通畅。

（6）建立家兔急性右心衰竭模型

①用2 mL注射器取温度为38℃的液状石蜡经耳缘静脉以0.1 mL/min速度缓慢注入，密切观察动脉血压和中心静脉压。当动脉血压明显下降（下降10~20 mmHg）或中心静脉压明显上升（增高20~30 mmH$_2$O）时停止注射液状石蜡。如上述指标又恢复到原对照水平，可再次缓慢注射液状石蜡，直至动脉血压下降或中心静脉压有明显上升为止（一般液体石蜡用量不宜超过1 mL/kg）。

②以80~100滴/分的速度快速经左侧颈静脉输入生理盐水直至动物死亡，观察动脉血压和中心静脉压的改变。

（7）打开胸腔和腹腔，观察肺、心脏、肠系膜血管、肠壁和肝脏的外观，观察动脉血压和中心静脉压的改变。

5. 注意事项

（1）麻醉时观察家兔的角膜和肌肉反射情况，使得麻醉的深浅适度。注射乌拉坦的速度要慢，过快会导致呼吸抑制引起动物死亡。如手术操作过程中动物仍有疼痛反应，可用少量的1%普鲁卡因作局部浸润麻醉。

（2）用0.3%肝素溶液填充中心静脉压测定仪和动脉导管，以避免凝血。

（3）耳缘静脉注入液状石蜡时，注入速度不宜太快也不宜太慢，要随时观察各项指标的变化。当其中有一项指标发生急剧变化时，应减慢注射速度。

（4）当输液量超过200 mL/kg，若各项指标变化仍不显著，可再次补注少量液状石蜡。

6. 相关问题

（1）本实验中有哪些指标可帮助判断急性右心衰竭的发生，为什么？

（2）影响中心静脉压的因素有哪些？试述右心衰竭时中心静脉压升高的机制？

（3）右心衰竭时，机体的主要病理生理变化有哪些？

（4）中心静脉压在诊断和治疗心衰中的临床意义有哪些？

实验十八 呼吸衰竭

1. 目的

（1）复制不同类型的呼吸衰竭动物模型（窒息、气胸和肺水肿）。 观察不同类型呼吸衰竭模型动物的血气和呼吸的变化。

（2）了解肺通气和换气功能障碍在呼吸衰竭中的发生机制。

2. 原理

呼吸衰竭指由于外呼吸功能严重障碍，导致在静息状态下，出现 PaO_2 降低伴或者不伴有 $PaCO_2$ 增高的病理过程。根据血气特点分为 I 型呼吸衰竭（低氧血症型呼吸衰竭，$PaO_2<60$ mmHg）和 II 型呼吸衰竭（伴有高碳酸血症型低氧血症呼吸衰竭，$PaO_2<60$ mmHg 同时伴有 $PaCO_2>50$ mmHg）。造成呼吸衰竭的主要原因有肺通气功能障碍（限制性和阻塞性通气不足）和换气功能障碍（弥散障碍、肺泡通气血流比例失调、解剖分流增加）。本实验中，通过夹闭气道引起窒息的方式造成全肺的通气障碍来复制 II 型呼吸衰竭模型；通过气管滴注 20% 葡萄糖造成肺间质水肿而阻碍肺换气过程来复制 I 型呼吸衰竭模型；通过人工方法造成家兔气胸，复制限制性通气障碍、肺泡通气 / 血流比例失调所致的急性呼吸功能不全模型。

3. 实验材料

（1）实验动物：家兔，2.0~2.5 kg，雌雄不限。

（2）实验器材：哺乳动物手术器械、兔台、BL-420 系统、呼吸换能器、动脉导管、Y 型气管插管、注射器、动脉夹、18 号针头、三通管、弹簧夹、血气分析仪。

（3）实验试剂：25% 氨基甲酸乙酯（乌拉坦）溶液、1% 普鲁卡因溶液、20% 葡萄糖溶液。

4. 实验步骤和观察项目

（1）术前准备：取 1 只家兔，称重后耳缘静脉注射 25% 乌拉坦溶液（4 mL/kg）麻醉，将麻醉后的家兔仰卧位固定在兔台上，清除颈部毛发。

（2）颈总动脉插管（附录 6）：颈部正中切口分离颈总动脉和气管。用动脉导管做颈总动脉插管，连接三通管后取 0.5 mL 动脉血进行血气分析。

（3）气管插管（附录 6）：在气管甲状软骨下 0.5~1 cm 处做 "T" 形切口（可酌情使用局麻），插入 Y 型气管插管并固定。通过呼吸换能器连接 BL-420 系统，记录呼吸频率和深度。

（4）复制窒息：用弹簧夹将 Y 型气管插管上端橡皮管完全夹闭，使动物处于完全窒息状态 30 s，描记呼吸曲线。打开弹簧夹使动物恢复正常呼吸。可重复多次。在夹闭 25 s 左右时取 0.5 mL 动脉血进行血气分析。

（5）复制气胸：局麻下于家兔右胸腋中线第 4 或第 5 肋间隙切开皮肤，用 18 号针头穿刺（有明显突破感即进入胸膜腔），该针头用三通管连接注射器。向胸膜腔内缓慢注入空气（30 毫升 / 次），家兔呼吸出现明显改变和口唇黏膜发绀后，采集血样行血气分析，同时用 50 mL 注射器将胸腔内空气抽尽，拔出针头。观察 10~20 min，待动物呼吸恢复正常。

（6）复制肺水肿：将家兔头端兔台垫高，从 Y 型气管插管一侧逐滴缓慢滴入 20% 葡萄糖溶液 2 mL，观察呼吸频率及幅度，并描记呼吸曲线，直至泡沫状液体随呼吸从气管插管冒出。若 20 min 后仍未见呼出泡沫状液体，可加注 20% 葡萄糖溶液 1~2 mL。

（7）动物安乐死：采用 2 倍剂量麻醉剂静脉注射，实施安乐死。打开胸腔，切开肺脏，观察有无泡沫样液体流出。

5. 注意事项

（1）气胸后胸腔内的空气一定要抽尽。

（2）复制肺水肿时，从 Y 型气管插管滴注葡萄糖溶液不能太快，以免造成窒息。

6. 相关问题

（1）实验中不同类型的呼吸衰竭模型血气变化有什么特点？请解释其可能的机制。

（2）本实验通过窒息、肺水肿或气胸复制了哪种类型的呼吸衰竭？

（3）可以观察到肺部有哪些病理变化？请解释其可能的机制？

实验十九　氨在肝性脑病发病机制中的作用

1. 目的

（1）复制急性肝功能不全动物模型。

（2）探讨血氨升高在肝性脑病发病机制中的作用。

2. 原理

肝性脑病（hepatic encephalopathy，HE）是指在排除其他已知脑疾病的前提下，继发于肝功能障碍的一系列严重的神经精神综合征，其发病机制尚不完全清楚。解释肝性脑病发生机制的学说主要有氨中毒学说、假性神经递质学说、血浆氨基酸失衡学说及 γ- 氨基丁酸学说等。本实验采用肝大部分结扎术复制急性肝功能不全动物模型，在此基础上经十二指肠插管分别灌注复方氯化铵溶液和复方氯化钠溶液；另一假手术组（不做肝大部分结扎术）家兔经十二指肠插管灌注复方氯化铵溶液，观察灌注前后家兔的反应（是否有抽搐、昏迷痉挛等类似肝性脑病的表现）和出现上述症状时所灌注的氯化铵的量，论证肝功能不全和血氨升高在肝性脑病发生中的辩证关系，加深对氨中毒学说的理解。

3. 实验材料

（1）实验动物：家兔，2.0~2.5 kg，雌雄不限。

（2）实验器材：哺乳动物手术器械、兔台、注射器、导尿管、粗棉线。

（3）实验试剂：1% 普鲁卡因溶液、2.5% 复方氯化铵溶液（氯化铵 25 g、碳酸氢钠 15 g、溶于 5% 葡萄糖溶液 1000 mL 中）、2.5% 复方氯化钠溶液（氯化钠 25 g、碳酸氢钠 15 g、溶于 5% 葡萄糖溶液 1000 mL 中）。

4. 实验步骤和观察项目

（1）术前准备：取 3 只体重相近的家兔仰卧固定于兔台上，剪去腹壁被毛，手术部位注射 5~10 mL 1% 普鲁卡因溶液，使家兔在局部浸润麻醉下分三组进行实验。

（2）肝叶大部分结扎术：家兔从胸骨剑突起，沿腹白线作长约 6~8 cm 的上腹正中切口。打开腹腔后，即可见位于右上腹的肝脏。用左手将肝脏往下压，右手持剪刀剪断肝与膈肌之间的镰状韧带；再将肝叶向上翻，用手剥离肝胃韧带。辨明肝脏各叶，用粗棉线沿着肝脏左外叶、左中叶、右中叶和方形叶的根部围绕一周并结扎。

（3）十二指肠插管：沿胃幽门向下找出十二指肠，用小圆针做荷包缝合。用眼科剪在荷包中央剪一小切口，将导尿管一端向十二指肠远端空肠方向插入约 4 cm，收紧缝线并打结固定插管。将肠管回纳腹腔，分层缝合腹壁。留导尿管（或头皮针管）另一端于腹外固定在兔耳上。

（4）松绑家兔，观察并记录动物呼吸、瞳孔大小、角膜反射、四肢肌张力及对疼痛刺激的反应。

（5）实验分组

①A 兔（模型组）：按照实验步骤（2）~（4）进行操作。每隔 5 min 向十二指肠插管中注入 2.5% 复方氯化铵溶液 5 mL，观察动物反应，直至痉挛、抽搐和强直（角弓反张）发作为止，记录所用的复方氯化铵溶液总量填入表 2-6，并计算出家兔每千克体重用量。

②B 兔（假手术组）：除了不结扎肝叶外，所有操作与 A 兔相同。

③C 兔（药物对照组）：按照实验步骤（2）~（4）进行操作。每隔 5 min 向十二指肠注入 2.5% 复方氯化钠溶液 5 mL，观察动物有无异常变化。

④在表 2-6 中记录各组家兔是否出现角弓反张以及出现角弓反张时的用药总量。

表 2-6　实验结果

家兔编号	肝叶大部分结扎术	灌注药物	用量	总量
A	是	复方氯化铵溶液	5 mL/5 min	
B	否	复方氯化铵溶液	5 mL/5 min	
C	是	复方氯化钠溶液	5 mL/5 min	

5. 注意事项

（1）为排除麻醉药对动物神经系统的影响，本实验采用 1% 普鲁卡因皮下注射的方法做局部浸润麻醉。

（2）剪断镰状韧带时，谨防刺破膈肌，造成气胸。游离肝脏时，动作宜轻柔，以免肝叶破裂出血。

（3）结扎肝叶根部，避免拦腰勒破肝组织造成大出血。

（4）荷包缝合应选在十二指肠壁血管分布稀疏的部位进行。插管结扎固定要可靠，以免复方氯化铵溶液漏入腹腔。

6. 相关问题

（1）结合实验结果，简述肝性脑病发病机制中氨中毒学说的基本观点。

（2）如何从复方氯化铵溶液的成分来理解肝性脑病的诱因及防治肝性脑病的病理生理基础？

（3）肝性脑病病人的临床表现和实验室检查有哪些？

实验二十　不同给药途径对药物作用的影响

1. 目的

观察药物在不同给药途径情况下，其药效动力学发生的变化及产生差异的原因。

2. 原理

通过不同给药途径给予动物药物，药物的吸收速度和吸收量有差异，药物效应因而产生差异，包括"量的差异"（即相同效应，但作用强度不相同）和"质的差异"（即出现不同的药理效应）。硫酸镁这一类药比较特殊，口服时基本不被吸收而仅发挥渗透性导泻作用，而注射给药则会进入血液循环，产生其真实的药理作用，因而在临床上通过注射用于治疗子痫。

3. 实验材料

（1）实验动物：小白鼠，18~22 g。

（2）实验器材：注射器、小鼠灌胃针、鼠笼。

（3）实验试剂：4% 硫酸镁溶液。

4. 实验步骤和观察项目

（1）取体重相近的 4 只小白鼠，随机分到两组中，每组 2 只，称重编号。1 号和 2 号鼠腹腔注射硫酸镁溶液 0.5 mL（或 0.2 mL/10 g 体重），3 号和 4 号鼠经口灌胃同样剂量的硫酸镁溶液。

（2）观察并比较两种给药方式的药物反应，填入表 2-7。

表 2-7　实验结果

编号	体重	药物剂量	给药途径	给药前		给药后		大便
				肌张力	呼吸	肌张力	呼吸	
1								
2								
3								
4								

5. 注意事项

（1）灌胃时注意操作要领，注意勿将灌胃针插入气管，以免造成动物窒息。

（2）腹腔注射时应掌握好注射部位（中下腹部）位和角度（30°~45°），避免伤及内脏。

（3）给药后如发现动物肌肉松弛明显，呼吸抑制严重，可腹腔注射氯化钙 0.2 mL 进行抢救治疗。

6. 相关问题

（1）当相同剂量的同一药物以不同给药途径给药时，动物为什么会出现不同的药物效应？

（2）硫酸镁的药理作用机制及临床应用如何？当硫酸镁过量中毒时如何进行解救？

实验二十一　药物的量效关系

1. 目的

以家兔离体空肠作为实验观察对象，研究乙酰胆碱（ACh）的量效关系。

2. 原理

离体肠管实验可用于观察药物对小肠平滑肌舒缩功能的影响。ACh可兴奋兔小肠上的M受体而使之收缩，且其收缩力随浓度的增加而有规律地增加，药理效应呈现出剂量依赖性，可定量分析相关的药效学参数，如 E_{max}（最大效应）和 EC_{50}（半数最大效应浓度，即在此浓度下，产生50%最大效应）。

3. 实验材料

（1）实验动物：家兔，2.0~2.5 kg。

（2）实验器材：哺乳动物手术器械、兔台、恒温平滑肌槽、张力换能器、BL-420系统、1 mL加样器、注射器、烧杯、培养皿、手术器械、氧气瓶等。

（3）实验试剂：氯乙酰胆碱溶液（10^{-7} mol/L、10^{-6} mol/L、10^{-5} mol/L、10^{-4} mol/L、10^{-3} mol/L、10^{-2} mol/L、10^{-1} mol/L）、台氏液、25%氨基甲酸乙酯（乌拉坦）溶液。

4. 实验步骤和观察项目

（1）实验前动物禁食12 h。

（2）实验前3 h启动恒温平滑肌槽，在浴槽内加适量水，保持水温37℃。

（3）制备空肠标本：取1只家兔，耳缘静脉注射25%乌拉坦（4 mL/kg）麻醉后，迅速打开腹腔，找到胃幽门与十二指肠交界处，以此处为起点取长约20 cm的肠管，沿肠缘剪去与该段肠管相连的肠系膜，迅速将标本放在4℃左右的台氏液中，并用台氏液将肠腔内容物冲洗干净，将肠管剪成2~3 cm长的肠段，置于4℃左右的台氏液中备用；剩下没有剪断的肠管放置于4℃冰箱中，12 h内仍可使用。

（4）悬挂标本：在浴管内加入台氏液20 mL，调节空气进入量，以每秒1~2个气泡为宜。用缝合线固定肠段两端，一端系于L型钩上，放入浴管，另一端用线连接于张力换能器，再与BL-420系统连接。在线完全松弛时，记录此时的肌张力大小（X g），然后调节线的松紧度，在逐渐拉紧线的同时观察张力大小，使肌张力值比完全松弛时所测的肌张力大2~3 g（X+2~3 g）。调好合适的肌张力大小后，将肠段置于标本槽内稳定10 min再继续下一步实验。

（5）打开BL-420系统，点击药理学实验模块（药物对离体肠的作用），启动描记。

（6）加药：描记一段给药前曲线作为对照，按下表滴加不同浓度的ACh，每加一次ACh待收缩曲线不再上升时，用台氏液冲洗三次，然后稳定5~10 min，再按顺序加下一个浓度的ACh，以此类推。

（7）列表绘图：测量小肠张力最大值（g），即收缩曲线上升最大幅度值，填入表2-8。以收缩幅度为Y，浴管中ACh浓度的对数（以10为底）为X绘制量效曲线，同时将数据输入已经制作好的Excel表中，生成相应的量效曲线。

5. 注意事项

（1）制备肠段时避免损伤，尽量在台氏液中操作，勿在空气中暴露过久。

（2）悬吊不宜过紧，采用合适的松紧度，且线和肠段不可与管壁相贴。

（3）加药量必须准确，要将药加在液面上，不能直接加在肠管上。

表 2-8　实验结果

加药顺序	ACh 浓度（mol/L）	ACh 容积（mL）	浴管中 ACh 浓度（mol/L）	X（g）	收缩幅度（g）
1	10^{-7}	0.2	10^{-9}		
2	10^{-6}	0.2	10^{-8}		
3	10^{-5}	0.2	10^{-7}		
4	10^{-4}	0.2	10^{-6}		
5	10^{-3}	0.2	10^{-5}		
6	10^{-2}	0.2	10^{-4}		
7	10^{-1}	0.2	10^{-3}		

（4）实验开始后不得随意调节换能器和各种参数。

6. 相关问题

量效曲线有哪些特征性参数，这些参数有什么意义？

实验二十二　肝功能对戊巴比妥钠催眠作用的影响

1. 目的

复制小鼠急性肝功能损伤模型，观察肝功能对药物药理作用产生的影响。

2. 原理

戊巴比妥钠主要在肝内代谢失活，肝功能状态直接影响其代谢过程，如血药浓度和持续时间，从而影响其药理作用的强弱和药理作用的时间，最终影响戊巴比妥钠的药理作用（即入睡时间和睡眠持续时间）。四氯化碳是一种无色、有毒、易挥发的液体，具氯仿的微甜气味，能溶解脂肪和油漆等多种物质；它对肝细胞有严重毒性作用，是建立中毒性肝损害动物模型的常用工具药。

3. 实验材料

（1）实验动物：小白鼠，18~22 g。

（2）实验器材：注射器、鼠笼、秒表。

（3）实验试剂：生理盐水、5% 四氯化碳油溶液、0.3% 戊巴比妥钠溶液、苦味酸。

4. 实验步骤和观察项目

（1）取 4 只健康小鼠，雌雄不限，称重后编号为 A1、A2 和 B1、B2。

（2）于正式实验前 48 h 在 A 组鼠皮下注射（皮下、腹腔或灌胃均可）5% 四氯化碳油溶液 0.1 mL/10 g 体重造模，B 组鼠皮下注射生理盐水 0.1 mL/10 g 体重作为对照。

（3）正式实验时 A、B 组小鼠均腹腔注射 0.3% 戊巴比妥钠溶液 0.15 mL/10 g 体重。

（4）观察给药后小鼠的反应，记录小鼠入睡的时间（从给药到翻正反射消失）和睡眠持续时间（翻正反射消失到恢复），将结果填入表 2-9，并综合各组结果作组间 t 检验。

（5）做完实验后，颈椎脱臼法处死小鼠，观察肝脏的病理变化。

表 2-9　实验结果

鼠号	体重	肝功能状态	药物剂量	给药时间	入睡时间	睡眠持续时间	肝脏外观
A1		四氯化碳					
A2		四氯化碳					
B1		生理盐水					
B2		生理盐水					

5. 注意事项

（1）室温如低于 20℃应注意给小鼠保暖，否则动物将因体温下降、代谢减慢而不易苏醒。

（2）四氯化碳可用植物油或甘油配制。

6. 相关问题

（1）为什么肝脏损害的小白鼠注射戊巴比妥钠后，其药理作用维持的时间会延长？

（2）请举例探讨论肝功能与临床用药的关系。

（3）四氯化碳中毒的小鼠的肝脏和正常小鼠的肝脏在肉眼观察时呈现什么病理上的区别，原因是什么？

实验二十三　传出神经系统药物对动脉血压的影响

1. 目的

在掌握直接测量动物血压方法的基础上，观察传出神经系统药物对动物血压的影响，加深对这些药物相互作用关系的理解，并根据受体学说初步分析其作用机制。

2. 原理

血压的大小受到心脏输出量、动脉血管张力和血容量等因素的影响。肾上腺素能药物能通过作用于心脏和血管上的 α、β 受体，影响心脏的输出量和动脉血管张力，进而对血压进行调节。肾上腺素为 α、β 受体激动药，对心脏和血管都有作用，升压明显；去甲肾上腺素主要为强 α 受体激动药，弱 β 受体激动，主要对血管张力影响大，外周阻力增强明显，升压非常显著，作用强而快；异丙肾上腺素主要为 β 受体激动药，对血管张力影响大，使外周阻力减弱，但同时增强心脏收缩力，心脏输出量增加，两者作用抵消，故而升压作用不明显，有可能略有降压作用。

3. 实验材料

（1）实验动物：家兔，2.0~2.5 kg。

（2）实验器材：哺乳动物手术器械、兔台、气管插管、动脉导管、动脉夹、头皮静脉注射针头、压力换能器、电脑及记录装置、注射器、铁支架、螺旋夹、棉线、药棉、纱布、三通管。

（3）实验试剂：25% 氨基甲酸乙酯（乌拉坦）溶液、50 U/mL 和 1000 U/mL 肝素溶液、

0.003% 盐酸肾上腺素溶液、0.125% 重酒石酸去甲肾上腺素溶液、0.005% 异丙肾上腺素溶液、1% 酚妥拉明溶液、1% 盐酸普萘洛尔溶液。

4. 实验步骤和观察项目

（1）取 1 只家兔，称重，耳缘静脉注射 25% 乌拉坦溶液（4 mL/kg），麻醉后，将动物背位固定于兔台上。

（2）采用三通管建立好耳缘静脉通道，缓慢而连续不间断地推注生理盐水。

（3）剪去颈部的毛，正中切开颈部皮肤，分离气管。在气管下穿一线，轻提气管，作一倒 "T" 形切口，插入气管插管，结扎固定。

（4）在气管一侧的颈动脉鞘内分离颈总动脉（注意有迷走神经伴行，应将其与颈总动脉分离），在颈总动脉下方近、远心端各穿一根线，远心端结扎；然后用动脉夹夹住近心端，在靠近结扎处用眼科剪剪一 "V" 形小口，向心方向插入装有枸橼酸钠溶液或肝素溶液的动脉导管，结扎并固定于动脉导管上。动脉导管与压力换能器相连并连接在 BL-420 系统上；慢慢松开颈总动脉夹，描记正常血压曲线。

（5）打开电脑，点击桌面上的 BL-420F 图标，选药理学实验模块（药物对兔血压的影响）。先描记一段正常血压曲线，然后依次由耳缘静脉注射不同药物，观察给药后所引起的血压变化。每次给药后再立即推入生理盐水 2 mL，将余药冲入静脉内。待血压恢复原水平或平稳后，再给下一药物。

（6）给药观察：依次从静脉注入下列药物，观察血压变化，并思考变化的原理。

①观察拟肾上腺素药的作用

- 耳缘静脉注射盐酸肾上腺素 0.2 mg/kg，待药物效应消失后，接着做下面一步。
- 耳缘静脉注射异丙肾上腺素 0.2 mg/kg，待药物效应消失后，接着做下面一步。
- 耳缘静脉注射重酒石酸去甲肾上腺素 0.2 mg/kg，待药物效应消失后，接着做下面一步。

②观察应用 α 受体阻断剂酚妥拉明后对拟肾上腺素药作用的影响

- 耳缘静脉缓慢注入酚妥拉明 0.5 mg/kg，用药 15min 后再给下列药物。
- 耳缘静脉注射盐酸肾上腺素 0.2 mg/kg，待药物效应消失后，接着做下面一步。
- 耳缘静脉注射重酒石酸去甲肾上腺素 0.2 mg/kg，待药物效应消失后，接着做下面一步。
- 耳缘静脉注射异丙肾上腺素 0.2 mg/kg，待药物效应消失后，接着做下面一步。

③观察应用 β 受体阻断剂普萘洛尔后对拟肾上腺素药作用的影响

- 耳缘静脉缓慢注入 1% 盐酸普萘洛尔 0.5 mg/kg，用药 15 min 后 再给下列药物。
- 耳缘静脉注射异丙肾上腺素 0.2 mg/kg，观察药物的作用效应。
- 耳缘静脉注射盐酸肾上腺素 0.2 mg/kg，待药物效应消失后，接着做下面一步。
- 耳缘静脉注射重酒石酸去甲肾上腺素 0.2 mg/kg，待药物效应消失后，接着做下面一步。

（7）结果与分析

① BL-420 系统记录、命名并保存数据于硬盘。打印原始血压曲线图。

②分析时读取数据，记录给药前后血压变化值（包括收缩压、舒张压、平均压），计算其变化值作表或作图。

③对实验结果作出正确的分析讨论，并得出简单的结论。

5．注意事项

（1）本实验用家兔进行，因家兔的耐受性较差，可能有些结果不很典型。

（2）实验中的剂量是按一般情况进行计算的，必要时可根据具体情况适当增减。

（3）为避免形成血栓，所建静脉通道在不给药时应连续、缓慢地推注生理盐水。

（4）激动药给药速度要快，两种阻断药给药速度要慢。

（5）每次给药时做好标记。

（6）家兔麻醉后注意保暖。

6．相关问题

拟肾上腺素药和抗肾上腺素药对血压各有何影响？他们之间有什么相互作用？机制如何？

实验二十四　地西泮对抗中枢兴奋药的致惊厥作用

1．目的

观察地西泮对抗戊四氮引起的惊厥反应的影响，了解小鼠惊厥动物模型的制作方法及表现特征。

2．原理

戊四氮为中枢兴奋药，剂量过大时可过度可兴奋大脑和脊髓并引起惊厥反应。表现为全身骨骼肌强烈的不随意收缩，引起阵挛性抽搐。其致惊厥的作用部位在大脑，发生机理可能是提高神经细胞膜外的 K^+ 浓度，使细胞膜部分去极化，减小兴奋的阈值从而提高兴奋性。因为 γ- 氨基丁酸（GABA）为中枢抑制性神经递质，而戊四氮可能抑制 GABA 的释放，因此戊四氮也可通过减弱中枢抑制而使兴奋性相对增强。安定促进中枢 GABA 与 GABA 受体结合，促进 Cl^- 内流，可使神经细胞超极化，抑制神经兴奋，因而具有抗惊厥作用。

3．实验材料

（1）实验动物：小鼠（也可用大鼠），18~22 g。

（2）实验器材：注射器、鼠笼。

（3）实验试剂：0.02％地西泮、0.5％戊四氮、生理盐水。

4．实验步骤和观察项目

（1）取4只小鼠，编号，称重后，随机分成2组，每组2只，分别腹腔注射（0.1 mL/10 g 体重）生理盐水和地西泮；30 min 后，全部动物腹腔注射 0.5％戊四氮（0.3 mL/10 g 体重），观察 30 min 内每组动物有无惊厥（如痉挛、肌肉强直、角弓反张、跳跃、跌倒）或死亡的现象，并记录发生次数。最后统计发生惊厥的动物数和死亡数，计算惊厥和死亡百分率，并比较给药组与对照组百分率的差异，以判断药物有无抗惊厥活性。

（2）结果与处理：将实验结果填入表 2-10，计算出惊厥发生率。

表 2-10　实验结果

组别	动物数	惊厥数	惊厥率	死亡数	死亡率
生理盐水组					
地西泮组					

5. 注意事项

（1）腹腔注射剂量必须准确，并且注射位置要确认在腹腔内。

（2）判断动物是否惊厥和发生次数以强直性痉挛出现与否为标准，细微震颤不作为惊厥的计算指标。

6. 相关问题

地西泮的抗惊厥作用机制及临床应用如何？

实验二十五　利多卡因的抗心律失常作用

1. 目的

（1）学习心律失常动物模型的制作方法。

（2）观察利多卡因的抗心律失常作用。

2. 原理

氯化钡可促进心脏蒲肯野纤维 Na^+ 内流，抑制 K^+ 外流，促进 4 相自动除极，使自律性增强，因而诱发室性心律失常。抗心律失常药物的分为四类，Ⅰ类阻断心肌和心脏传导系统的钠通道，具有膜稳定作用，根据药物对钠通道阻滞作用的不同，又分为三个亚类，即Ⅰa、Ⅰb、Ⅰc。Ⅱ类 β 受体阻滞药，抑制交感神经兴奋所致的起搏电流。Ⅲ类延长动作电位时程药，抑制多种钾电流。Ⅳ类钙通道阻滞药。利多卡因属于Ⅰb 类抗过速性心律失常药，是一种中度钠通道阻断剂，能减慢 0 相除极和 4 相自动除极，降低自律性，与氯化钡作用相反，可用于治疗心律失常。

3. 实验材料

（1）实验动物：家兔，2.0~2.5 kg。

（2）实验器材：BL-420 系统、哺乳动物手术器械、各种导管等。

（3）实验试剂：25% 氨基甲酸乙酯（乌拉坦）溶液、1% 氯化钡溶液（1 mL/kg）、0.5% 利多卡因溶液。

4. 实验步骤和观察项目

（1）称重后，耳缘静脉注射 25% 乌拉坦溶液（4 mL/kg）麻醉。

（2）将针形电极插入相对应导联肢体的皮下，红（右上肢）、黄（左上肢）、绿（左下肢）、黑（右下肢），各导联线分别插入并与 CH1 通道相连。

（3）选择 BL-420 系统中药理学实验模块（药物对实验性心律失常的作用），重点观察导联Ⅱ的心电变化。

（4）记录一段正常的心电图后，耳缘静脉注射 1% 氯化钡溶液 1 mL/kg（如需要可增大剂量），观察家兔心律变化，待心律失常出现后，立即静脉给予 0.5% 利多卡因溶液 1 mL/kg，1~2 min 内注完，持续观察家兔心律变化。

5. 注意事项

（1）注射氯化钡时，前一半药量快速注射，后一半药量缓慢注射，同时观察心电图的变化，出现心律失常后立即停药。

（2）利多卡因至少要稀释至 0.5%，且静脉注射要缓慢，否则可引起利多卡因中毒，造成动物死亡。

6. 相关问题

请分析利多卡因的药理作用及其抗心律失常的作用机制。

第三章　医学机能学实验中的人体实验

第一节　WebChart-400 人体生理实验系统介绍

一、系统主界面

选择桌面上的"WebChart-400"图标进入系统，启动系统可出现系统主界面（图 3-1）。本实验系统包含了人体心电图描记、人体呼吸运动、人体血压、人体脑电、人体心音、人体肌肉反应、反射与反应时间、人体感觉实验、人体眼电、人体肌电、人体肺功能、人体泌尿实验 12 种实验选项，通过鼠标选择进入不同的实验模块；点击左上角"人体生理常数"选项可显示常用的人体各类生理参数，包括血常规、肝功能、肺功能、心电图、心音，尿液等。

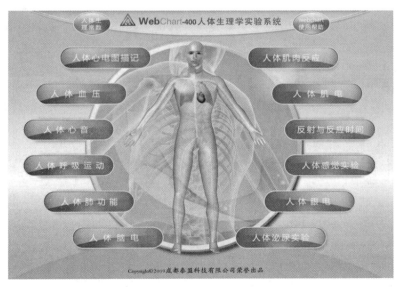

图 3-1　WebChart-400 人体生理学实验系统主界面

二、实验项目界面

下面我们以"人体心电图描记"项目为例，展示如何进入一个实验项目并且开始实验。

（1）点击主界面 人体心电图描记 选项，将会出现如图 3-2 所示界面：

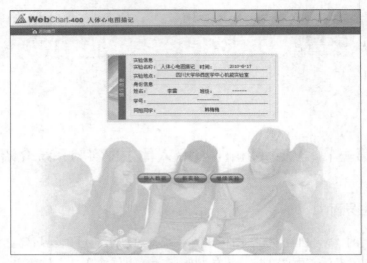

图 3-2　实验项目界面

这个界面用于选择如何开始您的实验。如果是新实验，填写实验者信息后，点击"新实验"按钮；如果是实验过程中不慎退出，以前的实验数据还保存在系统缓存中，可以选择"继续实验"以利用以前的数据继续实验；也可以选择"导入数据"，提供您以前的数据文件继续实验。

（2）点击"新实验"后会出现主实验界面，其中主功能选择区，如图 3-3 所示。

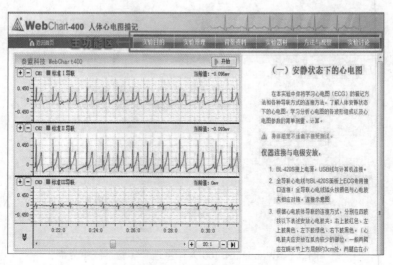

图 3-3　主功能选择区

点击不同的选项显示相应的网页内容，如"实验目的"、"实验原理"、"背景资料"、"实验器材"，可以显示本实验的相关内容（图 3-4）。

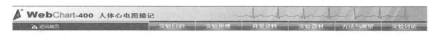

人体心电图描记 实验器材

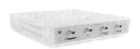

BL-420生物数据采集系统
用于人体生物信号的采集、放大和数据处理。

酒精或生理盐水
可增加皮肤导电性。

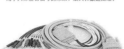

全导联心电线
连接BL-420系统和各心电肢夹的导线。

心电肢夹
用于采集心电信号的肢体夹子。

图 3-4　实验器材界面

　　将鼠标移动到"方法与观察"选项上，将会看到弹出的下拉菜单（图 3-5），这个菜单用于选择具体的实验模块。

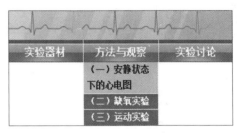

　　点击"（一）安静状态下的心电图"，会出现使用"安静状态下心电图"的实验步骤，如图 3-6 所示。根据出现的步骤，一步一步地完成实验。

　　可以按照上述步骤，选择需要的实验模块，

图 3-5　实验选择下拉菜单

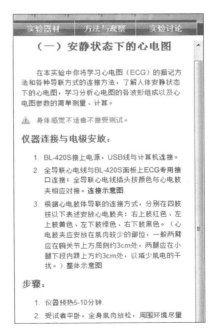

图 3-6　安静状态下的心电图实验步骤

完成所有的实验模块。

（3）在所有实验模块结束之后，点击"实验讨论"选项会出现本次实验的实验报告编辑界面，如图 3-7 所示。可以将波形数据调整到合适的显示方式，点击界面最下方的"保存"按钮，提示是否保存实验讨论，指定保存路径以及保存格式，最后出现提交电子实验报告的界面。

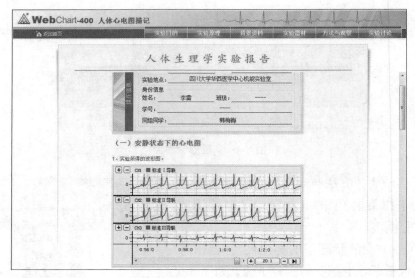

图 3-7　实验报告编辑界面

第二节　医学机能学经典人体实验

实验一　ABO 血型鉴定

1. 目的
鉴定人体 ABO 血型。

2. 原理
血液含有 55% 的血浆和 45% 的细胞成分，有四种类型的细胞，其中包括红细胞（red blood cells，erythrocytes）。红细胞表面含有抗原，称为凝集原（如 A 抗原和 B 抗原）；血浆中存在对应的抗体，称为凝集素（如抗 A 抗体和抗 B 抗体）。

（1）ABO 血型系统：卡尔·兰德施泰纳（Karl Landsteiner）于 1930 年因发现 ABO 血型系统而获得诺贝尔生理学或医学奖。图 3-8 总结了 ABO 血型中四

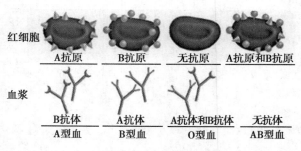

图 3-8　ABO 血型系统

种血型的特征。这些血型以红细胞表面是否存在抗原 A 和抗原 B 命名。编码这些抗原的基因位于第 9 号染色体上。

（2）Rh 血型系统：由于首先在恒河猴（Rhesus monkey）分离的抗原与抗原 A 和抗原 B 不同，它被命名为 Rh 因子。Rh 血液系统基于红细胞表面是否存在抗原 Rh 而进行分类，如果 Rh 因子存在于红细胞表面，则称为 Rh 阳性（Rh+），大多数人的血型是 Rh+；Rh 阴性（Rh-）是指红细胞表面缺乏 Rh 抗原。编码 Rh 因子的基因位于 1 号染色体上。

（3）ABO 血型鉴定：根据抗原、抗体免疫反应可以对 ABO 血型系统进行鉴定，将少量血液与抗 A 血清或抗 B 血清进行混合，根据是否产生凝集反应来判断血型。临床上进行输血时，供体指献血者，受体指受血者。万能献血者是指 O 型血的人，因为其红细胞表面不含 A 抗原和 B 抗原，所以他们的血液可以给任何血型的人；万能受血者是指 AB 型血者，因为其血清中没有抗 A 抗体和抗 B 抗体，因而他们可以接受任何其他血型的人的血液。

（4）交叉配血试验：临床输血前需要进行配血试验和交叉配血试验。血型鉴定是将受血者的红细胞与测试血清混合以鉴定血型，而交叉配血试验分成两种，将受血者的血清与供血者的红细胞进行配合试验，称主侧试验；而把受血者的红细胞与供血者的血清进行配合试验，称次侧试验；如果均没有发生凝集反应，称为配血相合，可以输血。

3. 实验材料

（1）实验对象：人。

（2）实验器材及试剂：血型鉴定用玻片，抗 A 血清，抗 B 血清，碘酒，75% 乙醇，无菌采血针，牙签，棉球，锐器收纳盒。

4. 实验步骤和观察项目

（1）准备一张血型鉴定用玻片（中间有两处圆形凹陷），分别标上 A 和 B。

（2）向标有 A 的一侧添加 1~2 滴抗 A 血清，向标有 B 的一侧添加 1~2 滴抗 B 血清。

（3）用碘酒和 75% 乙醇对手指进行消毒，用无菌采血针刺破手指，让血液自然流出。

（4）用干净的牙签取血，在玻片的两边各加入 1 滴新鲜血液。

（5）用牙签轻轻搅拌均匀，并来回倾斜玻片使液体充分混合。

（6）10 min 后检查是否发生凝集反应。若出现凝集反应，则表示测试结果为阳性，标记为 +。

（7）在表 3-1 中记录结果（凝集或无凝集）以及结论（血型类型）。

表 3-1　凝血试验结果

抗 A 血清	抗 B 血清	血型
+	−	A
−	+	B
+	+	AB
−	−	O

（8）将用过的采血针置于锐器收纳盒中，将玻片洗净并晾干。

5. 注意事项

（1）搅拌抗血清和血液时，一侧仅使用一个牙签，避免交叉污染。

（2）不要通过挤压手指来采血，以免检测结果不准确。

6. 相关问题

（1）和血型鉴定相关的诺贝尔生理学或医学奖是什么？

（2）第一个发现 ABO 血型的人是谁？ABO 血型鉴定在临床上的意义有哪些？

（3）世界献血者日是在哪一天？由来如何？

（4）如果受血者和献血者交叉配血试验的主侧试验结果为阴性，输血时是否就意味着绝对安全？

实验二　动脉血压测定

1. 目的

（1）理解间接测量血压的原理。

（2）利用血压计通过肱动脉测量收缩压和舒张压。

（3）理解收缩压、舒张压与心脏周期的关系。

2. 原理

血压为血液对单位面积血管壁施加的压力，通常情况下在动脉中测量。由于心脏交替收缩和舒张，导致每次心脏搏动时血压都发生升降，并且在整个心动周期中不断变化，因此，常常通过测量收缩压和舒张压来表示血压。收缩压（systolic pressure，SP）是心脏射血峰值时动脉内压力的最大值，而舒张压（diastolic pressure，DP）则反映了心脏舒张时血管内压力达到的最低值。血压常以毫米汞柱（mmHg）为单位，如 120/80 mmHg 表示收缩压为 120 mmHg，舒张压为 80 mmHg。脉压（pluse pressure，PP）是指收缩压与舒张压的差值，对于一个健康的成年人来说，脉压在 40 mmHg 左右。而平均动脉压（mean arterial pressure，MAP）只能通过微积分的方法得到，但可以使用以下经验公式进行粗略计算：平均动脉压 = 舒张压 +1/3 脉压（MAP=SP+1/3PP）。

正常情况下，血液在血管中平稳流动，不产生可辨别的声音（图 3-9A）。将袖带绕在手臂周围，并向袖带中充气直至其压力高于收缩压（如 160 mmHg），以阻断前臂的血液流动（图 3-9B）。当通过打开压力阀使袖带内压力逐渐下降时，检测者会通过听诊器听到一种特殊的声音，称为科罗特科夫（korotkoff）音，表明血液恢复流动，而此时检压计上对应的压力为收缩压（图 3-9C）。随着压力进一步降低，血流声音

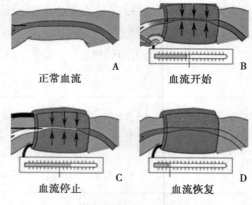

正常血流　　　A

血流开始　　　B

血流停止　　　C

血流恢复　　　D

图 3-9　听诊法间接测量血压的机制

变得更大，直到血液恢复自由流动（图 3-9D）时，科罗特科夫音突然减弱或消失，此时检压计上对应的压力为舒张压。

3. 实验材料

（1）实验对象：人。

（2）实验器材及试剂：听诊器（图 3-10），血压计（含气球、袖带及检压计，如图 3-10 所示），标记笔。

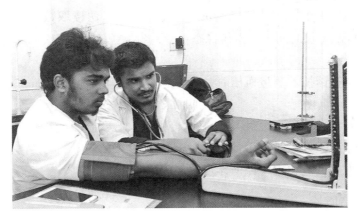

图 3-10　听诊器和血压计

4. 实验步骤和观察项目

（1）让受试者以舒适的姿势静坐 5 min，露出上臂，将手臂平放在实验桌上与心脏所在平面持平。

（2）检查是否能看清检压计的比例尺，确保听诊器正确、舒适地戴在耳朵上。

（3）测量动脉血压的方法

① 通过触摸找到手臂肱动脉搏动处，用标记笔小心标记，将听诊器的胸件膜片置于标记处。

② 将血压计的袖带置于上臂，在肘窝上方约 2.5 cm 处进行固定，并将听诊器的胸件置于袖带下。

③ 对气球迅速充气，使袖带内压力达到高于预计收缩压 20~30 mmHg（或高于使桡动脉脉搏消失所需压力 30 mmHg）以上，使上臂中的血流中断。

④ 轻轻转动压力阀门，以 2~5 mmHg/s 的速度缓慢释放袖带中的气体，同时仔细听血管音的变化。

⑤ 一旦袖带中的压力低于收缩压水平，血液流经过狭窄的动脉将发生湍流，这时通过听诊器就可以听到声音，而此时检压计指示的压力水平大约等于收缩压。

⑥ 继续缓慢释放袖带中的气体，当压力降至等于舒张压时，血管音突然变为低沉或者消失，此时检压计的读数为舒张压。

（4）进行两次血压测定，取两次结果的平均值作为最后结果。

5. 注意事项

（1）保持房间安静、舒适。

（2）测量时，不要和受试者交谈。

（3）血压袖带不应在衣服外固定，要和皮肤保持密切接触。

（4）手臂应与心脏在同一水平。

（5）双腿不能交叉。

（6）为实验对象选择最佳尺寸的袖带。

（7）袖带的充气时间不应超过 1 min，若在此期间无法读取数据，应该给袖带放气，等待 1~2 min 后再试（长时间干扰血压稳态可导致晕厥）。

6. 相关问题

（1）用听诊 - 触诊技术测量血压时，若你感觉到桡动脉在 175 mmHg 时消失，接下来该如何处理？

（2）若袖带对实验对象来说过大或过小，测出的血压值将会有何变化？

（3）为何建议脱去外衣露出手臂测量血压？

（4）在测量血压的过程中应如何体现人文关怀？

实验三 心音听诊

1. 目的

（1）练习心音听诊的方法。

（2）辨识第一心音和第二心音的特点。

2. 原理

心音听诊的目的是检查循环系统的功能和检测心脏活动的病理变化。听诊心音最常用的听诊器是声学听诊器，它的工作原理是将声音从听诊器的胸件通过充气的空心管传至检查者的耳朵。检查者将听诊器胸件放在受试者身上，身体产生的声音会使听诊器胸件上的振动膜发生振动，产生声压波，该声压波沿听诊器的管道向上传到检查者耳部而被听到，检查者根据结果进行进一步分析。

正常心动周期主要产生第一心音（S1）和第二心音（S2）。S1 在心室开始收缩推动房室瓣关闭时产生，它包括一系列低频振动，持续时间较长。S2 在心室开始舒张引起半月瓣关闭时可以听到，S2 的频率通常高于 S1，持续时间较短。在心室舒张期开始，心室快速充盈时，可能会听到第三种低频声音（S3）；第四心音（S4）则可能在心房收缩期的晚期听到。

总的来说，第一心音的特点是音低、持续时间长，第二心音的特点是音高、持续时间短（表 3-2）。

表 3-2　S1 和 S2 的比较

第一心音（S1）	第二心音（S2）
高频	低频
持久	短暂
Ⅰ—Ⅱ的间隔较短	Ⅱ—Ⅰ的间隔较长

注：Ⅰ指房室瓣关闭；Ⅱ表示半月瓣关闭。

心音听诊区（图 3-11）：通过在以下不同区域听诊，可以更容易、更清晰地检测出由瓣膜振动产生的心音。二尖瓣听诊区位于左第五肋间隙和锁骨中线交叉的内侧。三尖瓣听诊区位于第四肋间隙与胸骨交界的右边界。主动脉瓣听诊区位于第二肋间隙与中胸骨交界的右边界。肺动脉瓣听诊区位于第二肋间隙与胸骨交界的左边界。

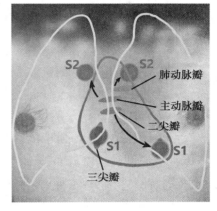

图 3-11　心音听诊区

3. 实验材料

（1）实验对象：人。

（2）实验器材：听诊器。

4. 实验步骤和观察项目

（1）根据图 3-11 确定心音的听诊区域。

（2）将听诊器的耳件插入外耳道，将听诊器的胸件按照图 3-11 所示放在各心音听诊区。

（3）在检测心音的同时，尝试同时触诊心尖冲动或颈动脉搏动。

（4）通过音调、持续时间、两声之间的时间间隔以及与心尖冲动的关系来区分第一心音和第二心音。

（5）比较各个区域的心音响度。

（6）检查心率及其节律。

（7）计算收缩期和舒张期的平均时间：测量第一心音和第二心音之间的间隔（收缩期）；再测量第二心音和下一个第一心音之间的间隔（舒张期），此过程重复 5 次，可计算出心脏收缩和舒张的平均时间。

5. 注意事项

（1）保持检测环境安静。

（2）找到正确的听诊区域。

（3）听诊器的胸件应放在受试者的胸部皮肤上。

（4）询问受试者的病史。

（5）同时触摸心尖冲动或颈动脉搏动，观察其与心音的关系。

6. 相关问题

（1）听诊器是谁发明的？心音听诊的机制是什么？

（2）如何区分 S1 和 S2？识别 S1 和 S2 的生理意义是什么？

（3）为什么在检测到心音时需要同时触摸心尖冲动或颈动脉搏动？

（4）如果听诊时听到 S1 和 S2 之外的心音，你该如何处理？

（5）如何在心音检测过程中实践人文关怀？

实验四　心电图检测

1. 目的

（1）学会人体体表心电图的检测与记录方法。

（2）了解正常心电图各波形的形成机制。

（3）学习如何阅读及分析正常的心电图。

2. 原理

心电图仪是记录心脏电活动的仪器。当心脏搏动开始并传播到整个心脏时，电流也从心脏传到周围组织，进而到达身体表面。心电图（electrocardiogram，ECG）是心电图仪记录的一个心动周期中传播到周围组织并扩散到身体表面的周期性电流的变化。正常的 ECG 由 4 个去极化波和 1 个复极化波组成（图 3-12）。去极化波包括 P 波和 QRS 波群。P 波是由心房在收缩开始前去极化时产生的电位引起的；QRS 波群（由 Q 波，R 波和 S 波组成）是由心室在收缩前去极化时产生的电位引起的。T 波又称复极化波，是心室从去极化状态恢复时产生的电位变化。

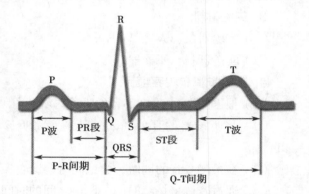

图 3-12　正常心电图的波形组成

ECG 各波之间存在正常范围的时间间隔，大于或小于该范围则表明心脏收缩可能存在异常。例如，P-Q 或 P-R 间隔是 P 波开始到 QRS 波群开始之间的时间，代表心房兴奋开始到心室兴奋开始之间的间隔。Q-T 间隔是从 Q 波开始持续到 T 波结束的时间间隔。心率是单位时间内心跳的次数，在成年人中，两个连续 QRS 波群之间的正常间隔约为 0.83 s，则心率为 72 次 / 分（60/0.83）。

任何信号传导方式的变化都可能在心脏周围引起异常电位，从而改变 ECG 中的波形。因此，可以通过分析心电图不同导联记录的波形及各波的间隔来诊断大部分严重的心脏疾病。

"导联"是指将两个电极与心电图仪连接起来的方式，包括标准的双极肢体导联，增强型导联和心前区导联。"双极肢体"导联是指从人体肢体表面上的两个电极记录心电图，电流总是从正极流向负极。导联Ⅰ：正极导线在左乳房上方或左臂上方，负极导线在右臂上方。心电图仪的负极通过一个电极连接到右臂，而正极通过另一个电极连接到左臂。导联Ⅱ：左腹部或大腿左端为正极，右臂为负端。心电图仪的负极通过一个电极连接到右臂，正极通过另一个电极连接到左腿。导联Ⅲ：左腹部或左小腿左端为正极，左臂为负极。心电图仪的负极通过一个电极连接到左臂，而正极通过另一个电极连接到左腿。如图 3-13 所示。

ECG 纸（图 3-14）是一个网格纸，水平轴表示时间，垂直轴表示电压。最小的分隔为 1 mm 长和 1 mm 高。横坐标上每个小方块的长度为 1 mm，代表 0.04 s；而较大的正方形长度为 5 mm，代表 0.20 s。纵坐标上每 10 mm 等于 1 mV 的电压。

心率可以很容易通过心电图计算出来。当节律规则时，心率是 300 除以 QRS 波群之间的大方块数或 60 除以 P-P 间期，例如，两个 QRS 波群之间有 4 个大方块，则心率是 75 次 / 分（300/4=75）。第二种方法适用于心跳节律不规则时估计速率，计算 6 s 条带中的 R 波数并乘以 10；例如，如果 6 s 条带中有 7 个 R 波，则心率为 70 次 / 分（7×10=70）。

3. 实验材料

（1）实验对象：人。

（2）实验器材及试剂：心电图仪、肢体导联、胸导联（图 3-15），75% 乙醇棉球，生理盐水棉球，电极膏。

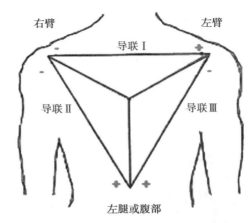

图 3-13　标准肢体导联

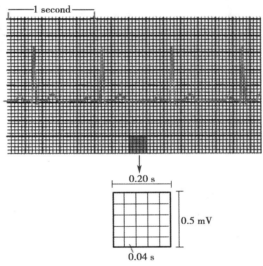

横坐标：25 mm/s，纵坐标：10 mm/mV，小方块 = 0.04 s，大方块 =0.20 s。

图 3-14　心电图图纸

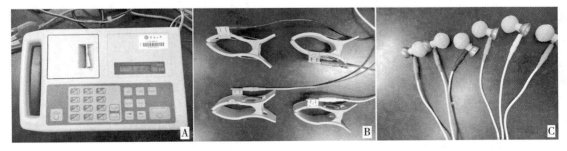

图 3-15　心电图仪（A）、肢体导联（B）、胸导联（C）

（参见彩插）

4. 实验步骤和观察项目

（1）将心电图仪连接电源，开机预热 3~5 min。

（2）受试者仰卧，全身放松。

（3）用 75% 乙醇棉球清洁皮肤，再用生理盐水棉球润湿皮肤。

（4）按如下方式将电极连接到 ECG 导联：4 根连接四肢肢体，6 根连接胸前区。确保电极与皮肤紧密接触（图 3-16）。

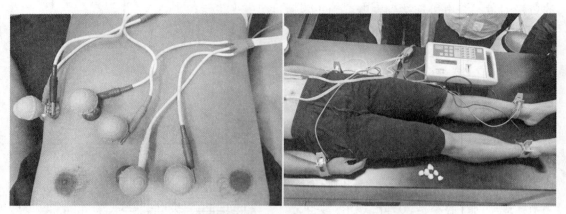

图 3-16　胸部导联（左）和肢体导联（右）的放置位置

（参见彩插）

① 标准双极肢体导联：红，右臂；黄，左臂；绿，左腿；黑，右腿。

② 胸导联：V1，红色，第四肋间，右侧边界；V2，黄色，第四肋间，胸骨左边界；V3，绿色，在 V2 和 V4 中间；V4，棕色，第五肋间，左锁骨中线；V5，黑色，腋前线，与 V4 相同水平；V6，紫色，腋中线，与 V4 和 V5 处于同一水平。

（5）调整心电图的标准电压：使 1 mV 的信号产生的偏转为 1 mm。

（6）选择手动或自动模式记录各导联心电图。

（7）关闭电源开关。从受试者身上取下电极和导联。

（8）读取心电图

① 浏览心电节律是否规则。

② 识别各波的组成，计算各波的波幅。

③ 测量 P-P 或 R-R 间隔，计算心率，心率 = 60 / R-R 间隔（s）。

④ 测量 Q-T 间隔和 ST 段。

5. 注意事项

（1）正确连接各电极。

（2）确保环境舒适以减少和避免骨骼肌收缩的干扰。

（3）受试者不得与金属物体接触（如不要戴手表、手链等金属装饰品）。

（4）检测时不要交谈。

（5）按读图规则对心电图进行分析。

6. 相关问题

（1）ECG 仪是由谁发明的？谁最先确定了心电图导联法和心电图纸的规格？

（2）ECG 与心脏细胞的 AP 有何不同？

（3）当心肌处于缺血、损伤和梗死状态时，心电图会有哪些变化？

（4）如何在心电图的记录过程中实践人文关怀？

实验五　人体呼吸运动的记录

1. 目的

（1）了解如何使用围带式呼吸换能器来记录正常的呼吸运动。

（2）根据波形读取相应的呼吸频率。

2. 原理

机体与外界环境之间的气体交换过程，称为呼吸。通过呼吸，机体从大气中摄取新陈代谢所需要的 O_2，排出所产生的 CO_2，因此，呼吸是维持机体新陈代谢和其他功能活动所必需的基本生理过程之一，一旦呼吸停止，生命也将终止。呼吸系统有 3 个主要部分：气道、肺和呼吸肌。气道包括鼻、嘴、咽、喉、气管、支气管和细支气管，在肺和外界之间运输空气。肺作为呼吸系统的功能单位，将氧气进入身体，将二氧化碳带出身体。呼吸肌包括横膈肌和肋间肌，充当泵的作用，在呼吸时推动空气进出肺部。

肺通气是指空气进出肺部以促进气体交换的过程。呼吸系统利用负压系统和肌肉收缩来实现肺通气。呼吸系统的负压系统涉及在肺泡和外部大气之间建立一个负压梯度。静息状态下，肺内压略低于大气压，所以空气会随着压力梯度进入肺部；当肺部充满空气时，肺内的压力就会上升，直到等于大气压。此时，通过横膈肌和外肋间肌的收缩，增加胸腔的体积，使肺压降低，当肺压低于大气压时，可以吸入更多的空气。呼气时，膈肌和外部肋间肌放松，而内部肋间肌收缩，减少胸腔的体积，增加胸腔内的压力，使压力梯度被逆转，导致气体向外排出，直到肺内、外的压力相等。这是因为肺的弹性性质使肺回退到静息容量，恢复了吸气时的负压。

外呼吸是指肺泡内的空气和肺泡壁周围毛细血管中的血液之间的气体交换。从大气中进入肺部的空气比毛细血管血液中的具有更高的氧分压和更低的二氧化碳分压。分压差导致气体顺着压力梯度通过肺泡上皮被动扩散。外呼吸的结果是氧气从空气中进入血液，最后被输送到身体各组织；而二氧化碳从血液中进入肺泡，最后被呼到大气中。

在正常的静息条件下，身体保持一定的呼吸频率和深度，称为平静呼吸。当身体对氧气的需求和二氧化碳的产生增加时，平静呼吸状态才会改变。人体的化学感受器可监测血液中的氧分压和二氧化碳分压的变化，并向脑干的呼吸中枢发送信号。然后，呼吸中枢调节呼吸的频率和深度，使气体分压恢复到正常的水平。

3. 实验材料

（1）实验对象：人。

（2）实验设备：BL-420 系统（图 3-17），围带式呼吸换能器（图 3-18）。

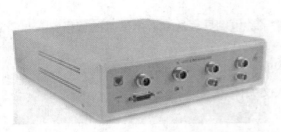

图 3-17　BL-420 系统

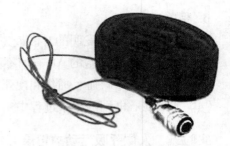

图 3-18　围带式呼吸换能器

4. 实验步骤和观察项目

（1）仪器连接（图 3-19）：将呼吸换能器连接到 BL-420 系统的 CH1 通道。

（2）记录呼吸运动

① 让受试者全身放松呈坐位。

② 将围带式呼吸换能器围绕于受试者胸部呼吸活动最明显的水平位置（图 3-20）。

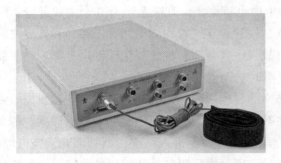

图 3-19　换能器与 BL-420 系统的连接方式

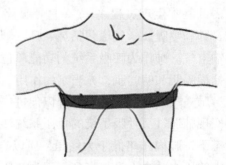

图 3-20　换能器的穿戴方式

③ 点击工具栏中的 ▶ 开始 按钮，开始采样，在 CH1 通道中可以看到常规的呼吸波。

④ 添加注释：在注释栏内输入受试者姓名，然后选择 添加注释 按钮。

⑤ 记录波形 1 min，点击 ■ 停止 按钮结束实验。

（3）呼吸运动的测量

① 按下滑动条 ＜ 按钮，向左移动波形到第一个姓名标记处。

② 按下滑动条 ＋ 20:1 － ▶| 的波形缩放 "+" "−" 按钮，调整呼吸波波形到比较稳定位置。

③ 点击此段波形中任何一点，其呼吸频率即可在数据读出框中显示。

④ 点击鼠标左键，选择数据读出框内的数据不放，拖拽到数据记录表（图 3-21）上所对应的位置中。

⑤ 重复以上步骤，完成所有波形数据的测量。

5. 注意事项

（1）保持环境安静。

（2）找到受试者的合适位置。

（3）感觉不舒服的人不应接受测试。

6. 问题

（1）哪些因素会改变呼吸的频率和呼吸深度？

（2）思考和计算等活动能改变呼吸频率吗？为什么？

记录数据		
记录频率	姓名	频率(次)

图 3-21 数据记录界面

实验六 视力测定

1. 目的

（1）理解使用国际视力表检查视力的原理。

（2）学会正确使用国际视力表检查视力。

2. 原理

视敏度是指眼睛的分辨能力或视力的清晰度，它取决于人能看清楚单词或图形所需的最小视角。视角是由来自物体两个边缘的光线定义的角度，可以区分两个不同点的最小视角称为视角极限，大约为 1 分（1′），这相当于健康的人眼从 5 m 处看到的物体落在视网膜上约为 1.5 mm。视敏度是实际的视角极限，与正常的 1′ 视角极限相比，以百分比或十进制分数表示。因此，视角为 1′ 的视力清晰度为 1（或 100%），而 2′ 的视力清晰度为 0.5（或 50%），以此类推。

在光学特性完美的眼睛中，最大的视觉清晰度取决于视网膜上感光细胞的密度。在视网膜的中央凹处，视锥细胞呈密集的蜂窝状分布，彼此之间的平均距离为 2 μm。如果两个点投影到视网膜上的图像大于一个视锥细胞的直径，则我们可以区分这两个点。在视网膜的外侧，视杆细胞的密度相近，但多个视杆细胞连接到同一神经节细胞（会聚），会导致此处光敏度较高。因此，黄斑部的视力最高（约 100%），由黄斑部到视网膜的边缘，视力逐渐降低。

我们使用国际标准视力表来测试视力。国际标准视力表中有 14 行字。第 11 行（由上至下排序）字母的每一侧发出的光仅形成 1 个视角。因此，人们在距单词 5 m 处能清晰地看到字母时的视敏度是正常的。

3. 实验材料

（1）实验对象：人。

（2）实验器材（图 3-22）：国际标准视力表，指示杆，挡眼板。

4. 实验步骤和观察项目

（1）让受试者站在距离国际视力表的 5 m 处。

（2）让受试者用挡眼板遮住自己一侧的眼睛，用另一侧眼睛观察图表。

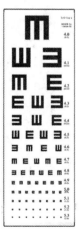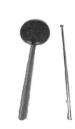

图 3-22 国际标准视力表，指示杆和挡眼板

（3）测试者指示某一字母，让受试者说出所指示字母的开口方向以表明是否清晰可见。

（4）从第一行最大的开始向下进行测试，直到受试者可以清楚最小单词所在的一行为止。

（5）重复步骤（2），检查另一侧眼睛的视敏度。

5. 注意事项

（1）使用世界公认的国际标准视力表。

（2）在进行测试时，确保所需的光线照射在视力表上。

6. 相关问题

（1）如何阅读国际标准视力表？视力为 1.0 是什么意思？

（2）近视的可能原因是什么？在日常生活中如何避免近视的形成？

（3）你如何看待近视的激光治疗？其原理是什么？

实验七　盲点检查

1. 目的

（1）验证视网膜上盲点的存在。

（2）测量和计算盲点范围。

2. 原理

供应视网膜的血管具有特征性分布，血管会聚点的颜色比视网膜的其余部分略浅，称为视盘。由于视神经通过的视盘上没有光感受器及感光细胞，因而没有视觉，所以称为盲点。在盲点的颞侧方向，可以找到一个颜色更深的点，称为黄斑。如图 3-23 所示。

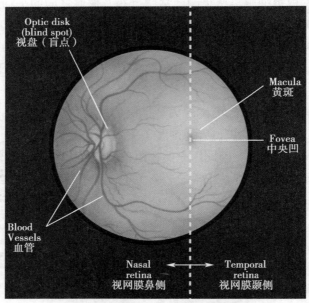

图 3-23　检眼镜下的视网膜结构

盲点的位置和范围可以根据成像的原理由其投影区面积确定。根据相似三角形原理，可计算盲点直径及其距视网膜中央凹的距离。

3. 实验材料

（1）实验对象：人。

（2）实验器材：白纸，铅笔，黑色小目标物，尺子，挡眼板，Webchart-400 系统。

4. 实验步骤和观察项目

（1）传统方法

① 在墙上贴一张白纸，让受试者站在离它 50 cm 的地方。在纸上画一个符号（如十字符号），符号要与受试者的眼睛在同一水平线上。让受试者用挡眼板遮住一侧眼睛，并用另一侧眼睛盯着符号。

② 将一个黑色小目标物从符号上慢慢移到符号的外侧，并在纸上标出受试者看不到黑色小目标物的位置。慢慢地将黑色小目标物移到符号更外侧，并在纸上标记出可以再次看到黑色小目标物的位置。

③ 将黑色小目标物从两个标记点的中心向各个方向移动，寻找能再次看到黑色小目标物的位置，依次将纸上的所有点连接起来，形成一个近似圆，称为盲点投影区。

④ 根据相似三角形原理，用下列公式可计算盲点直径及其距视网膜中央凹的距离。

$$盲点到中央凹的距离 = 盲点投影区中心到符号的距离 \times 15/500（mm）$$

$$盲点直径 = 盲点投影区直径 \times 15/500（mm）$$

（2）使用 Webchart-400 系统软件（盲点测试显示界面如图 3-24 所示）

① 闭上或遮住左眼，站在距屏幕 50 cm 处，用右眼盯着一个图标，当图标旁的圆点向右移动时，开始受试者可以看到圆点，后来圆点消失了，然后又出现了。请记录这两个点并在刻度尺上读取它们之间的距离，该值代表受试者视网膜盲点投影区的直径。

② 根据公式计算盲点直径，盲点直径=盲点投影区直径 ×15/500（mm），一般盲点直径为 1.5 mm 左右。例：在开闪光灯时，看到圆点时为 4 cm；消失时为 9 cm。那么，盲点投影区直径为 5 cm，根据上式，盲点直径=50 × 15/500=15/10=1.5 mm。当然，如果距离屏幕是 30 cm，公式中的 500 就应该改为 300。

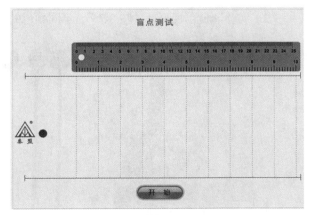

图 3-24　盲点测试显示界面

5. 注意事项

（1）测试时，受试者的眼睛必须始终注视符号，不得随黑色小目标物移动。

（2）受试者必须与白纸保持一定的距离（一般为 50 cm），不能随意变动。

6. 相关问题

（1）有人说检测不到他的盲点，你能帮忙分析一下原因吗？

（2）哪些因素可以决定盲点的大小？

（3）为什么用两只眼睛看物体时感觉不到盲点的存在呢？

实验八　视野测定

1. 目的

（1）理解视野的概念。

（2）了解如何使用视野计来检查正常人的白色、红色、黄色、绿色视野。

2. 原理

视野是当眼睛固定注视前方一点时所能看见的空间范围，是外部世界的一部分投射到视网膜表面的成像。在视野中，盲点位于从黄斑颞侧下方约 1.5° 处，与中心位置相距约 12°~17°。由于眼睛和视网膜的解剖结构，视野可能是规则的圆形或半球形，但脸部的不同结构（鼻子、眶上脊及颊骨等）会掩盖理论视野的某些部分。

在进行眼科和神经科检查时，常使用视野计确定视野。视野检查有助于发现视网膜的功能状态，查看视觉通路和视皮层是否存在问题。视野问题有多种原因，包括并非起源于眼睛而是起源于中枢神经系统或与视觉有关的脑区的疾病。视野测试中的信息有助于诊断以下疾病：青光眼、黄斑变性、视神经胶质瘤、脑瘤、多发性硬化症、中风、颞关节炎、垂体疾病以及高血压等。

3. 实验材料

（1）实验对象：人。

（2）实验器材：视野计（图 3-25），不同颜色的视标（图 3-26），视野图（图 3-27），铅笔。

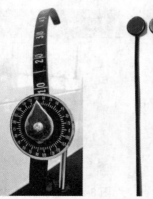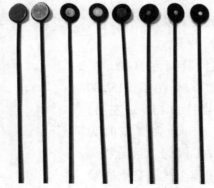

图 3-25　视野计　　　　　　图 3-26　不同颜色的视标

4. 实验步骤和观察项目

（1）观察视野计的结构，了解各部分组成。视野计的半圆形金属弧可绕其中心旋转 360°，圆弧内的小圆盘可以从中心向外移动到 90°（图 3-25）。

（2）将视野计放在光线充足的地方，让受试者的下颌紧贴在颌骨支撑件，并使受试者眼窝的下边缘紧贴眼窝支撑件。

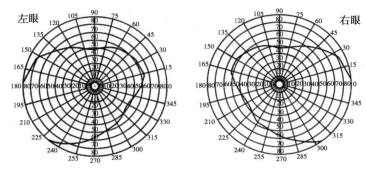

图 3-27　视野图

（3）调整下颌支撑架的高度，使受试者的眼睛和曲线架的中心点在同一水平线上。首先，将曲线架水平放置；受试者直接用被测眼注视其中心点，然后用手遮住另一侧眼。

（4）将白色视标从框架边缘缓慢移至框架的中央，并询问受试者是否能看到视标。若受试者能看到视标，则将视标向曲线架边缘移动一段距离；若受试者表示看不到视标，则再向曲线架中心移动，找到受试者能再次看到视标的位置，标记在视野图相应的经纬度上。用同样的方法测出对侧眼刚能看到视标的位置并标记在视野图相应的经纬度上。

（5）将曲线架旋转 45°，重复测试，得到刚才看到的两个点并将其绘制在图表上。

（6）测试共进行两次，在图表上总共获得 8 个点。依次连接这些点，所得区域即为白色的视野。

（7）重复上述步骤，以测试其他颜色的视野。

5. 注意事项

（1）要求受试者注视视野计曲线架的中心。

（2）确保受试者在测试过程中看到了视标。

（3）进行测试时，应缓慢移动视标。

6. 相关问题

（1）如何用视野计检测盲点？

（2）视神经损伤时人的视野会发生什么变化？

（3）黑白及彩色（绿色，蓝色或红色）视野在大小上是否有差异？为什么？

实验九　色盲检测

1. 目的

掌握用色盲检查图或 Stilling-Ishihara 平板检查色盲的方法，并作出正确诊断。

2. 原理

视网膜的感光细胞是视杆细胞和视锥细胞。视锥细胞负责明视觉，即日光下的色觉。在中央凹处只有视锥细胞，其数量由中央凹向视网膜外周急剧减少。视锥细胞根据其感光色素的类型可分为三组，三种不同的视锥色素分别存在于三种不同的视锥细胞中。感红细胞对红光波最敏感；感绿细胞对绿光波最敏感；感蓝细胞对蓝光波最敏感。当感光细胞的灵敏度降低或缺失时，它们将无法区分某些颜色，这种情况通常是互补出现的，如红绿、蓝黄。最常见的色觉障碍是红绿色盲。据统计，8% 的男性和 0.5% 的女性是色盲。编码红色和绿色视锥细胞色素蛋白的基因位于 X 染色体上，这就是为什么这种色盲在男性中更为常见。

通常使用 Stilling-Ishihara 平板检查颜色感知（图 3-28）。这些板块包含一个颜色与背景颜色不同的字符（字母或数字）或形状。图形和背景都由点组成，以消除图形的轮廓。图形和背景的点的平均大小和亮度相等，因而光对比或图案的感知无助于识别图形。因此，对于那些无法区分图形颜色和背景颜色的人来说，图形是不可见或难以看到的。这种检测红绿色盲的方法由日本的石原忍博士发明，称为"石原氏色盲检测"。我们在做色盲检查时，要求受试者观看石原氏色盲测试中的 8 个色板，看是否能识别数值。如果不能识别颜色，则认为他们是色盲。

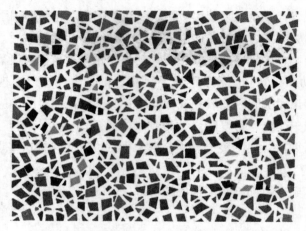

图 3-28　可视化图表（Stilling-Ishihara 平板）

（参见彩插）

3. 实验材料

（1）实验对象：人。

（2）实验器材：色盲检查图/册，Webchart-400 系统。

4. 实验步骤和观察项目

（1）观看每张图像，并在 5 s 内把你看到的数字写在图片上，然后点击"Opinion"按钮，它会告诉你是否选择了正确的答案，并显示正确的答案（图 3-29）。

（2）单击"Another"按钮开始下一个图像测试。

（3）如果答错，系统会自动出现另一张颜色相同的图片供你识别。如果连续答错，则得出"你是红/绿/蓝盲"的结论。

5. 注意事项

如果电脑屏幕太大或像素太高，需要降低浏览器的像素，并确保没有屏幕闪烁，否则会模糊整个视野。

6. 相关问题

（1）色盲患者能驾驶车辆吗？并解释原因。

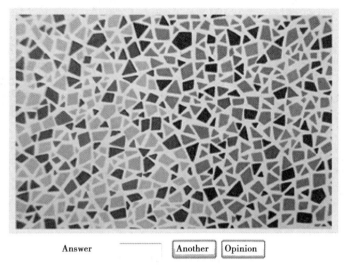

Answer _____ [Another] [Opinion]

图 3-29　色盲测试显示界面

（参见彩插）

（2）是谁首先发现了色盲的存在？他是怎么意识到这种色觉异常的？

（3）相比女性（0.5%），为什么红绿色盲在男性（8%）中更常见？

实验十　声音的传导方式

1. 目的

（1）用频率调谐音叉验证和比较声音的空气传导和骨传导。

（2）了解临床区分传导性耳聋和感觉神经性耳聋的简单方法和主要原则。

2. 原理

声波由外耳聚集，声波振动通过中耳鼓膜和三个听骨链时，声音得到放大，然后声波传播到前庭窗，引起耳蜗液流动，使基底膜螺旋器中的感觉毛细胞去极化，由此产生的动作电位，沿着前庭蜗神经（第八对脑神经）到达大脑。基底膜的每个区域在各自特定的频率下振动最剧烈，并引起大脑皮层特定听觉区域的兴奋，从而感知不同的声音。

传导性耳聋是由于到达内耳的声波被干扰而引起；感觉神经性耳聋是由毛细胞损伤或前庭耳蜗神经损伤引起的。

当音叉被敲击时，声音可通过空气和头骨进行传导。Rinne 试验（图 3-30）可对空气传导与骨传导进行比较。对正常个体而言，通过空气感知振动的时间是通过骨感知的两倍，因为在空气传导中，声波没有被组织吸收。如果有传导性耳聋，则骨传导表现正常的或轻微增强，而空气传导减弱。如果有感觉神经性耳聋，骨传导和空气传导均受到抑制。

Weber 试验（图 3-30）则用以比较双耳的骨传导。放置一个音叉在额头的中间，让受试者比较双耳的声音响度，这对正常人来说是相等的。将一个小棉球装进一只耳朵，重复上一步骤，询问受试者每个耳朵的音量；对一个正常人来说，填充棉球侧的耳朵能听到更响亮的声音，这是因为，在传导性耳聋中，环境声音到达被阻塞侧耳蜗的过程被阻止，

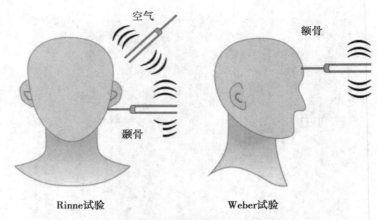

空气

额骨

颞骨

Rinne试验　　　　　　　　　Weber试验

图 3-30　Rinne 试验和 Weber 试验

这导致神经系统通过敏化耳蜗传导来放大一侧的声音。

3. 实验材料

（1）实验对象：人。

（2）实验器材：频率调谐音叉（图3-31），橡胶木槌（图 3-32），棉球。

4. 实验步骤和观察项目

（1）比较一只耳朵的空气传导和骨传导情况（Rinne 试验）

① 让受试者坐下，保持环境安静。

② 用橡胶木槌敲击音叉，将频率为512 Hz 振动音叉的手柄放到受试者的右侧颞骨乳突处，受试者开始可以听到音叉的声调，当听不到声音时，再把音叉放到右耳的前部，受试者很快可以再次听到声音。如图 3-33 所示。

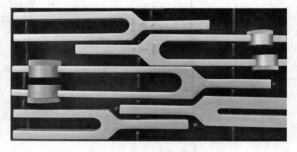

图 3-31　频率调谐音叉

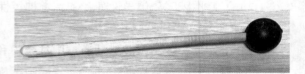

图 3-32　橡胶木槌

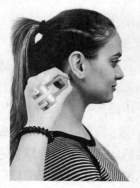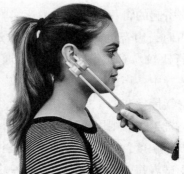

图 3-33　Rinne 试验

③ 用橡胶木槌敲击音叉，将振动音叉放在右耳前部直到受试者无法听到声音时，立即将其放置在颞骨乳突上，音叉的声调不再被听到。因此，在正常情况下，空气传导比骨传导更长，这在临床实践中被称为 Rinne 试验阳性（＋）。

④ 将一个小棉球塞入右耳，重复步骤②和③，如果空气传导等于或短于骨传导，这在临床实践中被称为 Rinne 试验阴性（－）。

⑤ 在左耳重复步骤①到④，将结果记录在答题纸上。

（2）比较双耳的骨传导（Weber 试验）

① 用橡胶木槌敲击音叉，并将手柄的尖端放在受试者额头的中线上，问受试者双耳听到的声音是否同样响亮。如果在头部中央听到声音，并且在两只耳朵上同样响亮，那么受试者的听力是正常的，或者受试者有对称的听力损失（传导性耳聋）。

② 用手指或棉球插入左耳，重复步骤①，描述结果；用手指或棉球插入右耳，重复步骤①，描述结果。

5. 注意事项

（1）在一个非常安静的房间里进行这些测试。

（2）避免在硬物上敲击调谐音叉以免损坏音叉。

（3）将振动音叉靠近外耳道时，不要触碰到耳垂和头发。

6. 相关问题

（1）获得诺贝尔奖的研究中哪些与听觉器官相关？在临床上有何应用？

（2）传导性耳聋和感觉神经性耳聋有什么区别？如何鉴别？

（3）助听器的原理是什么？目前有哪些研究进展？

实验十一　膝跳反射的引导和观察

1. 目的

（1）引导膝跳反射。

（2）测量反射时间。

2. 原理

反射是机体在中枢神经系统的参与下，对内、外环境变化做出的规律性反应。它是实现神经系统功能的基本方式。反射弧是能够接受刺激并产生反应的最小、最简单的通路。反射弧的结构包括：①感受器；②传入或感觉神经元；③神经中枢（中间神经元）；④传出或运动神经元；⑤效应器。大多数反射涉及的中枢是脊髓或脑干，而不是高级大脑中枢。与有意识的思考相比，反射能使人对刺激做出更快的反应，因而反射的保护作用是显而易见的。

反射时间是指施加刺激到反射动作开始之间的时间间隔。如果反射时间为 0.5 ms，那么这条反射弧只包含 1 个突触，所以这个反射是单突触反射。如果反射时间为 1.5 ms，那么这条反射弧可能包括 3 个突触，所以这是一个多突触反射。

膝跳反射是由于在髌腱上给予了一个有力的敲击而引起的腿部反射性伸展和上抬，膝跳反射的中枢在脊髓，是单突触反射，在临床上往往被用来检查上位和下位神经系统的损伤。

3. 实验材料

（1）实验对象：人。

（2）实验器材：叩诊锤（图 3-34），位移传感器（图 3-35），BL-420 系统（图 3-36）。

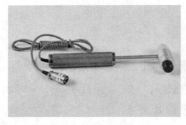
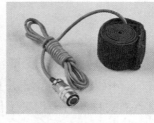
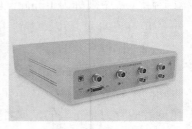

图 3-34　叩诊锤　　　　　　图 3-35　位移传感器　　　　　图 3-36　BL-420 系统

4. 实验步骤和观察项目

（1）设备连接：将叩诊锤连接到 BL-420 系统的 CH1 通道，位移传感器连接到 BL-420 系统的 CH2 通道（图 3-37）。

（2）膝跳反射的引导

① 让受试者坐下，提示受试者将左腿放在右腿上，让左小腿放松。检查左脚是否能自由活动。

② 将位移传感器绑在左小腿上。

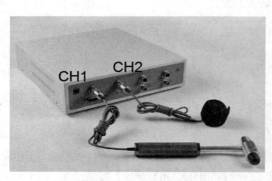
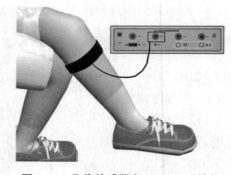

图 3-37　设备连接

图 3-38　位移传感器和 BL-420 系统的连接

③ 单击工具栏上的"start"按钮，看到两条移动的数据记录行。

④ 添加注释，输入个人信息并选择。

⑤ 实验者击打受试者左膝盖骨下的韧带。

（3）反射时间的测量

① 按下"滑块"按钮，将波形向左移动到第一个名字标签。

② 点击"滑块"按钮，将波形向右移动，直到 CH1 通道出现第一个刺激信号，点击左下角的"M"标记，拖动至刺激信号波形的峰值。

③将光标从 CH1 通道向右移动到 CH2 通道的第一个信号峰值，然后单击左键。

④数据读出框中显示的数据是从刺激到反应（肌肉收缩）的时间间隔。

⑤用左键拖动数据读出框中的数据，将数据拖放到数据记录表中相应的位置。

⑥重复上述步骤，测量所有波形数据。

5. 相关问题

（1）屈肌反射和膝跳反射有什么不同？

（2）如何分析膝跳反射在临床上的诊断意义？

（3）膝跳反射的反射弧是怎样的？和其他反射的反射弧相比有什么特点？

实验十二　人类听觉和视觉反应

1. 目的

（1）通过叩诊锤和事件标记开关测量听觉响应时间。

（2）根据闪光信号测量听觉反应时间。

2. 原理

反应时间（潜伏期）是指从刺激开始到反应开始的时间间隔，其长短因人而异。反应时间消耗的时间由三部分组成：刺激沿感觉神经传导的时间，中枢处理信息的时间（最长）以及效应器产生反应的时间。

3. 实验材料

（1）实验对象：人。

（2）实验器材：叩诊锤（图 3-34），事件标记开关（图 3-39），BL-420 系统（图 3-36）。

4. 实验步骤和观察项目

（1）设备连接：将叩诊锤连接到 BL-420 系统的 CH1 通道（左侧），事件标记开关连接到 BL-420 系统的 CH2 通道（右侧）。如图 3-40 所示

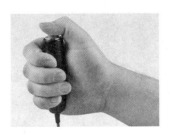

图 3-39　事件标记开关

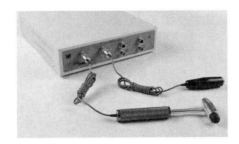

图 3-40　设备连接

（2）测量听觉反应时间

①让受试者背对着实验者坐下，让受试者用拇指轻轻按住按钮上的事件标记开关。

②点击工具栏上的按钮开始记录，可以看到两条移动的数据记录线。

③在评论区添加注释，然后输入主题名称，加以选择。

④实验者用叩诊锤敲击实验台，受试者听到声音后立即按下事件标记开关。

⑤ 按下"滑块"按钮，将波形向左移动直到第一个名称标签。

⑥ 单击"滑块"按钮，将波形向右移动至 CH1 通道中的第一个刺激信号，单击左下角的"M"标记，将其拖动到刺激信号波形的峰值处。

⑦ 在 CH1 通道内向右移动光标直到 CH2 通道中的第一个信号峰值，单击左键。

⑧ 数据读出框中显示的数据是从刺激到反应的时间间隔。

⑨ 用左键将数据读出框中的数据拖放到数据记录表（图 3-41）中的相应位置。

⑩ 重复上述步骤，测量所有波形数据。

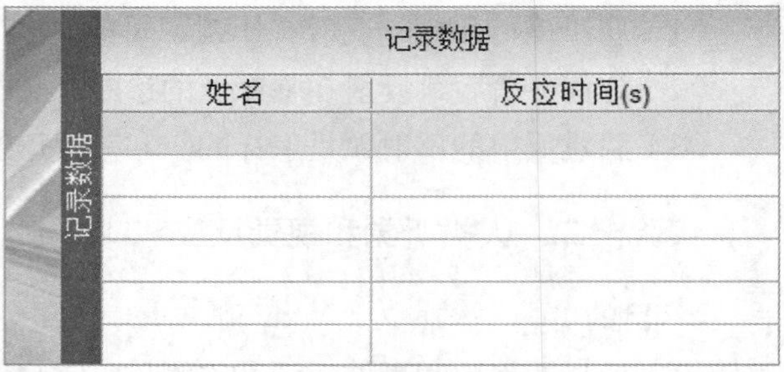

	记录数据	
	姓名	反应时间(s)
记录数据		

图 3-41　数据记录界面

（3）测量视觉反应时间：当测量视觉反应时间时，请在播放卡通时将注意力集中在屏幕上。当看到红球出现时，立即按鼠标左键，即可获得视觉反应时间。当球出现之前切勿按鼠标左键。视觉反应时间测量界面如图 3-42 所示。

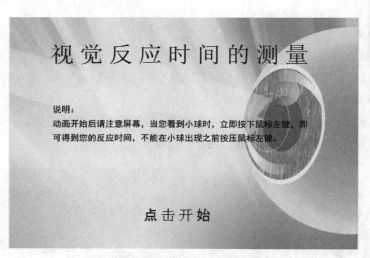

图 3-42　视觉反应时间测量界面

5. 相关问题

（1）反应时间和反射时间有什么区别？

（2）听觉反应时间和视觉反应时间，哪个更长？

第四章　医学机能学实验研究

随着医学的不断发展，为顺应国家对创新型人才的迫切需求，医学机能学实验已经从单纯验证性实验发展到设计性实验、综合性实验和创新性实验。近年更加注重对学生科研思维和科学创新能力的培养和训练，因而创新性实验的比例有所增加。创新性实验一般仅针对学有余力的学生开设，他们在掌握了基本实验技能的基础上，在教师的指导下确定感兴趣的科研课题，而后通过文献检索进行实验设计，一般需经过开题报告论证其可行性之后再进行实验，这些实验往往是融合了形态学、机能学、分子生物学的整合性实验，其创新性是第一位要考虑的因素，因此难度比较大。为了有效地开展综合性及创新性实验，有必要对医学机能学实验研究进行介绍。

第一节　医学实验研究的基本原理

一、医学实验研究方法与实验设计

医学实验研究方法是在医学研究领域中应用的科学方法，例如，当我们观察到可能影响疾病发生或明显影响健康的因素时，首先可以从临床实践或实验室研究甚至理论推测中提出一个科学问题；其次，我们需要确定重要的自变量和因变量，如实验对象暴露于某一实验条件，这一条件可能是危险因素，也可能是保护因素或某种治疗方法，其结果可能是导致疾病也可能是治疗疾病；再次，我们可以提出一个具体的假设以回答有关暴露于某一实验条件与结果之间关系的具体问题；最后，设计一个实验来检验该假设是否有效，包括体内实验和体外实验，而人体实验主要是指在体实验。可见，在科学研究中做实验非常重要，这是科学研究中至关重要的一步，适用于所有科学领域。要做实验，我们首先需要设计一个实验。从狭义上讲，实验设计是指一个准备充分的研究计划，而研究计划是对具体实验操作的描述，侧重于问题陈述、实验目的和科学假设。

二、实验设计的一般规则

要设计一个好的实验，必须严格遵守以下方法及规则。

1. 样本量

为了确保实验结果有统计学意义，应该验证每组实验对象的数量是否合适。组的大小应设计为能帮助研究人员检测实验组内的统计学显著性差异。分配给每个实验组的实验对象数量，通常由特定的统计方法根据每个组预期结果之间的差异程度来确定。例如，在比较两个组时，影响样本大小的主要因素是：①能够检测到的偏差程度；②实验因素的变化程度；③代表统计学"显著性"标准的"p"值大小。

2. 分组方法

设计实验最常用的方法可能是将实验对象分成两组：实验组和对照组。然后对实验组改变实验条件并与对照组进行比较。研究人员必须决定如何将这些样本分配到不同组。例如，如果有 10 个实验对象，所有实验对象是否会同时处于这两个条件（例如重复测量）中，或者实验对象是否被分成两组，每个实验对象仅参与一种情况？基本上，有三种类型的样本分配方法。

（1）独立分组：自变量的每个条件都使用不同的实验对象。这意味着实验的每个条件都包括一组不同的实验对象。这应该通过随机分配来完成，可确保每个实验对象有平等的机会被分配到一个组或另一个组，并且各组是相似的。独立措施包括使用两组独立的实验对象，每个条件一组。例如表 4-1。

表 4-1　独立分组的样例

自变量		因变量
蹲起运动（20 s）	蹲起运动（40 s）	血压、呼吸变化
10 位学生	10 位不同的学生	

① 优点：避免顺序效应（指条件的顺序对实验对象的行为有影响）。如果实验对象遇到几种情况，当他们遇到第二种情况时，他们可能会感到无聊、疲倦和厌倦，或者意识到实验的要求。

② 缺点：需要更多的实验对象和更多的重复测量设计（即更耗时）。群体实验对象之间的差异可能会影响结果，例如年龄、性别或社会背景的差异。

（2）重复分组：相同的实验对象参与自变量的每个条件，这意味着实验的每个条件都包括同一组实验对象。

① 优点：在参加所有条件时，需要的实验对象更少（即节省时间）。由于在每个条件中使用相同的实验对象，实验对象变量（即个体差异）会减少。

② 缺点：可能有顺序效应。第二种情况中的表现可能更好，因为实验对象知道该怎么做（即练习效果）。或者，在第二种情况中，他们的表现可能更糟，因为他们累了（即疲劳效应）。

（3）配对分组：每个条件都使用不同但相似的实验对象。对任何可能影响行为或表现的因素，如性别、年龄、智力。在每种条件下，这些因素相同的实验对象应被配对，每组配对必须随机分配，一个分配到实验组，另一个分配到对照组。

① 优点：减少实验对象的个体差异，因为研究人员试图配对实验对象，使每个条件

都有相似的能力和特征，也因为避免了顺序效应，因此不需要进行平衡。

② 缺点：除非是同卵双胞胎，否则不可能与其他实验对象完全匹配；而且在尝试查找最合适的配对组合时，也非常耗时。

3. 随机规则

随机化是随机地将实验对象分配给对照组或实验组的过程。为了实现随机化，必须从定义种群开始，同质种群中的个体可能并不相同，但可能具有一些共同特征（如性别、年龄、体重）。可以给每个实验对象贴上标签，然后使用随机数表或用计算机生成的数字来实现随机化。也可以使用骰子或卡片将实验对象随机分配给实验组。

4. 重复规则

如果重复实验不能产生相同的结果，则意味着原始结果可能是错误的。因此，对单个实验进行多次重复是很常见的，尤其是当存在不受控制的变量或其他实验误差时。对于重大的结果，特别是当这些结果对科学家们的工作很重要的时候，他们也可能尝试自己重复实验以验证该结果。

5. 对照规则

对照观察是任何实验设计的重要组成部分，特别是在研究不稳定的生命系统时。对照观察的目的是确定由研究人员直接操纵的变量是否是控制反应变化的变量。从实验变量来看，还有一些因素可能影响实验的结果，如遗传、环境、传染性因素。为了最大限度地减少这些无关变量的影响或确定不需要的变量，应该安排与实验组直接对比的对照组。对照组包括阳性对照组、比较对照组、阴性对照组、假手术/治疗对照组和溶剂对照组等。时间是不受研究人员控制的变量。每一次观察都会在不同的时间发生，重要的是要知道反应的差异仅在多大程度上反映了时间的流逝。为了评估这种影响，可以设计一个对照组，在实验中定期重复测定特定的测量值。

（1）阳性对照：所谓的阳性对照组是能预知其变化的组。用阳性对照组与实验组进行比较。例如，在测试新抗生素对细菌培养的影响时，可以使用一种经证明是有效的既定抗生素。如果除阳性对照外所有样品均失败，则所测试的抗生素可能无效；阳性对照也用于证明可以检测到反应，从而对实验方法进行质量控制。

（2）比较对照：通常是采用已知治疗方法的阳性对照，用于与其他治疗方法进行直接比较。例如，在评估癌症动物模型中的新化学预防药物方案时，人们希望将这一方案与目前被视为"公认做法"的化学预防药物方案进行比较，医学上的比较对照可以称为黄金标准。例如，磁共振血管成像（magnetic resonance angiography，MRA）是主动脉解剖的"黄金标准"测试，灵敏度为95%，特异性为92%。

（3）阴性对照：目的是确保未知变量不会对实验组造成影响，使研究人员能够证明其研究结果的有效性。阴性对照的预期结果是在正常状态下不会产生任何变化。例如，设置不含抗生素的培养皿为阴性对照组，如果所有的新药都起作用，而阴性对照组也表现出对细菌生长的抑制，那么可以确定可能有其他的变量对结果产生了影响。

（4）溶剂对照：并非所有药物或试剂都是水溶性的，有些需要溶解在特定的溶剂中，如广泛使用的乙醇或二甲基亚砜（DMSO）就是溶剂，也称为媒介物。在这种情况下，为了排除溶剂本身对结果的影响，必须设置溶剂对照。盐水或矿物油等溶剂可能无害，使用方式与实验试剂或药物相同，但对于乙醇或 DMSO 这样可能会损害细胞的溶剂，则需要将其稀释至安全剂量。通常，乙醇或 DMSO 的浓度应调整到复合溶液的 0.5% 以下。与未处理的对照相比，媒介物对照将确定媒介物是否会单独引起任何影响。

（5）假手术 / 治疗对照：用于模拟手术或治疗程序，而不实际使用可能诱发变化的关键步骤或测试物质。安慰剂是药物研究中最使用的例子。另一个例子是假手术，它被广泛用于外科动物模型。在使用假手术对照组时，我们模仿实验组的处理程序，但实际上并没有执行会产生实验效果的实质性步骤。例如，在外科脑损伤的研究中，研究人员要对实验组大鼠切开头皮，钻开颅骨，打开硬脑膜，并对脑组织进行切割损伤；而对假手术组大鼠则只切开头皮，钻开颅骨，打开硬脑膜，但并不损伤脑组织，这样就排除了手术过程本身对实验结果的影响。

三、实验设计的基本要点

从广义上讲，实验设计需要遵循的规则和制定科研计划的规则是基本相同的。在设计实验时，我们需要仔细设计并记录要解决的科学问题、实验目的和验证假设所需的实验操作等，基本要点如下。

（1）标题：体现某自变量对某因变量的影响。

（2）实验变量（自变量，IV）：在初步学习设计实验的阶段，最好选择一个独立的变量进行操作。

（3）实验测试参数（因变量，DV）：选择能够准确评估实验变量造成的影响的测试参数。

（4）实验假说：你对将要发生的情况的猜想是什么？把猜想用"如果……那么……"写出来，清楚地写出自变量对因变量的影响。例如，如果自变量发生 XX 变化，则因变量将会有 XX 变化。

（5）样品采集方法及分组方法：确定样品采集的最适方法以及分组方法。

（6）数据采集及统计方法：获取测试数据的最适方法，在实验设计阶段确定用何种合适的方法进行数据统计，以对各实验组之间的差异进行比较。

（7）实验步骤：详细说明实验步骤，但不要重复常识性或通用性的信息，例如，无需复制本实验室手册或课本中的文字和图形等，只需标注参考来源。

（8）给药方法：假设在动物实验中，动物要接受化学或生物处理，此时应明确恰当的给药方法（例如饮食、灌胃、注射、渗透泵）。注意事项：如有已知或潜在的危险，要提前做好适当的预防措施。

（9）时间因素：考虑时间的限制，如在一个下午或 180 min 内进行几次实验，能够完成实验并作记录。

第二节 研究论文的撰写及发表

我们投入了大量的时间、精力和经费来设计一个严谨的研究计划，并实施该计划来检验已提出的科学假设，而所有科学研究的最后一步就是面向公众发表研究论文。撰写和发表论文至少有两个目的。首先，它可传播科学成果，可以为科学的发展进步作出贡献；其次，它可促进个人的职业发展。当我们试图撰写论文并在学术期刊上发表时，熟悉一些简单的原则是非常有用的，这也是本节的期望与目的。

一、研究论文的基本结构

尽管不同的学术期刊有其独特的风格和要求，但大多数文章仍然采取大致相似的部分，通常包括：标题、摘要、引言、主体、讨论与结论、参考文献。研究论文的简短部分包括摘要、引言和结论。而将摘要、引言和结论部分称为"简短"部分意味着这三个部分应足够简洁，只包含必要的信息以概括研究工作的重要发现，借此来吸引读者阅读整篇论文。通常，读者会先浏览一下摘要，找出论文中真正重要的内容；如果摘要是足够吸引人的，读者会看看结论。如果他们觉得很有趣，将查看引言，了解作者开展了什么样的实验项目，然后他们将阅读文章的其余部分以获取更多细节内容。

1. 标题

标题是论文的一部分，通常是读者最开始阅读的部分。电子索引服务非常依赖于标题的精确性，使读者能够寻找到对其有价值的论文。1983 年，罗伯特·戴（Robert A. Day）将一个恰当的标题描述为"尽可能少的、足以描述论文内容的词语"。标题不应包含太多不相关的词或过于笼统的词语，合适的标题反映了论文所要探究的基本问题。

要点：

① 准确、明确、具体和完整。

② 从论文主题开始。

③ 不要包含缩写，除非读者已知缩写的具体内容。

④ 要足够吸引读者的眼球。

研究论文的标题主要有四种，表 4-2 列出了相应的类型、定义和示例。

2. 摘要

摘要的目的是让读者了解到文章的概要，以便读者能够迅速决定是否继续阅读该篇文章。一个好的摘要对于正在研究某一领域的读者快速找到相应的文献具有重要意义。摘要是整篇论文的缩影，它通常以小字体出现在文章标题和作者列表下方。摘要作为独立的一部分，其传播范围比文章本身更加广泛。随着电子出版数据库成为当今检索特定领域文献的基本方法，摘要的撰写变得越来越重要。

摘要有两种基本类型。虽然格式和内容不同，但每种类型的摘要都应概述要解决的问题、结果以及可以从中得出的结论是什么。信息性摘要概括了论文中的所有内容，例如，

表 4-2 四种标题类型的比较

类型	定义	示例
描述性标题	描述什么对论文真正重要	跑步 30 min 对心肺功能的影响
声明性标题	对论文的结果留下印象	跑步 30 min 有利于心肺功能的增强
疑问句标题	提出一个问题	跑步 30 min 有利于心肺功能的增强吗？
复合型标题	合并以上几种类型并用冒号或问号分隔开	跑步 30 min 对心肺功能的影响：增强还是递减？

旨在达到的研究目标、解决问题的策略、获得的结果和得出的结论，这种摘要基本上是文章结构的一个缩影。相反，指示性或描述性摘要只是对文章内容进行概括，不具体描述文章中的目标、方法、结果和结论。

摘要概括了整篇论文，包含了文章研究的线索。摘要虽然是论文的第一部分，但由于它是整篇论文的概要，因此经常最后才被撰写。

要点：

① 问题：需要解决的问题是什么？

② 动机：我们为什么要做这项研究？

③ 解决方案：已经做了什么来解决问题？

④ 结果：问题的答案是什么？

⑤ 启示：对于研究结果应该给出的建议是什么？

3. 引言

在引言部分，我们需要回答两个至关重要的问题：研究试图解决的科学问题是什么，回答该问题的意义是什么？通常，引言开始于对以前相关研究的简要概述（即所谓的文献综述），接着简要描述本研究中所提的科学问题以及为解决该问题而设计的实验。引言的目的是引导读者从一般学科领域进入特定的研究领域，使读者在阅读完这一部分之后，能够了解这个研究领域的最新成果，而无需阅读以前关于该领域的文献。这部分应该吸引读者的眼球，并向他们强调你正在做的事情是至关重要的，值得认真阅读的。虽然引言位于论文的第二部分，但许多作者在论文完成后才撰写引言部分，并在此之前已进行了实验，得出了结论。

要点：

① 对研究主题作一般性陈述。

② 对当前主题的研究进展进行回顾。

③ 提出需要研究的科学问题。

④ 概述当前工作的意义。

⑤ 提炼当前研究的特色和创新。

4. 主体

论文主体由材料和方法以及结果两部分组成，它们解释了论文中的实验内容，旨在回答引言中提出的研究问题。告诉我们研究的问题是如何解决的（即材料和方法）以及研究的发现是什么（即结果），这也是论文主体的两个目的。

（1）材料和方法：介绍用于研究的仪器和试剂，以及用于解决研究问题的方法或实验步骤，并提供足够的信息，以便其他研究人员将其应用于相关问题时能够重复该实验步骤。实验步骤部分应让读者相信研究者已经认真进行了实验并掌握了足够的知识。在撰写实验步骤时，最好把读者看作是一个对你的结果持怀疑态度，且保持严谨态度的人。

对实验程序的典型描述一般从对设备进行列表和描述开始。大型设备应按制造商的名称、型号和序列号进行描述。好的实验方法部分应有足够的细节，以便让其他研究人员能够复制你的实验，但不需要过度描述非关键性的步骤；当然，如果你在一些看似通常的程序中做了一些改良并显著提高了结果的准确性，那一定要写出来。

要点：

① 列出实验所需的主要设备和器材，并提供相关信息。

② 描述所有步骤，并按正确的顺序排列。

③ 确定适当的给药方法。

④ 列出为减少实验不确定性而采取的任何措施，以尽量减少实验误差。

⑤ 确定已知或潜在的危险因素，并采取适当的预防措施，以尽量减少实验风险。

（2）结果：以逻辑顺序和各种形式来显示实验所得的数据，包括文字描述、表格、图表、图形、图片甚至视频。所有表格、统计图和图片应该使用通用的标准化格式。例如，条形图有助于比较两个或多个组或条件，图题应准确地解释正在绘制的内容，要标注度量单位，并根据有无统计学意义来解释实验数据。

结果部分应简单地说明事实结果，而不作出评论和解释，与这些结果相关的解释和意见应包含在讨论部分。数据的客观性是十分重要的，尽量避免诸如"我们的结果证明某某理论是正确的"这样的语句，相反，"我们的结果与某某理论一致（或不一致）"更容易让人接受，没有那么强的主观性。

要点：

① 简要描述数据，包括图表。

② 简单地说明事实结果，而不作出评论和解释。

③ 指出实验中所有的不确定性，需说明样本量。

5. 讨论与结论

讨论部分有时表述为"讨论和结论"，或简单地称为"结论"。在这一部分应回顾实验目的并总结实验结果的含义，也就是说，引言中所提出的基本问题应该从结果中以某种方式或在某种程度上得到回答。而在评估实验时，不应基于实验结果与公认的结果或理论一致或不一致来评判实验的"成功"或"失败"。一般来说，应该直接讨论研究结果的意义，对不可预见结果的影响力的讨论更能展示作者的功底。

结论在文章结尾处作为引言的对应部分出现，所以它应该给人以文章快要结束的感觉，将强调从数据分析中得出的推论，比摘要更详细地描述最初的实验推论，并以这种方式推动读者将具体结果上升到一般结论。

要点：

① 简要介绍研究背景和研究目的。

② 突出最重要的结果；重点讨论结果如何回答引言中提出的科学问题，而不是重述结果。

③ 将结果与先前发表的研究进行比较。

④ 说明结果的重要性和影响。

⑤ 通过总结实验数据，从结果中得出结论或假设。

⑥ 指出这项研究的局限性，提出后续的研究问题和建议，以便今后改进。

⑦ 结论应回到引言中，并与开头涉及的最初目的进行比较，以形成一个闭环。

6. 参考文献

研究大多是以前人的研究工作为基础的。如果使用别人的想法而不指出信息的来源，会因为剽窃或书面造假而受到指责，这在科学界被视为一种严重的犯罪。因此，在使用他人的想法、意见、假设或数据时，应该在引言、主体和讨论部分中提及他们的相关工作，然后在论文末尾的参考文献中列出。

不同的出版社需要不同格式或样式来发表论文和参考文献，尽管参考文献的格式不尽相同，但基本原则是相同的，可向想投稿的各个期刊网站下载相关的投稿须知，里面有详细的参考文献格式要求和样例。

要点：

① 要检查参考文献列表，并确保文本中引用的每个参考文献都在参考文献列表中，反之亦然。

② 根据期刊"投稿指南"中的要求统一参考文献的格式。

③ 可借助一些文献检索和阅读工具来添加文献，如 EndNote 和 NoteExpress 等。

二、在期刊上发表论文

什么样的论文值得发表？在奥康纳看来，一篇"记录了重要的实验性、理论性或观察性的新知识，或已知原理在实际应用中有进展"的论文是值得发表的。显然，为了准备一份专业出版的研究论文，我们至少要走两步。首先，应该通过做实验来精确地回答需要研究的科学问题；其次，实验应遵循公认的标准，记录研究工作的过程应得到业内的认同，即使所做的实验研究适合出版，清晰、简洁、连贯的写作风格也是论文被接受和发表的基本前提，语言的组织和优化也是决定性因素。大多数情况下，待发表的论文需要经过许多次修订才能通过严格的同行评审过程。事实证明，与他人讨论和撰写论文对研究是非常有帮助的。

1. 选择投稿期刊并符合其要求

在选定合适的期刊后，作者必须按照期刊编辑的说明提交论文。为了熟悉论文的组织、格式和写作风格，认真阅读目前发表在该刊物上的论文是一条捷径。现在，通过期刊网站的提交管理系统提交论文变得越来越普遍和流行。在提交论文阶段，如果您不想直接被拒稿，您的论文必须满足说明中列出的所有要求。即使论文有科学贡献，质量高，如果出现以下任何错误，编辑仍可能立即拒绝该论文。我们在此提出一些论文投稿阶段常见的错误：

① 论文的主题不在期刊主题范围之内。

② 不遵守书写格式和页面布局等规则（如字体大小，行间距，页码，参考文献样式，图形和表格，页面布局准则）。

③ 超过了最大篇幅［字数和（或）页数］。

④ 与其他期刊已经发表的研究相似。

2. 外部评审和同行审查

提交的论文首先由各自领域的专家审阅，这个过程被称为同行评议，这是科学质量管理的主要机制。同行评审的过程包括专家对实验的客观评价，专家匿名发表意见。通常，编辑会选择至少三名评审人，他们是该主题的专家，以便对论文进行同行审阅。在高度专业化的领域中，有时期刊要求作者提供可能的同行评审人名单。同行评审的做法可以是盲审，作者不知道评审人的身份，或者是更严格的双盲审阅，评审人也不知道论文的作者。评审人对论文提出建议，有时他们要求作者添加新的实验数据，这在影响编辑者的创作能力方面也起着关键作用。如果论文通过同行评审，它将被发表在同行评审的科学杂志上，表明该论文的质量受到了好评。决定一篇论文是否适合发表的一般要点如下。

要点：

① 论文的原创性、贡献及意义。

② 与期刊主题的相关性。

③ 相关文献的覆盖度。

④ 相关写作风格（写作的清晰度、合适的标题和摘要、精心设计的图表、合理的结论和讨论）。

⑤ 合适的论文篇幅相对于其用处而言。

⑥ 可增加论文被接收机会的论文特征：作者的良好声誉，引用期刊上发表的论文。

3. 审查过程的三个结果

评审专家完成审阅后，编辑收集他们的意见并做出决定。通常有三个结果，由编辑发送给相应的作者。

（1）接收：论文未经修改直接发表在期刊上，这种情况很少发生。

（2）修改：为了保证论文的出版，作者必须根据审稿人和编辑的建议对论文进行修改。修改完论文后，作者将修改后的稿件连同一封带有回复评审人和编辑建议的信件一并提交给编辑。收到修订版后，编辑会提出接受或拒绝修改的建议。有时，论文会转到另一轮评审中，通常包括那些对原始论文最挑剔的评审人。通常，作者会尽力使论文符合编辑的建议，直到被接受为止。有时，如果作者真的不同意审阅者的修改建议，他们可能会告知编辑自己将放弃修订，并将论文投送到另一家合适的期刊。

（3）拒绝：这实际上是最常见的结果。

由编辑转达评审人的建议。一个或多个评审人对下面提到的任何一个条件有严重反对意见时，一般会被拒稿：

① 论文不属于期刊的刊登范围。

② 论文缺乏相关参考文献和意义。

③ 论文有原则性错误。

④ 修订后的版本相比于原始提交版本没有改进。

⑤ 抄袭他人作品中的短语、句子或段落（剽窃）。

为了避免稿件被拒，并提高论文被发表的机会，除了上述问题之外，在撰写和提交论文需时记住以下要点：

① 遵循提交的专业期刊所需的样式和格式。

② 绝大多数参考文献应该是原创研究文章，而不仅仅是来源于综述或教科书。

③ 通过用自己的语言总结相关信息来表达对问题的理解，即使确实引用了参考文献，也切勿直接复制他人作品中的短语、句子或段落。

④ 抄袭已发表的文章构成剽窃罪的，作者将受到纪律处分。

第三节　医学机能学实验设计与实施

我们已经讨论了实验作为科学方法周期中一个关键步骤的重要性，并阐述了在进行科学研究时应遵循的基本原则和要点。此外，我们也学习了撰写科研论文并将其发表在科学期刊中的相关知识和要点。有了这些知识技能，现在我们就可以运用它们并开始设计自己的实验并书写实验报告了。

实验设计是提高一个小组或团队中学生科研能力的好方法。为设计和执行一个优秀的实验，通常需要进行连续两个下午的实验课程。在第一堂课上，教师将简要说明设计实验的方法，并提供一些可备选主题；然后，学生选定一个主题（或自定主题），以小组为单位分工合作，通过查阅文献完成一份实验设计报告（也称实验前报告）。在第一次实验课中，各组派学生代表进行汇报，通过其他学生的提问和教师评点，最后确定具体的实验步骤，并与实验技术老师落实可用的实验器材和试剂等。在第二次实验课中，学生将按照自己的实验设计方案进行正式实验，以证明他们的假设并完成实验目标；实验结束后，学生需要写一份完整的实验报告并按时提交。

一、实验设计报告（实验前报告）的格式

（1）标题：构思一个适当的标题，体现出要检验和验证的因素。

（2）目的：1~2 个目的。

（3）原理：提供实验要解决的关键问题或要验证的关键假设的背景信息及理论基础。

（4）实验对象：包括对照组和实验组。

（5）器材和试剂：根据需要确定。

（6）方法/步骤和观察项目：列出详细的实验步骤，以便他人重复实验。此外，还应说明将收集哪些数据以及如何分析数据。

（7）注意事项：指出为保证实验安全和结果准确性应采取的所有预防措施。

（8）预期结果：根据所学知识预测可能的结果。

（9）参考文献：格式应以期刊出版物的标准格式为准。

二、完整实验报告（实验后报告）的格式

（1）标题：构思一个适当的标题，体现出要检验和验证的因素。

（2）目的：1~2个目的。

（3）原理：提供实验要解决的关键问题或要验证的关键假设的背景信息及理论基础。

（4）实验对象：包括对照组和实验组。

（5）器材和试剂：根据需要确定。

（6）方法/步骤和观察项目：详细列出实验步骤，便于他人重复实验。此外，还应说明将收集哪些数据以及如何分析数据。

（7）注意事项：指出为保证实验安全和结果准确性应采取的所有预防措施。

（8）结果：使用各种数据和统计图详细展示结果。

（9）讨论：基于结果做出合理而具体的分析。

（10）结论：从结果和讨论中提炼出高度概括的结论，用简洁的语言表达。

（11）参考文献：格式应以期刊出版物的标准格式为准。

三、期刊论文形式的实验报告格式

试着把实验报告当作要发表在正式期刊上的文章那样去写，而且要假设期刊的读者对研究的话题比较熟悉，故书写时要采用研究论文的标准格式。

（1）封面页：应注明实验的标题和作者的姓名（按照各位作者对此篇论文的贡献大小排序）。

（2）摘要：包括研究目的、主要方法、主要结果和主要结论。一个好的摘要可以让读者无需通读全文，仅仅通过摘要就能理解整个报告。一般在完成文章其他部分的写作后，再进行摘要的写作。

（3）其他部分请参考本章第二节。

实验三 刺激频率对肌肉收缩的影响

1. 目的

观察刺激频率与肌肉收缩方式之间的关系。

2. 原理

当 AP 沿着运动神经传到肌细胞时，它会引起肌细胞膜发生去极化并产生 AP，AP 沿着肌膜传到三联管，可使肌质网释放钙离子，启动肌肉收缩过程，而钙离子泵通过主动转运恢复胞浆中的钙离子水平，此时肌肉收缩停止，转为舒张。

肌肉单收缩是指一次刺激引起一次收缩，包括潜伏期、缩短期和舒张期。通过频率总和可以增加肌肉收缩的幅度，在较低频率的刺激下，单收缩相继发生，不发生重合；随着刺激频率的增加，新的收缩将在前一次收缩结束之前发生，导致第二次收缩被部分地加到第一次收缩上，因此肌肉收缩强度随着刺激频率的增加而增加，在较高频率的刺激下，连续的收缩融合在一起，但可以区别开来，收缩曲线呈锯齿形，称为不完全强直收缩；当频率继续上升到某一临界水平时，肌肉的连续收缩将融合在一起，收缩曲线看上去是完全平滑和连续的，称为完全强直收缩。因此，有效刺激的频率决定了肌肉收缩的形式（图 1），且刺激频率越高，肌肉收缩的幅度也越大。

3. 实验材料

（1）实验动物：青蛙。

（2）实验器材：电子刺激器、万能支架、青蛙解剖装置、机械 - 电换能器、BL-420 系统。

（3）实验试剂：任氏液。

4. 实验步骤和观察项目

（1）制备坐骨神经 - 腓肠肌标本。

（2）用机械 - 电换能器将标本与 BL-420 系统的输入孔相连。

（3）把刺激电极放在坐骨神经或肌肉上，并使其密切接触。

（4）用 BL-420 系统的电输出对坐骨神经进行电刺激，调整频率刺激，记录骨骼肌收缩曲线。

5. 实验结果

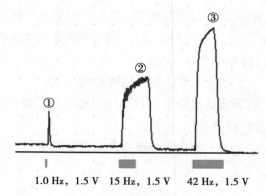

| 1.0 Hz，1.5 V | 15 Hz，1.5 V | 42 Hz，1.5 V |

①单收缩；②不完全强直收缩；
③完全强直收缩。

图 1 肌肉收缩随刺激频率变化模式

6. 讨论

当刺激频率为 1.0 Hz 时，单一的低频率刺激引起肌肉产生单收缩，单收缩曲线包括三个成分，潜伏期、缩短期和舒张期。潜伏期是刺激产生的 AP 沿着肌膜和横小管流向肌浆网的时间，在这一时期，肌肉长度没有变化。AP 引起肌浆网中的钙离子释放到细胞质中，启动横桥循环而产生肌丝滑行，引起肌肉缩短，进入缩短期。随着钙离子被钙泵主动地运回终末池，横桥循环减少并终止，肌肉恢复到原来的长度，进入舒张期。

随着刺激频率的增加，新的刺激引起的收缩将在前一次收缩的舒张期产生，导致第二次收缩的缩短期叠加在前一次收缩的舒张期，而第三次收缩的缩短期叠加在第二次收缩的舒张期，以此类推，因此肌肉收缩曲线呈现锯齿状，称为不完全强直收缩，且肌肉收缩强度随着刺激频率的增加而增加；当刺激频率进一步增加时，可出现第二次刺激引起的收缩在第一次收缩的缩短期的现象，而第三次刺激引起的收缩落在第二次收缩的缩短期，以此类推，最终产生连续的收缩，外观上难以区分开来，收缩曲线看上去是平滑和连续的，这种现象称为完全强直收缩。

7. 结论

刺激频率决定了肌肉收缩的形式，且随着刺激频率的增加，肌肉收缩的幅度也增加。

8. 参考文献

［1］HALL J E. Guyton and Hall textbook of medical physiology［M］. 13th ed. Philadelphia（PA）：Elsevier Science Publishers，2016.

附录2 实验设计报告样例

这里我们以运动对人体心血管和呼吸活动的影响为例，向大家展示一个好的实验设计样例。然后，您将了解如何使用前面所描述的实验设计原则和步骤设计一个合理的实验。

运动对人体心血管和呼吸活动的影响

1. 目的
（1）观察并解释运动对人体心血管和呼吸活动的影响。

（2）练习基本实验设计程序设计一个遵循基本原理的实验。

（3）学习记录心率、动脉血压和呼吸频率的方法。

2. 原理
心血管系统由心脏和血管组成，与呼吸系统（肺和呼吸道）配合使用。这些系统将氧气带到身体各处的肌肉和器官处，并带走代谢废物和多余的二氧化碳。在持续运动的情况下，心肺系统的能力将增强，为骨骼肌肉提供比静息状态时更多的氧气。有许多指数和测量方法可以用来评估心脏、血管和肺的功能。鉴于当前实验需在一个下午内用有限的仪器完成，本实验将采用以下指标进行评估：心率、血压（包括收缩压，舒张压、脉压）和呼吸速率。

（1）心率：运动消耗了葡萄糖氧化所产生的能量。葡萄糖和氧气必须经由血液输送，这意味着在运动时心脏必须更加努力地向全身泵送更多的血液。为了达到更高的搏出量，心脏必须加快跳动速度。静息状态的人心率约为 70 次 / 分。在剧烈运动期间，心率会显著增加，人的最大心率是 220 次 / 分，这将导致血流量增加。

（2）血压：随着心率的增加，心脏的收缩力在运动时也会增加，因此每次跳动都会泵出更多的血液，这将会升高血压。然而，在运动过程中，供应肌肉的血管将扩张，使得增加的血液流向肌肉，而不会对血管壁施加过多的压力。因此，当我们在运动过程中血压升高时，其升高幅度远小于心率的升高幅度。在停止锻炼几分钟后，我们的血压和心率就会恢复到静息水平。

（3）呼吸频率：当我们锻炼时，体内的肌肉细胞会消耗更多的氧气，产生更多的二氧化碳。肺必须增加呼吸频率，提供更多的氧气，并除去二氧化碳。因为身体会尽可能摄取更多的氧气，并尽量减少氧债。在运动后或当身体必须偿还身体的氧债时也会有上述的现象发生。呼吸频率指的是一个人直立和静息时每分钟的呼吸次数。健康人静息时平均每分钟呼吸 12~18 次。当呼吸频率超过或少于每分钟 25 次时，呼吸频率被视为异常。

3. 实验材料

（1）实验对象：人。

（2）实验仪器：血压计，听诊器，计时器，秒表。

4. 步骤和观察

（1）确定运动类型及其强度：以 3 min 台阶测试为例，按照节拍器的节奏直接上 / 下台阶，或在两个台阶之间先左脚迈向上一台阶，右脚再迈向上一台阶，之后左脚迈向下一台阶，右脚再迈向下一台阶，以 24 步 / 分为一个周期行进，共走 72 步。

（2）将受试者随机分成不同的组别。

（3）让受试者安静地坐 3 min，然后在运动前测量血压、心率和呼吸速率（作为参照值）。呼吸速率通常是在人处于静息状态时测量的。测量时只需计算 1 min 内胸部上升的次数，即可得知呼吸次数。重复三次实验进行测量并取其平均值。

（4）按计划进行不同强度的锻炼

① 安排受试者以相同的节奏做 20 s 上下台阶运动，让指定的人立即测量并记录他们的心率（HR）、动脉血压（BP）和呼吸频率（BF）。20 min 之后再重复测量受试者的心率、动脉血压和呼吸频率，填入表 1。

② 让另一组的受试者做 40 s 的上下台阶运动（保持相同的节奏），同一个记录员立即测量并记录他们的心率、动脉血压和呼吸频率。20 min 之后再重复测量受试者的心率、收缩压、舒张压和呼吸频率，填入表 1。

5. 预期结果

根据所学的理论知识，预期的实验结果可能是：

（1）运动会提高心率。运动强度越大，心率越大，直至达到最大心率。

（2）在运动过程中，血压也会上升，但与心率相比，血压的上升幅度要小得多。在停止运动的几分钟后，血压和心率会恢复到静息水平。

（3）当我们从静息状态转变为运动状态时，呼吸频率会迅速变化。刚开始锻炼时会有初始反应，此时呼吸频率将迅速增加。在初始反应或最初几分钟之后，呼吸频率会趋于平稳。此后若增加运动强度，呼吸频率也会相应地增加，但增加幅度不会和初始反应一样剧烈。

6. 参考文献

［1］HALL J E. Guyton and Hall textbook of medical physiology［M］. 13th ed. Philadelphia（PA）: Elsevier Science Publishers，2016.

［2］朱大年，王庭槐 . 生理学［M］. 8 版 . 北京：人民卫生出版社，2013.

表 1　不同程度的运动对心率、动脉血压和呼吸频率的影响

学生信息		运动前				运动 20 s				运动 40 s			
性别	学生姓名	心率（次/分）	收缩压（mmHg）	舒张压（mmHg）	呼吸频率（次/分）	心率（次/分）	收缩压（mmHg）	舒张压（mmHg）	呼吸频率（次/分）	心率（次/分）	收缩压（mmHg）	舒张压（mmHg）	呼吸频率（次/分）
男生	学生 1												
	学生 2												
	学生 3												
	学生 4												
女生	学生 5												
	学生 6												
	学生 7												
	学生 8												

蹲起运动对青年学生呼吸频率、心率和血压的影响

1. 目的

（1）学习测量记录心率和动脉血压的方法，了解运动对心血管系统的影响。

（2）学习呼吸频率的记录方法，了解运动对呼吸系统的影响。

（3）观察运动对呼吸频率、心率和血压的影响。

2. 原理

机体在运动时，心脏、血管、肺、肌肉、大脑、神经以及骨骼等器官组织协调工作。因此，我们可以通过研究这些器官、系统进而观察运动对它们产生的影响。例如，运动使得心血管系统、呼吸系统（尤其是肺）和肌肉骨骼系统发生短期变化，大脑发出的信息可以对这些变化进行调控。在运动的前后可对这些变化参数进行测量，并对运动前后各参数的变化进行比较。

（1）无氧运动和有氧运动：运动需要能量。有氧运动是指能量来自细胞中的有氧代谢，而无氧运动是指能量来自无氧糖酵解。在有氧代谢中，1分子的葡萄糖完全氧化可以产生38个ATP，但1分子葡萄糖无氧糖酵解只产生2个ATP。

① 有氧运动动用了较大的肌群，使得身体比静息状态时消耗更多的氧气。有氧运动可以增强心血管耐力。骑自行车、游泳、快走、跳绳、划船、徒步旅行、打网球、连续训练和长距离慢速训练等都属于有氧运动。

② 无氧运动包括力量训练和阻力训练，可以使肌肉变得紧实、强壮，还可以增强骨骼的力量、平衡能力和协调能力。力量运动包括俯卧撑、引体向上、弓步和哑铃运动等。此外，重量训练、机能训练、偏心训练、间歇训练、短跑等高强度间歇训练无氧运动都可以在短期内增加肌肉力量。

（2）运动对心率的影响：运动消耗了葡萄糖氧化所产生的能量。葡萄糖和氧气必须经由血液输送，这意味着在运动时心脏必须更加努力地向全身泵送更多的血液。为了达到更高的搏出量，心脏必须加快跳动速度。静息状态的人的心率约为70次/分。在剧烈运动期间，心率会显著增加，人的最大心率是220次/分，这将导致血流量增加。

（3）运动对血压的影响：随着心率的增加，心脏的收缩力在运动时也会增加，因此每次跳动都会泵出更多的血液，这将会升高血压。然而，在运动过程中，供应肌肉的血管将扩张，使得增加的血液流向肌肉，而不会对血管壁施加过多的压力。因此，当我们在运动过程中血压升高时，其升高幅度远小于心率的升高幅度。在停止锻炼几分钟后，我们的血压和心率就会恢复到静息水平。

（4）运动对呼吸的影响：当我们锻炼时，体内的肌肉细胞会消耗更多的氧气，产生更多的二氧化碳。肺必须增加呼吸频率，提供更多的氧气，并除去二氧化碳。因为身体会尽可能摄取更多的氧气，并尽量减少氧债（氧债指从剧烈运动中恢复时肌肉组织所需要的额外氧气量）。静息状态时呼吸频率为每分钟 14 次左右，运动时呼吸频率可增至每分钟 32 次。

3. 实验材料

（1）实验对象：人。

（2）实验器材：秒表、听诊器、血压计。

4. 实验步骤和观察项目

（1）首先，让受试者休息 5 min，确保身体处于平静放松状态。指定的测量者记录受试者的呼吸频率、心率和血压。

（2）受试者保持频率不变做 20 个蹲起运动后，指定的测量者记录心率、动脉血压和呼吸频率。

（3）待以上指标恢复正常后，受试者再保持相同频率做 40 个蹲起运动，指定的测量者立即测量并记录心率、动脉血压、呼吸频率。

（4）详细测量方法

① 间接测量动脉血压：将血压袖包裹在肘部正上方的手臂上，打气使之膨胀，直至前臂的血液流入停止，无法感觉到或听到任何臂压。逐渐放气使袖口中的压力降低，同时检查者用听诊器听肱动脉的声音。当听到第一个轻轻敲击的声音时（小股喷射的血流经过收缩的血管时发出的第一个声音），此时的压力被记录为收缩压。随着压力不断降低，这个声音会变得更明显、更响亮。但是，当动脉不再受到限制，血液自由流动时，就再也听不到声音了。声音消失时对应的压力被记录为舒张压。

② 正确计算呼吸频率：为了在运动前准确测量呼吸频率，应让受试者坐直。至少休息 10 min，再开始测量。记录受试者在 1 min 内胸部上、下起伏的次数。测量三次取平均值，以提高结果的准确性。也可以测量 15 s 内的呼吸次数，然后将结果乘以 4（这接近每分钟的呼吸，在紧急情况下很有用）。

5. 结果

表 1　蹲起运动对心肺功能的影响

状态	收缩压（mmHg）	舒张压（mmHg）	脉压（mmHg）	平均动脉压（mmHg）	心率（次/分）	呼吸频率（次/分）
静息	106.9 ± 6.52	64.6 ± 8.15	42.3 ± 9.53	78.7 ± 6.19	82 ± 11.35	21.4 ± 3.01
锻炼（20 个）	121.4 ± 11.14	66.7 ± 10.08	54.7 ± 6.66	84.93 ± 9.96	92.5 ± 19.31	29 ± 3.38
静息	106.7 ± 5.62	65 ± 4.84	41.7 ± 4.94	78.9 ± 4.55	83.2 ± 12.2	22.3 ± 3.13
锻炼（40 个）	125.9 ± 7.34	63.2 ± 12.97	62.7 ± 10.69	84.1 ± 10.23	102.4 ± 24.96	32.9 ± 5.92

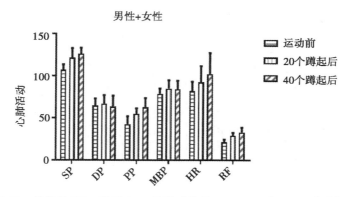

收缩压 SP；舒张压 DP；脉压 PP；平均动脉压 MBP；心率 HR；呼吸频率 RF。

图 1　蹲起运动对心肺活动的影响

表 2　男性组蹲起运动对心肺活动的影响

状态	收缩压 （mmHg）	舒张压 （mmHg）	脉压 （mmHg）	平均动脉压 （mmHg）	心率 （次/分）	呼吸频率 （次/分）
静息	106.4 ± 8.62	63.6 ± 10.98	42.8 ± 12.17	77.87 ± 8.5	72.8 ± 6.88	19.2 ± 2.48
锻炼（20 个）	114.8 ± 7.76	57.6 ± 3.44	57.2 ± 6.14	76.67 ± 4.42	83.6 ± 15.72	27.6 ± 3.88
静息	108.4 ± 7.09	66.4 ± 4.96	42 ± 4.56	80.4 ± 5.34	75.2 ± 11.97	20 ± 2.76
锻炼（40 个）	123.8 ± 5.53	53.6 ± 6.25	70.2 ± 5.31	77 ± 5.47	90.6 ± 24.06	31.6 ± 6.97

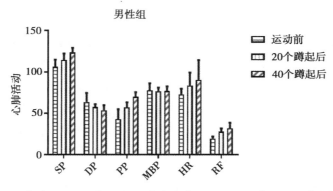

收缩压 SP；舒张压 DP；脉压 PP；平均动脉压 MBP；心率 HR；呼吸频率 RF。

图 2　男性组蹲起运动对心肺活动的影响

表 3　女性组蹲起运动对心肺活动的影响

状态	收缩压 （mmHg）	舒张压 （mmHg）	脉压 （mmHg）	平均动脉压 （mmHg）	心率 （次/分）	呼吸频率 （次/分）
静息	107.4 ± 3.2	65.6 ± 3.2	41.8 ± 5.74	79.53 ± 1.71	91.2 ± 6.4	23.6 ± 1.5
锻炼（20 个）	128 ± 10.04	75.8 ± 5.08	52.2 ± 6.21	93.2 ± 6.5	101.4 ± 18.46	30.4 ± 1.96
静息	105 ± 2.68	63.6 ± 4.27	41.4 ± 5.28	77.4 ± 2.89	91.2 ± 5.15	24.6 ± 1.2
锻炼（40 个）	128 ± 8.27	72.8 ± 10.63	55.2 ± 9.37	91.2 ± 8.87	114.2 ± 19.7	34.2 ± 4.26

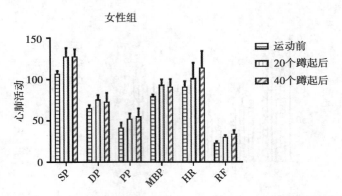

收缩压 SP；舒张压 DP；脉压 PP；平均动脉压 MBP；心率 HR；呼吸频率 RF。

图 3　女性组蹲起运动对心肺活动的影响

6. 讨论

蹲起运动是一种无氧运动，可以产生比有氧运动更多的乳酸，使肌肉更加疲劳。这可能刺激神经系统增强心血管和呼吸活动。

（1）运动对呼吸速率的影响

从表 1 和图 1 中观察发现，运动可以使心率增加。随着运动强度增大，心率也增加，直至达到最大心率。

当我们从静息状态转为运动状态时，呼吸频率会马上发生变化。刚开始运动时会有初始反应，此时呼吸频率将迅速增加。在初始反应或最初几分钟之后，呼吸频率会趋于平稳。此后若增加运动强度，呼吸频率也会相应地增加，但增加幅度不会和初始反应一样剧烈。在运动过程中，身体组织会消耗能量。正常情况下，能量的来源是有氧呼吸中一系列分解葡萄糖的反应。当运动强度增加时，能量需求增大。由于氧气的吸收量低于耗氧量，血液中的 PO_2 降低，而 PCO_2 和 H^+ 升高。这将会刺激周围的化学受体，如颈动脉体、主动脉体以及位于延髓的中央化学受体，传递信号至呼吸中枢，促进肺通气，提高呼吸频率。

此外，当组织缺氧时，机体通过无氧呼吸获得能量并产生乳酸。乳酸会进一步降低 pH 值，提高 H^+ 离子的水平，刺激外周化学感受器和中枢化学感受器，进而促进肺通气，提高呼吸速率。乳酸积累越多，刺激的效果越强，呼吸频率增加得越多。

高强度运动结束后的呼吸速率高于运动开始时静息状态的呼吸速率。这是因为乳酸在体内积累，发生氧债，必须有额外的氧气才能将乳酸代谢成葡萄糖，使得所有系统恢复正常状态。在运动结束后的很长一段时间内，呼吸速率仍会增加。

（2）运动对心率的影响

所有脊椎动物的心脏由副交感神经抑制系统和交感兴奋系统支配。在正常情况下，心率由窦房结调节。当身体开始运动时，骨骼肌收缩会刺激心肌交感神经使之兴奋。迷走神经通过向窦房结细胞释放乙酰胆碱，向心脏输送副交感神经信号。因此，交感神经的刺激使心率加快，而迷走神经刺激使心率减慢。运动强度越高，交感神经分泌的去甲肾上腺素就越多，心率升高越快。由于心肌细胞中化学受体的数量有限，运动强度越高，人体代谢掉大量去甲肾上腺素的时间就越长。

在高强度运动后，受试者的心率总体上高于低强度运动心率，这是因为肌肉中乳酸的积累会导致血液中 pH 值降低，从而导致心跳加快。

（3）运动对血压的影响

平均血压在运动时升高，但其升高幅度小于心率的升高幅度。在停止锻炼几分钟后血压和心率就会恢复到静息水平。

由图 1 可知，随着运动强度的增加，机体对血液供应的需求增加，故收缩压急剧升高。然而，由于无氧运动中产生的乳酸发生沉积，舒张压将随着运动强度的增加而降低，这是因为体内的乳酸会使血管扩张，从而降低舒张压。

（4）性别差异对运动的影响

对比表 2 和表 3 以及图 2 和图 3，可以发现相同条件下男性组和女性组蹲起运动的效果存在差异。首先，我们可以观察到，女性组在第一轮运动（20 个蹲起）和第二轮运动（40 个蹲起）时所达到的心率平均值均高于男性组，表明女性的心室肌能力低于男性。这可能是因为女性的耐力不如男性，因此女性才会更快地达到最大心率。其次，在两次蹲起运动后，男性的舒张压下降，而女性的舒张压上升。造成这种差异的原因之一可能是女性产生乳酸的能力弱于男性，使得乳酸扩张血管的能力减弱，因此血管外周阻力增大导致女性舒张压升高。

7. 结论

由于运动产生了额外的能量需求，运动时心血管和呼吸系统活动增加。

8. 参考文献

［1］HALL J E. Guyton and Hall textbook of medical physiology［M］. 13th ed. Philadelphia（PA）：Elsevier Science Publishers，2016.

［2］MARIEB E，HOEHN K. Human anatomy & physiology［M］. 7th ed. New York：Pearson Education，2007.

［3］GOOTMAN P M，COHEN H L，GOOTMAN N. Autonomic nervous system regulation of heart rate in the perinatal period［J］. Pediatric and Fundamental Electrocardiography，1987(56)：137-159.

［4］DI DONATO D M，WEST D W，CHURCHWARD-VENNE T A，et al. Influence of aerobic exercise intensity on myofibrillar and mitochondrial protein synthesis in young men during early and late post exercise recovery［J］. American Journal of Physiology-Endocrinology and Metabolism，2014，306(9)：E1025-E1032.

［5］FISHER J P，ADLAN A M，SHANTSILA A，et al. Muscle metaboreflex and autonomic regulation of heart rate in humans［J］. The Journal of physiology，2013，591（15）：3777-3788.

［6］朱大年，王庭槐. 生理学［M］. 8 版. 北京：人民卫生出版社，2013.

［7］TANAKA H，SEALS D R. Endurance exercise performance in Masters athletes：age-associated changes and underlying physiological mechanisms［J］. The Journal of physiology，2008，586（1）：55-63.

1. CO 发生装置

本实验中利用化学方法来获取 CO。CO 发生装置如图 1 所示，取 4 mL 甲酸放入试管内，再缓慢加入浓硫酸 2 mL，塞紧胶塞。反应产生的 CO 通过塑料胶管与装有小鼠的缺氧瓶相连（缺氧瓶与外界相通）。其反应原理如下：

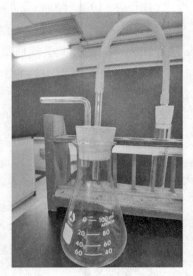

图 1　CO 发生装置

$$HCOOH \xrightarrow{H_2SO_4} CO+H_2O$$

2. 钠石灰作用机制

钠石灰（NaOH·CaO）是一种粉红色颗粒，具有吸收 CO_2 的功能。其反应式如下：

$$NaOH·CaO+H_2O+CO_2 \rightarrow NaHCO_3+ Ca（OH）_2$$

3. 亚甲蓝的解毒机制

亚甲蓝是一种无毒性的染料，它的氧化型呈蓝色，还原型呈无色。在 6- 磷酸葡萄糖脱氢过程中产生的氢离子经还原型辅酶Ⅱ（三磷酸吡啶核苷）传递给蓝色亚甲蓝，使之转变为无色亚甲蓝。无色亚甲蓝能迅速将 Hb-Fe^{3+} 还原为 Hb-Fe^{2+}，同时又被氧化成蓝色亚甲蓝，如此反复。亚甲蓝本身为氧化剂，当大量亚甲蓝进入人体，还原型辅酶Ⅱ不能迅速将其全部还原为无色亚甲蓝，此时则会生成更多的高铁血红蛋白。因此，治疗高铁血红蛋白血症时，应采用小剂量亚甲蓝注射。

附录5　小鼠耗氧量测定

1. 原理

小鼠在密闭的缺氧瓶内不断消耗氧气，产生 CO_2。CO_2 可以被钠石灰所吸收，反应如下：

$$NaOH \cdot CaO + H_2O + CO_2 \rightarrow NaHCO_3 + Ca(OH)_2$$

由于小鼠不断的消耗瓶内氧气，使缺氧瓶内氧分压逐渐下降并形成负压。当缺氧瓶与耗氧量测量装置相连时，移液管内液面因缺氧瓶内的负压而上升，量筒液面则下降，量桶内液面下降的毫升数代表总耗氧量。再根据 67 页式（2-1）计算出小鼠耗氧量。

2. 方法与步骤

（1）耗氧量测量装置如图 1 所示。

（2）量筒内加水至 100 mL 刻度，将耗氧量测定装置一端的乳胶管接头与缺氧瓶上的乳胶管相连。

（3）打开乳胶管上的弹簧夹，待移液管内液面上升稳定后，从量筒上读出液面下降的毫升数，即为小鼠的总耗氧量。

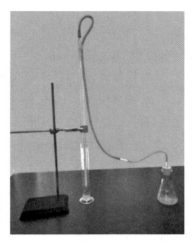

图 1　耗氧量测量装置

附录6 哺乳类动物实验基本操作技能

1. 实验动物的麻醉

实验动物麻醉的基本任务是消除实验操作所致的疼痛和不适感觉，保障实验动物的安全，使动物在实验中服从操作，确保实验顺利进行。

（1）常用局部麻醉剂及麻醉方法：利用局部麻醉药的组织穿透作用，透过黏膜来阻滞表面的神经末梢，称表面麻醉。在口腔及鼻腔黏膜、眼结膜、尿道等部位手术时，常把麻醉药涂敷或喷于表面上使用。常用的局部麻醉剂有普鲁卡因和利多卡因。

① 普鲁卡因：0.5%~1%的普鲁卡因常用于局部浸润麻醉，此药毒性小，见效快。

② 利多卡因：1%~2%利多卡因常用于大动物神经干阻滞麻醉，此药见效快，组织穿透性好。0.25%~0.5%的利多卡因溶液也可用作局部浸润麻醉。

（2）常用全身麻醉剂及麻醉方法

① 异氟烷：是实验室最常用吸入性麻醉药。先将动物放入2%~3.5%的麻醉诱导罐中诱导麻醉，然后用合适浓度的异氟烷（小鼠1.5%~2%的浓度，大鼠用2%~3%的浓度）维持麻醉。

② 戊巴比妥钠：使用时用生理盐水配置成3%溶液静脉或腹腔注射，有效时间可持续3~5 h，家兔使用剂量及方法为：耳缘静脉注射30 mg/kg；大、小鼠常用腹腔注射的方法，使用剂量为50 mg/kg。

③ 氨基甲酸乙酯（乌拉坦）：是比较温和的麻醉药，安全系数大，多数实验动物都可使用。使用时配成25%溶液，家兔使用剂量及方法为耳缘静脉注射100 mg/kg；大、小鼠常用腹腔注射的方法，使用剂量为140 mg/kg。

在注射麻醉药物时，先用麻醉药总量的2/3，密切观察动物生命体征的变化，如已达到所需麻醉的深度，余下的麻醉药则不用，避免麻醉过深抑制呼吸导致动物死亡。

2. 动物实验的常用插管术

（1）气管插管：家兔颈部手术部位剪毛备皮，在麻醉状态下沿颈部正中线切开皮肤4~5 cm，用止血钳逐层钝性分离肌肉组织，暴露并分离出气管。在气管下穿线备用，在甲状软骨下约0.5~1 cm处两软骨环之间横向切开气管前壁（气管口径的一半），作倒"T"形切口，如气管内有血液或分泌物，应先用棉签擦净，将Y型气管插管由切口处向胸腔方向插入气管腔内并用线扎紧，再将余线绕气管插管的分叉处结扎固定。

（2）颈总动脉插管：家兔颈部手术部位剪毛备皮，在麻醉状态下沿颈部正中线切开皮肤4~5 cm，用止血钳钝性逐层分离肌肉组织，暴露气管后即可见在气管两侧纵行的左、右颈总动脉鞘，在鞘内，颈总动脉与迷走神经、降压神经伴行在一起。可先将颈总动脉鞘分离出来，再从鞘内分离出颈总动脉，剔尽周围结缔组织，游离出长 3~4 cm 长的颈总动脉。在动脉下穿 2 根线，用其中一根结扎远心端，用动脉夹夹住其近心端。用动脉导管或 22G 静脉留置针刺入颈总动脉进行插管，固定插管以备后续使用。

（3）颈总静脉插管：家兔颈部手术部位剪毛备皮，在麻醉状态下沿颈部正中线切开皮肤 4~5 cm，用止血钳钝性逐层分离肌肉组织，可清晰地看见位于颈部皮下、胸锁乳突肌外缘的颈静脉。沿血管走向，用玻璃分针或止血钳钝性分离颈总静脉两侧的浅筋膜，游离出 3~4 cm 长。在血管的远心端穿线结扎后用眼科剪剪一小口迅速插入静脉导管并结扎固定。

（4）股动脉和股静脉插管：股动脉和股静脉插管与颈总动脉插管类似，所不同的是位置的区别。先在大腿根部近腹股沟处摸到股动脉搏动点，局部剪毛，以搏动最明显处为起点沿血管走行的方向作长约 4 cm 的切口，股动脉、股静脉、股神经行走于同一鞘内，位置比较表浅，向下分离后很快就能见到。股动脉和股静脉与颈总动脉插管方法相同。

动物实验常用插管术的操作视频

附录7 BL-420N生物信号采集与分析系统简介

1. 主界面介绍

BL-420N 生物信号采集与分析系统，后文简称 BL-420N 系统，其主界面中包含 4 个主要的视图区，分别为功能区、波形显示区、实验数据列表区、刺激参数调节区以及其他信息显示区，参见图 1。

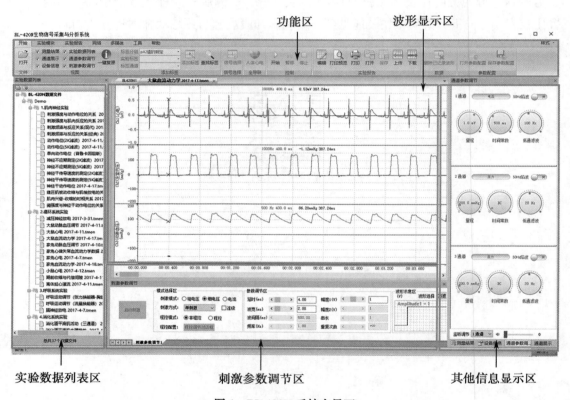

图 1　BL-420N 系统主界面

视图区是指一块独立功能规划的显示区域，这些区域可以装入不同的视图。在 BL-420N 系统中，除了波形显示视图不能隐藏之外，其余视图均可显示或隐藏。除波形显示区和顶部的功能区之外，其余视图还可以任意移动位置。其他信息显示区包括测量结果视图、设备信息视图、通道参数调节视图、通道信息视图等。

打开软件，对应图 1 找到各个视图。耐心认识系统主界面将有助于您使用软件。表 1 为主界面上主要功能区划分的说明。

表 1　主界面上主要视图划分说明

序号	视图区名称	功能说明
1	功能区	位于主界面顶部，是功能按钮选择区
2	波形显示区	位于主界面正中间区域，显示采集和分析后的通道数据波形
3	实验数据列表区	位于主界面左侧，用于快速选择并打开已存贮实验数据文件
4	刺激参数调节区	位于主界面的底部，是调节刺激参数并给予刺激的控制区
5	其他信息显示区	位于主界面右侧，可切换显示测量结果视图、设备信息视图、通道参数调节视图、通道信息视图

注意：

进入 BL-420N 系统后，您看到的主界面可能会和图 1 所显示的主界面有所不同，这是由于 BL-420N 系统的很多视图都可以隐藏和移动，而且视图之间还可能会相互覆盖，造成主界面有所变化。

如果您进入 BL-420N 系统后显示的主界面与图 1 不一致，请不要担心，接下来我们将简单介绍主界面各视图的操作和使用。

（1）主界面各个视图的显示和隐藏

BL-420N 系统中多个视图的位置和显示状态都可以改变，这是为了适应不同用户的使用习惯，但这种变化有时候会造成系统的主界面变得让我们无法理解。但是万变不离其宗，只要掌握了其变化规律，就可以轻松应对这种变化，而且还可以更方便地完成实验。

1）功能区的最小化和恢复：功能区位于主界面的最上方，可以被最小化。在功能区的分类标题位置单击鼠标右键，会弹出功能区相关快捷菜单，选择"最小化功能区"命令，则功能区分类标题下面的功能按钮被隐藏。如果要恢复被隐藏的功能按钮，则需要再次在功能区分类标题上单击鼠标右键弹出快捷菜单，然后选择打勾的"最小化功能区"命令，则可恢复最小化的功能区。参见图 2。

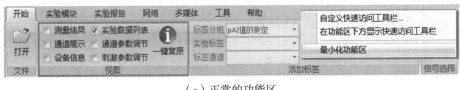

（a）正常的功能区

开始　　实验模块　　实验报告　　网络　　多媒体　　工具　　帮助

（b）最小化的功能区

图 2　BL-420N 系统顶部功能区的最小化和恢复

2）视图的隐藏和显示：BL-420N 系统中包含多个视图，除波形显示视图之外，其余视图都可以被隐藏或显示。这些视图的隐藏显示状态显示在"功能区"→"开始"分类栏下面的"视图"选项中，参见图 2（a）。当"视图"选项中的某一个视图前面的方框中有一个小勾，表示该视图被显示，比如实验数据列表视图。

由于视图在某一个区域中会相互覆盖，因此即使该视图处于显示状态，但是它可能被其他视图所覆盖而无法显示。如果要显示这些被覆盖的视图，最简单的方法就是在视图区的下方单击该视图的名称即可。

（2）主界面各个视图的移动

在 BL-420N 系统中，除波形显示区和功能区之外，其余视图都可以按需移动位置或改变大小。每个视图都具有两种状态，一种是紧挨主界面边缘的停靠状态，这是视图的默认状态，另一种是以独立窗口形式存在的浮动状态，参见图 3 和图 4。

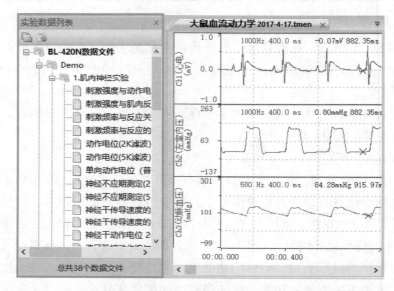

图 3　BL-420N 实验数据列表视图的停靠状态（和主视图紧挨排列）

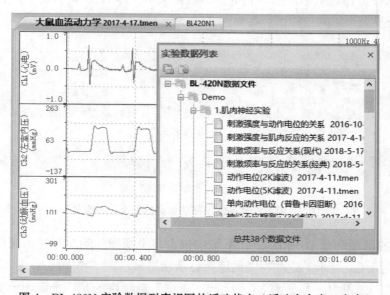

图 4　BL-420N 实验数据列表视图的浮动状态（浮动在主窗口上方）

1）停靠状态和浮动状态的切换：在视图标题栏上双击鼠标左键就可以在停靠状态和浮动状态之间切换。

2）停靠状态和浮动状态的移动：在视图标题栏上按下鼠标左键不放，然后移动鼠标，就可以按需移动视图位置。

当在视图标题栏上按下鼠标左键不放时，主界面上会出现停靠位置透明指示按钮（后文简称停靠按钮），参见图5。视图可以停靠在主视图的上下左右，为了精确停靠视图，需要将鼠标位置移动到这些停靠按钮上，当鼠标移动到停靠按钮上之后，选择视图就会出现在主视图的相应位置，确认好位置之后松开鼠标左键就会将选择视图停靠在指定位置；如果不将鼠标移动到停靠按钮上，而是直接在任意位置松开鼠标左键，则窗口浮动在鼠标指示位置。

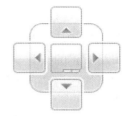

图5　选择视图停靠位置透明指示按钮

BL-420N 系统会自动记录用户最近一次移动视图的位置，这样在下次打开软件的时候所有视图仍然保持原来的位置和大小。因此当您移动过视图之后软件的主界面会呈现出与图1不同的情形。

2. 开始实验

BL-420N 系统提供三种开始实验的方法，分别是从实验模块启动实验、从信号选择对话框进入实验或者从快速启动视图开始实验。接下来就简单介绍开始实验的三种方式。

（1）从实验模块启动实验（适用于学生的教学实验）

选择功能区"实验模块"栏目，然后根据需要选择不同的实验模块开始实验，比如，选择"循环"→"期前收缩 - 代偿间歇"，将自动启动该实验模块，参见图6。

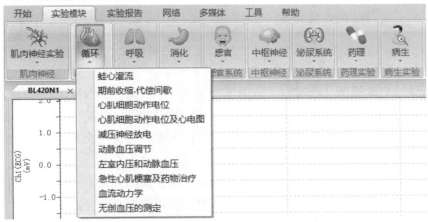

图6　功能区中的实验模块启动下拉按钮

从实验模块启动实验时，系统会自动根据用户选择的实验项目配置各种实验参数，包括：采样通道数，采样率、增益、滤波、刺激等参数，方便用户快速进入实验状态。

实验模块通常根据教学内容配置，因此通常适用于学生的教学实验。

（2）从信号选择对话框启动实验（适用于科研实验或新的学生实验）

选择工具区“开始”→“信号选择”按钮，系统会弹出一个信号选择对话框，参见图7和图8。在“信号选择”对话框中，实验者可根据自己的实验内容，为每个通道配置相应的实验参数，这是最为灵活的一种启动实验的方式。

信号选择对话框是一种最灵活、通用的开始实验的方式，主要适用于科研工作。对于灵活配置的实验参数在将来的BL-420N版本中也可以存贮为自定义实验模块，帮助科研工作者快速启动自己的实验。

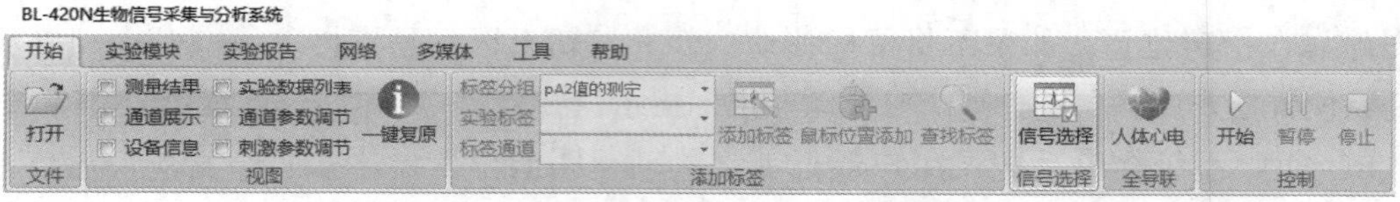

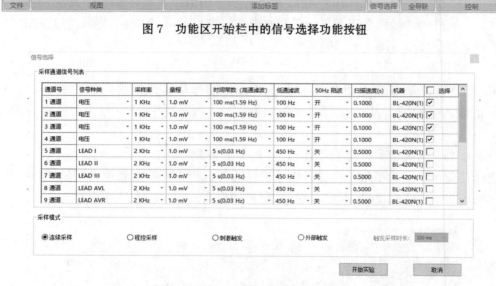

图7　功能区开始栏中的信号选择功能按钮

通道号	信号种类	采样率	量程	时间常数（高通滤波）	低通滤波	50Hz 陷波	扫描速度(s)	机器	选择
1 通道	电压	1 KHz	1.0 mV	100 ms(1.59 Hz)	100 Hz	开	0.1000	BL-420N(1)	☑
2 通道	电压	1 KHz	1.0 mV	100 ms(1.59 Hz)	100 Hz	开	0.1000	BL-420N(1)	☑
3 通道	电压	1 KHz	1.0 mV	100 ms(1.59 Hz)	100 Hz	开	0.1000	BL-420N(1)	☑
4 通道	电压	1 KHz	1.0 mV	100 ms(1.59 Hz)	100 Hz	开	0.1000	BL-420N(1)	☑
5 通道	LEAD I	2 KHz	1.0 mV	5 s(0.03 Hz)	450 Hz	关	0.5000	BL-420N(1)	☐
6 通道	LEAD II	2 KHz	1.0 mV	5 s(0.03 Hz)	450 Hz	关	0.5000	BL-420N(1)	☐
7 通道	LEAD III	2 KHz	1.0 mV	5 s(0.03 Hz)	450 Hz	关	0.5000	BL-420N(1)	☐
8 通道	LEAD AVL	2 KHz	1.0 mV	5 s(0.03 Hz)	450 Hz	关	0.5000	BL-420N(1)	☐
9 通道	LEAD AVR	2 KHz	1.0 mV	5 s(0.03 Hz)	450 Hz	关	0.5000	BL-420N(1)	☐

图8　信号选择对话框

（3）从快速启动视图开始实验（适用于快速打开上一次实验参数）

用户可以从启动视图中的快速启动按钮开始实验，也可以从功能区“开始”菜单栏中的“开始”按钮快速启动实验，参见图9。这两种快速启动实验的方法完全相同，之所以有两种相同的启动方法是为了方便用户的操作。

在第一次启动软件的情况下快速启动实验，系统会采用默认方式，即同时打开4个心电通道的方式启动实验。如果在上一次停止实验后使用快速启动方式启动实验，系统会按照上一次实验的参数启动本次实验。

3. 暂停和停止实验

在“启动视图”中点击“暂停”或“停止”按钮，或者选择功能区开始栏中的“暂停”或“停止”按钮，就可以完成实验的暂停和停止操作，参见图10。这两种操作方式

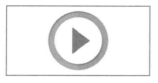
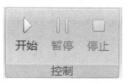

启动视图中的开始按钮　　　　　功能区开始栏中的开始按钮

图 9　快速启动实验按钮

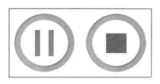
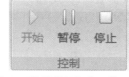

启动视图中的暂停、停止按钮　　　功能区开始栏中的暂停、停止按钮

图 10　暂停、停止控制按钮区

完全相同，提供两种操作方式是为了方便用户的操作。

暂停是指在实验过程中停止快速移动的波形，便于仔细观察分析停留在显示屏上的一幅静止图像的数据，暂停时硬件数据采集的过程仍然在进行但数据不被保存；重新开始，采集的数据恢复显示并被保存。

停止是指停止整个实验，并将数据保存到文件中。

4. 保存数据

当单击停止实验按钮的时候，系统会弹出一个询问对话框询问是否停止实验，如果确认停止实验则系统会弹出"另存为"对话框让用户确认保存数据的名字，参见图 11。文件的默认命名为"年_月_日_Non.tmen"。用户可以自己修改存贮的文件名，点击"保存"即可完成保存数据操作。

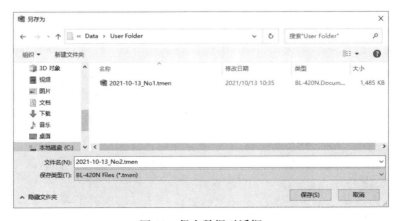

图 11　保存数据对话框

5. 数据反演

数据反演是指查看已保存的实验数据，有两种方法可以打开反演文件：

1）在"实验数据列表"视图中双击要打开的反演文件，参见图3。

2）在功能区的开始栏中选择"文件"→"打开"命令，将弹出与图11相似的打开文件对话框，在打开文件对话框中选择要打开的反演文件，然后单击"打开"按钮。

BL-420N系统可以同时打开多个文件进行反演，参见图12，最多可以同时打开4个反演文件。

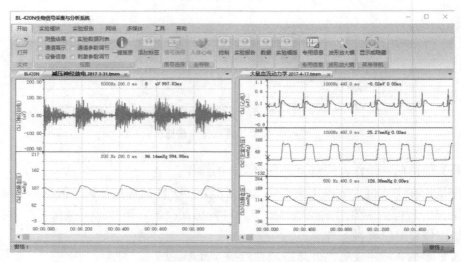

图12　同时打开两个反演文件进行数据反演

6. 实验报告编辑和打印

实验完成后，用户可以在软件中直接编辑和打印实验报告，对于编辑后的实验报告可以直接打印，也可以存贮在本地或者上传到NEIM-100实验室信息化管理系统（需要实验室独立配置）。实验报告的相关功能可以在"功能区"→"开始"→"实验报告"分类中找到，这里包括5个与实验报告相关的常见功能，参见图13。

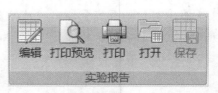

图13　功能区开始栏中与实验报告
相关的功能

1）编辑实验报告：选择图13中的编辑按钮，系统将启动实验报告的编辑功能，参见图14。实验报告编辑器相当于在Word软件中编辑文档，参见图14。

用户可以在实验报告编辑器中输入用户姓名，实验目的，方法，结论或其他信息，也可以从打开的原始数据文件中选择波形粘贴到实验报告中。实验报告默认将当前显示的波形自动提取到实验报告"实验结果"显示区中。

2）打印实验报告：单击"功能区"→"开始"→"实验报告"→"打印"功能按钮，将打印当前编辑好的实验报告。

3）存贮实验报告：单击"功能区"→"开始"→"实验报告"→"保存"功能按钮，将存贮当前编辑好的实验报告。

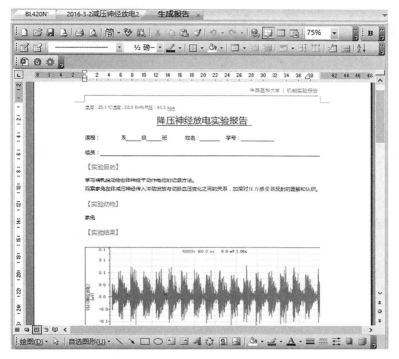

图 14　实验报告编辑器

4）打开已存贮实验报告：单击"功能区"→"开始"→"实验报告"→"打开"功能按钮，打开已存贮在本地的实验报告。

附录8 HPS-102人体生理实验系统介绍

1. 主界面

HPS-102 人体生理实验系统，后文简称 HPS-102 系统，其主界面主要由"工具栏"和"主工作区"构成，参见图1。在工具栏上有丰富的功能按钮，比如：打开文件，添加标签，信号选择，采样控制按钮等。主界面的正中间是主工作区，用于波形数据的绘制、实验标签和刺激标记的显示，还可以对波形在水平和垂直方向上进行调节。在主工作区的右侧是硬件参数调节、仪器连接状态展示视图停靠区；在主工作区的左侧是实验数据列表停靠区；在主工作区下方是刺激器和数据测量结果视图停靠区，通过单击这些视图缩略图可以展开对应的界面。

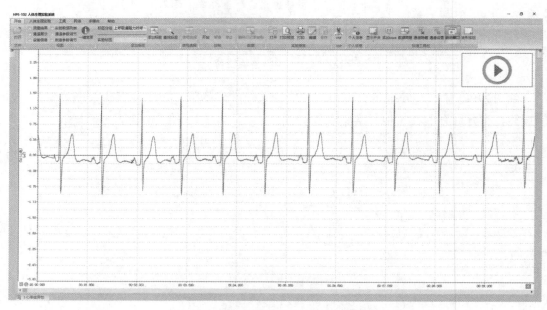

图1 HPS-102 系统主界面示意图

2. 首页

HPS-102 系统默认提供 20 个实验模块，这些实验模块按人体器官系统分为：循环系统实验，呼吸系统实验，中枢神经系统实验等 10 类。进入 HPS-102 系统后，其主界面将展示这些实验模块的分类，参见图2。不同的分类下面有不同数量的实验模块，具体的实验模块涵盖了实验概述、实验项目、实验测验、实验拓展四个部分的电子多媒体内容。同时还设置了正确的采样通道、采样率、量程、滤波等实验参数。使用者在学习完成实验相关知识后可以直接开始实验。

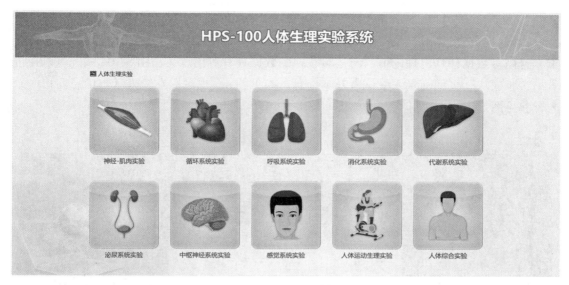

图 2　HPS-102 系统首页

3. 实验模块界面

具体的实验模块页面主要包括：实验概述、实验项目、实验测验、实验拓展，参见图 3。实验概述包括实验目的和实验原理；实验项目包含器材与药品、实验准备和观察项目，详细描述了整个实验的完整步骤，也是本教材中讲解实验过程的主要内容；实验测验是对该实验相关知识的考核；实验拓展是对该实验相关知识的拓展，包括发展历史、原理拓展、临床应用和参考文献。

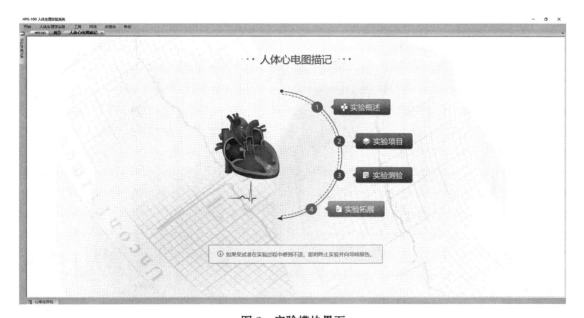

图 3　实验模块界面

4. 受试者基本信息界面

受试者基本信息对于人体生理实验有重要意义。部分人体生理指标可以根据个人的体重、身高等数据计算出理论值，与实验获取的数据具有对比意义。HPS-102 系统可以在进入"实验模块"页面前录入受试者基本信息，参见图 4，也可以在个人基本信息窗口中录入，参见图 5。

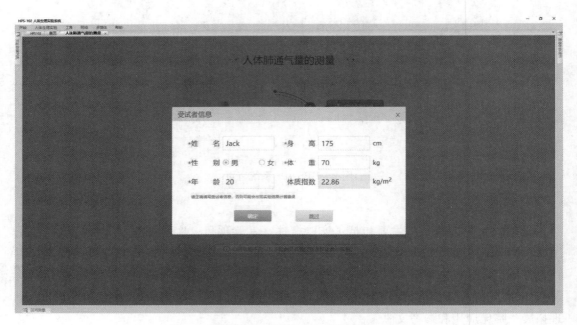

图 4　实验模块中受试者基本信息界面示意图

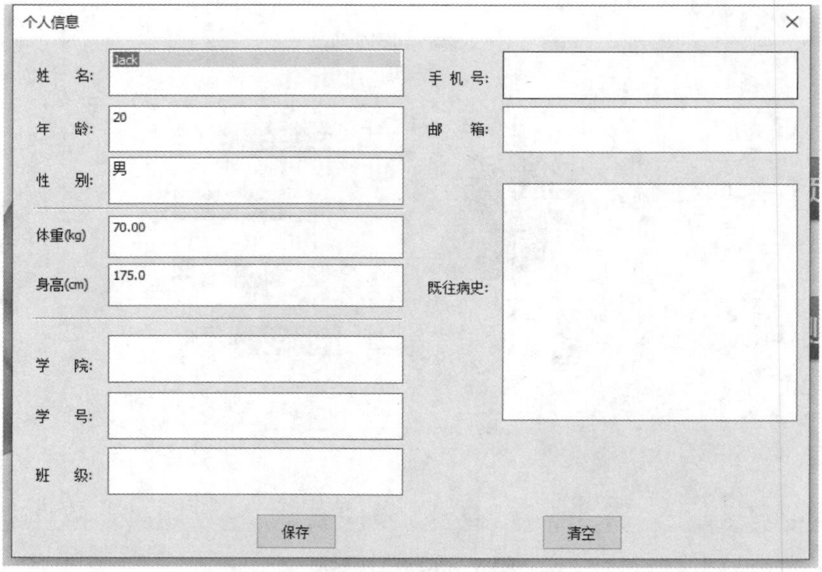

图 5　受试者个人基本信息窗口示意图

5. 实验步骤界面

在"实验项目"界面中单击"开始实验"按钮，将进入实验操作指南界面，参加图 6。实验操作指南界面由实验列表导航区、实验操作步骤展示区和实验控制区三个部分组成。其中实验列表导航区可以切换本次实验的全部实验观察项目；实验操作步骤展示区通过图文或视频指导实验的全部操作过程；实验控制区中的"开始 / 暂停"、"停止"按钮是对实验采样的控制，"上一步"、"下一步"是对操作指南步骤的导航控制，"编辑报告"是指进入到实验报告的编辑界面。

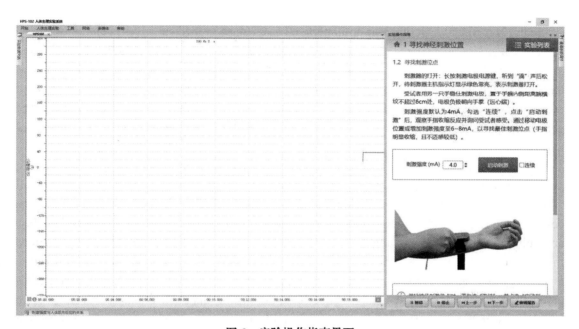

图 6　实验操作指南界面

Chapter I   Introduction to Medical Functional Experiment

Medical functional experiment is an important basic course in medical colleges and universities. It mainly includes physiology, pathophysiology and pharmacology, and also includes cellular and molecular biology generally. In order to adapt to the development trend of medical education and teaching in the information era, with the establishment and development of modern new type of medical mode, the experimental teaching content, experimental methods and technology in the above disciplines are selected, combined and integrated to form an independent medical functional experiment.

Medical functional experiment is designed primarily for medical students or students in medical related majors, including clinical medicine, pharmacy, nursing, stomatology, traditional Chinese medicine, preventive medicine, biomedicine and other disciplines and specialties. The course objectives include acquisition of knowledge and skill, development of ability and quality, and cultivation of emotional values. Firstly, through the basic training of functional experiments, the students can use the general experimental instruments correctly, master the basic operation technology, and grasp the scientific methods of acquiring knowledge of functional experiments gradually. Secondly, it can help students understand the writing and publication process and acquire skills of research papers from the training of experiment design and reports writing, establish the scientific thinking and problem awareness, improve the capacity to find, analyse and solve problems. Meanwhile it can enhance students' competence of cooperation, communication and scientific spirit. Finally, it can cultivate students' reverence for life, care for animals, pursuit for medical ethics and the will to serve the country and the people. Overall, it is an important basic course of medical colleges, which lays a solid foundation for the study of subsequent courses at the level of theoretical and experimental skills. It is also helpful to cultivate new comprehensive medical talents with international vision, innovative spirit and job competence.

This guideline consists of 4 chapters and 37 experiments including animal experiment, human experiment, design experiment, integrative experiment and innovative experiment. The determination of experimental contents is mainly based on the following aspects: not only help students better understand and grasp the basic principles and skills of medical functional experiment (like brain and spinal pithing, endotracheal intubation, common carotid artery intubation, superficial carotid vein intubation, femoral artery intubation, left ventricular intubation, ureteral intubation, gavage, and external intestinal perfusion, etc.), but also train and improve the students' scientific research ability, meanwhile, guide students to establish correct world outlook, scientific view and values. For example, follow the realistic and innovative scientific spirit in the experimental design, pay attention to animal protection and animal welfare during animal surgery, conduct humanistic care in human physiology experiments.

This guideline keeps the classic and core experiments carried out for many years by the departments of physiology, pathophysiology and pharmacology in the school of Basic Medicine of Jinan University. The experiments have been arranged according to the order of physiological, pathophysiological and pharmacological experiments. But there are a greater flexibility when we use the book. The specific experiment content and teaching progress in each semester are different, it can be arranged by various combination according to the specific requirements of the training program and teaching syllabus of each major. For example, for the nursing major students, we can focus on human experiments; and for the clinical medicine students, in addition to the retained animal experiments and human experiments, comprehensive and innovative experiments should be added. In Jinan University, according to the different places where the students come, the difficulty of experimental design and the proportion of comprehensive and innovative experiments should also be adjusted. The comprehensive experiment is planned mainly based on the concept of organ system integration where two or more experimental skills should be used to study the activities of two or more organ systems in one experiment. For example, in studying the influence of hypoxia on cardiovascular system activities, endotracheal intubation and carotid artery intubation are used. And in the experiment of influence of blood pressure change on urine formation, tracheal, carotid and ureteral intubations are needed. Innovative experiments are mainly conducted by the outstanding students who have grasped the basic experimental skills, they design the experiment under the guidance of their tutors which is often a part of their scientific research project. It is likely an integration experiment on the basis of morphology, function and molecular biology. And the innovation is the primary consideration, only when the feasibility has been passed in thesis proposal, can it be actualized. The difficulty of innovative experiments is quite bigger, so the proportion should be reasonable.

In line with the teaching concept of "student-centered, output-oriented", starting from the actual needs of students, combining with the characteristics of Jinan University "overseas Chinese university + prestigous high-level univesity" and the existing experimental conditions, we edited this concise bilingual experimental guidance, the distinguishing features are list as follow: concise, easy to carry, easy to grasp, and useful for the readers when they continue the subsequent study and further scientific research.

Section 1　The Development and Basic Types of Medical Functional Experiment

1. The development of medical functional experiment

How do human beings understand the objective world and how do they acquire knowledge? The history of science is a powerful demonstration of the importance of human practice. From the fourth century BC. to the third century BC., Aristotle, the founder of ancient Greek biology, applied anatomical techniques to demonstrate the internal differences of various animals, which is the first western literature on animal experiments. In ancient Rome, Dr. Galen made a study of the physiological function of the human body by preliminary living anatomy of a variety of animals, which had a great impact on the development of medicine. He thought experiment plays a significant role in the progress of science. In the seventeenth century, William Harvey, a British physician, used an autopsy method to conduct many experiments on several animals. In this way, he clarified the pathways of blood circulation and pointed out that the heart is the center of the circulatory system. In 1628, he published his work 《On the Motion of the Heart and Blood》 (De Motu Cordis). It is the first book on physiology based on experiments and marked the appearance of modern physiology. The discovery of the blood circulation has made physiology develop into a subject, and establish the scientific research method of physiology, which has created a new era for experimental physiology. In the nineteenth century, people began to realize that only clinical observations and autopsies could help them get comprehensive and profound understanding of the diseases. Therefore, they began to produce human diseases in animal models to investigate the causes and conditions of diseases, and the dynamic changes of function and metabolism during the diseases course. They further revealed the internal relationship between various clinical manifestations and changes in the body, clarified the mechanism and development of diseases, and rationally understood the essence of diseases. In 1865, Claude Bernard, a French physiologist, is the first advocator to use living animals as the main objects to study various diseases. He created "experimental medicine", which is now called animal experimental research, referring to using animals instead of human beings to do experiments. At that time, the experimental methods such as animal experiments were extremely powerful and opened the golden age of medicine.

With the development of natural science, medical science has made remarkable achievements in the past few centuries, and gradually formed many branches, in which experimental science is one of the important branches. Moreover, with the progress of various branches of medicine, a lot of experimental techniques for the study have emerged. At present, medical experimental techniques are generally divided into four categories: morphology, functional science, molecular biology and cell biology. However, in the field of medical education and scientific research, the vast majority of basic experimental research in medicine usually depends on the cooperation of a number of experimental techniques because in the complicated natural environment, by only one experimental technique, the knowledge of facts and objective laws is onesided and has great contingency. In the era of rapid development of science and technology, the comprehensive application of medical laboratory technology is particularly important; and functional experimental technology has been widely used in the study of medical branches. At the same time, the experimental techniques of other branches also have been widely applied to the experimental study of functional subjects. In recent years, the integration of function and morphology, the connection among different organ systems and the development of virtual imitation training system from basic medicine to clinical medicine become the trend of medical functional experiment reform. Professor Gong Yongsheng from Wenzhou Medical University put forward that experiment leads the medical integration and innovation, whereas function experiment guides the integration of basic medical experiment. He also hopes to promote medical functional experiment from course to subject, deepen the fusion between the information technology and education teaching, and build scientific innovation platform and medical science popularization platform based on the teaching platform, etc. In the tide of national education and teaching reform, we will surely usher in the unparalleled beautiful future of medical functional experiment.

2. Basic level and types of medical functional experiment

(1) Basic levels of medical functional experiment

1) **Molecular and cellular level:** Cell is the basic unit of the living body, and each organ is an aggregation of many different cells held together by intercellular supporting structures, and cellular level research is to understand the function of the organ. The physiological characteristics of cells depend on the physical and chemical features of the large molecular substances consisting of the cells. Therefore, molecular level research is to study the functions of cells, for instance, contraction of muscle cells and excretion of endocrine cells.

2) **Organ and system level:** The goals of study at organ and system levels are to explore the basic functions, activities and the influencing factors of organs and systems. For example, what is the function of respiratory system? What is the exchange mechanism between O_2 and CO_2? What factors can influence respiratory activities?

3) **Integral level:** The goals of study at integral level are to study interactions among organs and systems, and interactions between human body and environment. Human being has complex emotional activities and psychological activities that can affect many somatic activities and visceral activities, and lead to the corresponding behavioral manifestations. Human being lives in various families and societies，and the information from the external environment can affect the emotions, feelings and wills, etc. thus further causing positive or negative effects on the body.

Therefore, medical functional experiments are mainly carried out at the molecular, cellular, organ and integral level. For the specific experiments, there are several basic types as below.

(2) Types of medical functional experiment

1) **Human experiments and animal experiments:** The theoretical knowledge of medical functional experiments comes from the experimental research on dogs, cats, rabbits, rats, mice, frogs and other animals. With the development of experimental medicine, more and more experiments can be carried out on the human body. According to different objects, medical functional experiments can be divided into human experiments and animal experiments. The human experiments include blood pressure and heart rate measurement, electrocardiogram and ECG records which are related to clinical observation, while animal experiments often use a variety of animal models, such as disease animal model or transgenic animal models.

2) **In vivo experiments and in vitro experiments:** The main methods of medical functional experiments are in vivo studies and in vitro studies. In in vivo studies, experiments are conducted on intact animals, there are acute and chronic experiments, the former are performed on animals under anesthesia or on brain-damaged animals, and the latter are performed on conscious animals for long periods of time. In in vitro studies, experiments are performed on cells, isolated

tissues, or organs. Sophisticated experiments can be performed to gain a deeper insight into the mechanism of life activities at the cellular and molecular levels. In vitro studies, compared to studies of whole organisms, show their simplicity, species specificity, and convenience. Another advantage of the in vitro study is that human cells can be studied without "extrapolation" from the cellular responses in experimental animals. Last but not least, in vitro studies can be miniaturized and automated, yielding highthroughput screening methods for testing molecules in pharmacology or toxicology.

The primary disadvantage of in vitro studies is that it may be challenging to extrapolate from the results of in vitro works back to the biology of the intact organism. Investigators doing in vitro experiments must be careful enough to avoid overinterpretation of the results, which can lead to erroneous conclusions about organisms and systems biology.

3) Acute experiments and chronic experiments: Acute experiments can be subdivided into in vitro experiments and in vivo experiments with the following advantages: Experiment condition is easy to be controlled and the results are easy to be analyzed. Many experiments require to be observed and detected for a long time dynamically, they belong to chronic experiments with the following advantages: It is possible to observe continuously the activities under conscious conditions and the findings are similar to physiological state. But the shortcoming is that the conditions in the body are so complicated that it is hard to analyze the results.

Section 2 The Basic Code and Safety Rules of the Functional Laboratory

Given the importance of functional experiments, everyone should cherish the opportunity to conduct experiment in the laboratory to ensure the smooth progress and the objective, authenticity and reliability of the results. We formulate the following basic laboratory codes, which need to be strictly followed and implemented.

1. Requirements of experimental class
(1) Pre-class requirements
1) Preview the teaching schedule and know which experiment will be done.
2) Read the experimental guide carefully, and know why and how to do this experiment.
3) Preview related theoretical information and try to predict the results and raise questions.
(2) In-class requirements
1) Enter the laboratory on time. Students who leave the laboratory ahead of time or cannot show their leave permits in class will be identified as absent.
2) Wear a white coat to enter the laboratory, and wearing opentoe shoes is not allowed.
3) Remember to set the phone to mute during class; do not make noise in class.
4) Listen to the teacher at the beginning of the course, with particular attention to the do's and don'ts that determine whether the experiment can be completed successfully.
5) Look carefully as the instructor demonstrates.
6) Remove unrelated articles out of the workbench in order to keep the experimental area clean

and tidy, and prevent errors and accidents.

7) Use the equipment and software correctly under the guidance of the teacher. If the equipment goes wrong, tell the teacher to check it out.

8) Do experiment step by step following the procedure. Observe the experimental phenomenon patiently, and take notes timely and accurately, keep a full record of all the data. Correlate the collected data with the pertinent material in your textbook.

(3) After-class requirements

1) Tide up the laboratory bench, clean the experimental apparatus and return them as required. Each team member should cooperate and perform his own duties.

2) Separate the specimen from facial tissue and plastic gloves. Specimens should be placed in yellow plastic bags and then stored at the designated places, and the non-medical waste should be put in regular trash can.

3) The monitor arranges a group of students to clean the entire laboratory, including cleaning the floors and emptying the trash.

4) Collect and organize the original recordings, write experimental reports according to the required format and requirements, and submit the reports on time.

2. Laboratory code and safety guideline

1) When going inside the laboratory, a white coat must be worn. Never wear sandals, shorts and short skirts. The students should tie back hair that is chin-length or longer.

2) When going inside the laboratory, make sure you know fire control pass-way, fire auxiliary and position of sharping container.

3) Do not eat and play in the laboratory. During the experiment, no activities unrelated to the experiment may be performed. Also keep quiet in the laboratory. If you leave for some reason during the experiment, you should ask your teacher for leave.

4) When using experimental equipment and reagents according to the experimental operating procedures, pay attention to personal protection, use scissors, blades, needles and other sharp tools carefully, and avoid breaking glass instruments.

5) Discarded sharp tools and broken glass must be placed in the sharping container. Strong acids and alkalis are highly corrosive, so be careful not to splash them on clothes, skin and laboratory benches.

6) Assuming that all laboratory chemicals are potentially hazardous sources, use as instructions; do not touch any chemicals or pipettes by mouth, and goggles must be used for experiments involving chemical solutions. If you spill any chemicals on yourself accidentally, tell your teacher immediately.

7) In the laboratory, each group shall use their own instruments and equipments. To avoid confusion, shall not be exchanged with other groups. If the instrument is damaged or malfunctioning, you should report to your teacher or technician for repair or replacement.

8) Do not touch computer switches, keyboards, mice, equipment switches, desks, chairs, door handles and window handles with gloves that have been in contact with reagents and

animals.

9) Anaesthetics are available as needed and must not be taken out of the laboratory without permission.

10) Master correct catch method of experimental animals to avoid being bitten. If bitten, you need to rinse with plenty of water, disinfect with iodophor, tell your teacher, and go to the hospital immediately.

11) Cherish experimental animals, follow "3R" principles of animal experiments strictly, treat them humanely, reduce unnecessary waste, reduce pain and suffering, and experimental animals need to be euthanized before disposal.

12) In human experiments, if you have heart or respiratory diseases, do not volunteer to be subjects. If the subject feels discomfort during experiment, you should stop experiment immediately and inform your teacher. If the subject is taking special medicines or is pregnant, inform your teacher.

13) After the experiment, clean and return the used instruments and equipment, dry metal instruments with a dry towel; at the same time, clean the experimental bench and return the experimental chair. Students on duty are responsible for cleaning the cages and trays of experimental animals, sweeping the floor, taking out the garbage.

Section 3　Preparation of Common Reagents for Medical Functional Experiment

The solutions most commonly used in medical functional laboratory mainly include: normal saline, Ringer's solution and Tyrode's solution, which are suitable and useful for human, amphibious animals and mammal animals respectively.

1. Normal saline

Normal saline (NS) is 0.9% sodium chloride sterile aqueous solution. Its osmotic pressure is similar to the human blood and tissue fluid. NS can prevent the rupture of cells, it won't cause cells dehydration or let the cells absorb too much water. In order to correct the dehydration and acidosis, some mixed solution with different saline in proportion is applied clinically. NS is also used for sterile purposes. Intravenous drip (IV) is frequently used in patients who are not able to take oral liquid drugs.

So how do we prepare the saline solution? First, we need to prepare the sodium chloride crystal (NaCl) and the distilled water (H_2O) and the weighing devices. The preparation of the normal saline solution of 0.9% requires that 9 g of sodium chloride be dissolved into the 1000 mL distilled water, and the concentration of sodium chloride in the solution is 0.154 mol/L. Sodium chloride is ionized to produce sodium and chloride ions, both of their molar concentration is 0.154 mol/L. The permeability coefficient of the solution is 286.44. The plasma osmotic pressure is 280~310 mOsm/L (average 300), < 280 mOsm/L for low osmosis, > 310 mOsm/L for high osmosis, so the osmotic pressure of NS is close to the plasma osmotic pressure.

2. Ringer's solution

Based on saline, Ringer's solution contains the sodium chloride, potassium chloride, calcium chloride and sodium bicarbonate, known as the compound sodium chloride injection, which is invented by the British physiologist Ringer. Ringer's solution is similar to the normal saline, and sometimes it is better, when regulating electrolyte and acid-base balance of body fluid. Ringer's solution added with sodium lactate can often be used in clinical treatment for dehydration cases of acidosis or acidosis tendency. Because the sodium ion, potassium ion, calcium ion and chloride ion can maintain the physiological activity of amphibian's body tissues and organs in the experiment, for example, the frog's heart can be kept beating for long in vitro, etc, it is relatively close to the amphibian animal environment fluid.

To prepare Ringer's solution, you need to follow the following table (Table 1-1) and procedures:

Table 1-1   Formula of Ringer's solution

Substance	Concentration (g/L)
KCl	0.14
NaCl	6.50
$CaCl_2$	0.12
$NaHCO_3$	0.20
NaH_2PO_4	0.01

1) Dissolve sodium chloride, potassium chloride, sodium bicarbonate, and sodium dihydrogen phosphate in 800 mL of distilled water.

2) Diluted with distilled water to 980 mL.

3) Dissolve calcium chloride in 20 mL of distilled water.

4) Add calcium chloride solution to the above solution, dropping while stirring, lest it produces insoluble calcium phosphate precipitation.

5) Adjust the pH to 6.50 with 1 mol/L hydrochloric acid or 1 mol/L sodium hydroxide.

3. Tyrode's solution

Compared with Ringer's solution, Tyrode's solution is used in the in vitro experiment on mammals, which contains magnesium, some glucoses as the energy source and uses bicarbonate and phosphate as a buffer instead of lactate. It's necessary to keep feeding oxygen in the solution to maintain the normal physiological function of the intestinal muscles of the body. Besides, Tyrode's solution is often used to feed and clean the tissue of mammals. Tyrode's solution needs to be prepared according to Table 1-2.

Table 1-2 Formula of Tyrode's solution

Substance	Concentration (g/L)
KCl	0.20
NaCl	8.00
$CaCl_2$	0.20
$MgCl_2$	0.1
$NaHCO_3$	1.00
NaH_2PO_4	0.05
Glucose	1.00

Section 4 Formats and Requirements of Medical Functional Experiment Reports

Writing experimental reports is the last but maybe the most important step of the whole experiment. It describes all the works done by the experimenter and also reflects the authors' understanding and thinking on the experiment by presenting the results, discussion and conclusions properly. It is one of the important dimensions for teachers to assess the students' comprehensive abilities. An experimental report is different from a scientific paper, but the basic elements are the same. So, it is also a key process to make it easier for the students to write and publish scientific papers successfully in the future.

1. General requirements

1) Use the required report paper format (see below and Appendix 1~3 for details).

2) Complete each blank and mark your name and student number clearly.

3) Follow the standard format to write all parts of experimental report.

4) Provide accurate charts, tables, diagrams or pictures if possible.

5) Use legible handwriting or type.

6) Write your report by yourself (if you copy each other's, both or all of you will get zero).

7) Hand in the report on time.

2. Basic format of experiment reports

Some medical functional experiments stress operational skills or surgical methods, such as the nerve-muscle preparation, others emphasize the detection of changes in phenomenon, such as gastrointestinal motility, while still others lay particular emphasis on the results and analyses, such as the influence of factors on urine formation. Most experiments include all three dimensions.

In a typical functional experimental report, the following contents should be included: aim, principle, experimental material, procedure and observation, result, discussion, conclusion, and reference.

(1) Aim

State the purpose of experiment (*One or two*) briefly, i.e.what principles you are trying to test and which techniques you want to learn in the experiment, etc.

(2) Principle

Briefly introduce the related theoretical knowledge.

(3) Experimental material

List experimental materials briefly, including subjects (animals or human being), equiments, reagents, etc.

(4) Procedure and observation

Describe the procedure in detail, and you will follow to complete the experiments step by step.

(5) Result

If possible, present the results in the form of charts, tables, diagrams or pictures.

1) The chart, diagram or picture should include at least title and illustration which are normally placed below the chart, diagram or picture . Stimulus marks are also needed in the chart, diagram or picture (Figure 1-1).

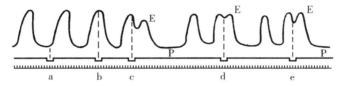

E: extrasystole   P: compensatory pause.

Figure 1-1   Extrasystole and compensatory pause of frog heart

2) The tables should have a title on the top of the table and notes are below the table (Table 1-3 and Table 1-4).

Table 1-3   Observations of flexor reflex on a spinal frog

Observation	Flexor reflex (+/−)
Normal right leg	
Take off the skin of right foot	
Normal left leg	
Cut off the left sciatic nerve	
Stimulate the left peripheral end	
Stimulate the left central end	
Destroy the spinal cord	

+ stands for positive flexor reflex, − means negative flexor reflex.

Table 1-4　Heart beat of a frog's heart under different conditions (times/minute)

Observation	Sinus venosus	Atrium	Ventricle
Control			
Tie off 1			
Tie off 2			

Tie off 1: block the conduction from sinus venosus to atrium. Tie off 2: block the conduction from atrium to ventricle.

3) When designing a table, you can put items of observation on the left side (from top to bottom) (Table 1-3) and set the results on the right side (Table 1-4).

4) For quantified data, you should determine the correct units and amounts of results, such as weight, speed, length, height, heart rate, blood pressure, respiratory rate, etc.

(6) Discussion

1) Discussion requires us to analyze the results step by step according to the known theoretical knowledge detailedly.

2) It serves to interpret the results. Anything irrelevant to the results shouldn't be covered.

3) Consider the following aspects when analyze and evaluate the data: ① Compare the data with the anticipated result that can be found in reference books. ② Analyze the reasons and mechanisms for the various phenomena using medical knowledge. ③ Explain why your results are different from the results found in the textbook and how to avoid the errors induced by uncontrolled variables or unexpected factors?

4) Give suggestions for further experimentation.

(7) Conclusion

1) Conclusion should be drawn from the results and discussion synoptically. It is commonly expressed by one or two sentences.

2) It is quite different from results themselves, and never just list the results in a simple way instead of conclusion.

(8) Reference

A minimum of one references are suggested to be included. They should be kept in an uniform format or style.

Section 5　Clinical Case Discussion in Medical Functional Experiment

Functional experiment derived from three disciplines (physiology, pathophysiology and pharmacology) is a bridge from basic medicine to clinical medicine. Physiology focuses on how the body under the regulation of the nervous system and endocrine system to maintain the environmental homeostasis, once the physiological function of the organ system can not cooperate with each other, the body will produce disease.The main task of pathophysiology is to study the causes and conditions of disease, the function of disease process, metabolism, and the mechanism of disease occurrence, development and transformation on the basis of physiology and pathophysiology. The functional experiment not only requires students to verify the theoretical knowledge, but also to develop the clinical thinking and job competence of the disease (including replicated animal disease models and clinical practical cases).Therefore, appropriate case discussion can not only combine teaching content with actual cases to achieve "early clinical and multiple clinical" , but also sensitized and contextualized the abstract theoretical knowledge to stimulate students' interest in learning, and cultivate students' medical humanistic care ability in case analysis.

1. Basic steps for case discussion in medical functional experiment

(1) Select typical cases carefully

Generally, after teaching the theoretical knowledge related to a chapter, students have a case analysis after a preliminary understanding of the cause of disease, pathogenesis, body function and metabolic changes, clinical manifestations and prevention and control principles. The main source of cases are the previous cases from the affiliated hospital or other hospital of the school, the literature and the cases reported in magazines and so on. But no matter what form the case comes from, it must include a true description of the general condition, medical history, physical examination and of other auxiliary examinations. Through case discussion, students can deepen their systematic understanding of the disease, and achieve a comprehensive and systematic grasp of the content of this chapter, so that the theoretical knowledge is learned and used alive.

(2) Arrange case discussion content

The classic cases can be sent to students through class WeChat group or network teaching platforms one week in advance. Students will consult textbooks and relevant information and make group disscussion. Analyze the direct and indirect causes based on the information provided by the cases.

(3) Conduct case discussion

In class, the group will select representatives to summarize the discussion results of the group and put forward the unsolved or newly discovered problems that cannot be solved. When the opinions are inconsistent, the whole class can also have a debate, and the instructor will give appropriate guidance in the discussion process.

Key points of the classroom case discussion:

① Diagnostic results and diagnostic criteria of the disease

② The evolution process and the occurrence principle of the course of the disease

③ The possible mechanism of the main symptoms, development and diagnosis

④ Optimal scheme and mechanism of clinical drug treatment

(4) Make a summary

The teacher will give a brief summary of the simple problems that are unified and give an explain in detail of the complex problems that students have divergence of views in order to deepen students' understanding.

2. The main principles followed in case discussion

(1) Orientation

During the discussion, teachers need to guide the discussion around the theme and explain in time to help students get their points.

(2) Enlightening

During the discussion, teachers should put forward some enlightening questions to enable students to focus on the key points and give the correct conclusions in the end.

(3) Mutuality

During the discussion, teachers and students should discuss about the cases mutually rather than teachers only explain the cases.

3. Example of case discussion

(1) Simple case discussion

Medical history and chief complaint: A 25-year-old female was admitted into the hospital with complaints of pain, dizziness and weakness after the left quarter rib was hit by a car half an hour ago.

Physical examination: The face of the patient was pale and the limbs felt cold. body temperature (T) 35 ℃, heart rate (HR) 115 times/min, blood pressure (BP) 70/45 mmHg. There was slight tenderness and muscle tension in the whole abdomen, especially in the left upper abdomen. The shifting dullness was also found and the bowel sound was weakened.

Auxiliary examination: There was non-coagulated blood in the abdominal puncture.

Question:

1. What was the patient's initial diagnosis?

2. How did the process of the disease develop?

3. How to rescue the patient according to the treatment principles?

(2) Complex case discussion

Medical history and chief complaint: A 38-year-old male was admitted into the hospital with complaints of palpitation, chest distress, shortness of breath, hyposarca and sleep in flat position with difficulty. Half a year ago the patient had palpitation and shortness of breath after exertion. Since the past last month, he was frequently suffering from palpitation, dyspnea, breath holding, chest tight feeling, and swelling of ascending lower extremities was observed, which developed to general dropsy in a week. No myocardial infarction and heartstroke was noted.

Physical examination: The patient was in orthopnea with tachypnea, could not sleep on flat position. Distention of jugular vein was obvious. BP 130/86 mmHg and HR 110 beat/min. The border of cardiac dullness was enlarged to both left and right sides. A systolic blow murmur was heard at the region of cardiac apex. Scattered moist rales were heard over the entire extent of both lungs. The abdominal bulge with shifting dullness was positive. The liver edge was palpable 6 cm below the costal margin in the mid-clavicular line and was sensitive to percussion. Pitting edema was observed in all the body below the breasts.

Results of electrocardiogram: Sinus tachycardia, HR 110~130 beat/min. Bigeminal premature ventricular beat were occasionally observed.

Results of ultrasonic imaging: Pleural effusion and ascites were detected. The heart chambers were enlarged obviously. Valvular incompetence of mitral valve and tricuspid valve was observed. Left ventricular end-diastolic internal diameter was 77 mm (normal value 49 ± 4 mm) and left ventricular end-systolic internal diameter was 67 mm (normal value 30 ± 5 mm), left ventricular ejection fraction was 28% (normal value 50%~70%).

Diagnosis: chronic heart failure, bigeminal premature ventricular beat.

Treatment: Intravenous drip of deslanoside injection 0.4 mg + furosemide 20 mg was given immediately and the therapeutic strategy for heart failure and fluid retention was taken orally as follows:

1) Control the fluid retention:	Hydrochlorothiazide	50 mg qd
	Furosemide	20 mg qd
	Spironolactone	40 mg tid
2) Increase the myocardial contractility:	Digoxin	0.125 mg qd
3) Anti-ventricular remodeling:	Enalapril	2.5 mg bid

Questions:

1) How did the process of the disease develop? Why cardiac enlargement occurred?

2) Why could systolic blow murmur at the region of cardiac apex be heard? How did it happen?

3) What types of water and electrolytes disorders would happen and what steps should be taken during the treatment?

4) What therapeutic measures made the dilated heart growing downwards? What aspects should be paid special attention to during the treatment?

Chapter II   Animal Experiments in Medical Functional Experiment

Section 1   The Classification and Selection of Laboratory Animals

1. Classification of laboratory animals

The laboratory animals are artificially cultivated with clear genetic background, controlled microorganisms and parasites, which are used for scientific research, teaching, testing and verification. Based on the genetic background, they can be classified into inbred strain, closed colony (outbred stock) and hybrid etc. According to a number of different microbiological qualities, laboratory animals can be classified into conventional animal, clean animal, specific pathogen free (SPF) animal, and germ free (GF) animal.

(1) Classification by genotype

1) Inbred strain: In an animal population, when the alleles above 99% in the genome of any individual are homozygous, it is defined as an inbred strain. The classic inbred strain is produced after a minimum of 20 successive generation of brother-sister mating. All individuals in the stain can be traced back to a pair of common ancestors at the 20th or subsequent generation. The inbred stains are high homozygosity of gene loci, homology of genetic composition, uniqueness, discernibility of genetic characteristics, phenotypic homogeneity and long-term genetic stability. But because of "inbreeding depression, the stains are decreased vigour and a negative effect upon growth, survival and/or fertility)". Common inbred stains in the experiment include BALB/c mice, C57BL/6J mice, F344 rats, Lewis rats, etc.

2) Closed colony (outbred stock): A closed colony is a group of laboratory animals in which mating occurs in a non-inbreeding manner for at least 4 consecutive generations without introducing new individuals. This stocks animals has high heterozygosity of genetic composition, stability of genetic characteristics, reproductive rate, and disease resistance, and there are many valuable mutant genes. They are widely used in drug screening, toxicology experiment and teaching some common stocks include KM mice, ICR mice, NIH mice, Wistar rats and New zealand rabbits.

3) Hybrid: The offspring animals are produced by the cross of two different inbred stains, also called F1 animals. Although the animals is not homozygous for their genes, the individuals are the same genotype, with high genetic and phenotypic homogeneity, while overcoming the phenomenon of inbreeding decline, with hybrid vigor, adaptability and disease resistance Therefore, they are widely used in the biological evaluation of nutrition, drugs, pathogens and hormones, etc.

(2) Classified by microbiological qualities

1) Conventional animal: Do not carry the pathogens which could lead to zoonotic diseases and severe animal infectious diseases. Such animals are generally housed in an open environment. Common conventional animals include guinea pigs, hamsters, cats, rabbits, dogs and primates. In 2003, the conventional mice and rats were be canceled.

2) Clean (CL) animals: Clean animals are laboratory animals that exclude pathogens that should be excluded from conventional animals and do not carry pathogens that are harmful to animals and interfere with scientific research. They are usually kept in a barrier environment. The clean animals are products of Chinese special national conditions. With the improvement of the economic, there are few clean animals on the market. And they have been canceled in the local standards of some provinces and cities.

3) Specific pathogen free (SPF) animals: Specific pathogen free (SPF) animals, are laboratory animals that do not carry major potential infections or conditionally pathogenic pathogens and major interference to scientific experiments, except for the pathogens that should be excluded from clean animals, referred to as SPF animals.These animals are raised in barriers or isolation systems and are widely used in scientific research, mainly including rats, mice, and guinea pigs.

4) Germ-free animals: Germ-free animals are laboratory animals with no detectable living organisms. If the GF animals were implanted with one or several known microorganisms, they will be call gnotobiotics animals. Both germ-free animals and gnotobiotics animals must be kept in an isolated environment, and the items they contact with must be strictly sterilized. They are widely used in research on the relationship between microecology and diseases, nutrition and metabolism, and anti-tumor research.

2. Selection of laboratory animals

Medical functional experiment is an objective observation and analysis of life phenomena under the specific conditions of manual control, so as to obtain the knowledge of physiology, pathophysiology and pharmacology. The research of medical function is inseparable from laboratory animals. The selection of laboratory animals is an important part of animal experimental research. Each experimental research has different purposes and requirements, and the selected animals are also different. The main factors considered as follow.

(1) Select standardized laboratory animals

The quality of laboratory animals includes genetic and microbiological quality. The animal users should have the ability to select the strains/stocks suitable for the purpose of the animal experiments. Microbiological quality control aims to produce animals that meet with their requirements of the animal protocols. Most viral, bacterial and parasitic infection do not lead to overt clinical symptoms, but have a considerable impaction the results of animal experiments. Only selecting standardized laboratory animals which are bred under the control of genetics, microbiology, nutrition, and environmental hygiene, the effects of bacteria, viruses, parasites and potential diseases on experimental results can be excluded. It can rule out the inconsistencies of individual responses to experiments due to individual genetic and microbiological differences, in order to facilitate the communication of experimental results internationally.

(2) Select laboratory animals according to the purpose and requirements of the experiment

Difference species of animal have their own special anatomical and physiological characteristics. To have the basic knowledge about these characteristics could help to choose the right animal models. It could also help to handle animals during the animal procedure, reduce the difficulty of experiment preparation and operation, and make the experiment easy of succeed. For example, the rats (without gallbladder) can be used to intubate the bile duct, to collect bile, and for their search on digestive function. The rabbits are ideal animal models for repeated intravenous injections, because of their moderate size, docile temperament, large ears and clear blood vessels. Therefore, they are widely used in the study of physiological experiments of various systems, such as acute experiments in the blood pressure or respiration study. The isolated frog heart can maintain activity for a long time, which is often used to study the physiological function of the heart. The sympathetic nerves, vagus nerves and depressor nerves in the neck of rabbit are independently. Therefore, it can be used to observe the influence of depressor nerves on cardiovascular activities. If dogs or chickens are selected incorrectly, it is difficult to find the depressor nerve from the gross anatomy, so that the experiment cannot be carried out.

(3) Select laboratory animals that are easy to obtain and raise

Although the choice of animals used in physiological search is quite wide, it is necessary to consider the availability of the animal models, as far as the economic issue and management. In general, mice, rats, rabbits and toads have a large number of sources, and are easy to manage. So they are the most commonly used laboratory animals in medical physiology research.

(4) Select the appropriate individual of the animal

When choosing laboratory animals, the age, sex, and weight of the animals should also be taken into consideration. Adult animals are generally used for experiments. For example, it is better to choose the younger ones among adult animals for the endocrine gland experiments. During the juvenile period, most of the endocrine of the body is still developing, and has not reached the standard state or mature stage. If a juvenile animal is selected in the study, the results obtained are unscientific. In addition, animals of different sexes have different sensitivity to drugs. For example, when rats are anesthetized with sodium pentobarbital, the sensitivity of females is 2.5 to 3.8 times that of males. In the acute toxicity test of table salt, female mice are more sensitive, while male mice are more sensitive to chronic toxicity. Therefore, if there is no special need, the number of male and female individuals should be roughly equal and the individual size should be moderate in the experimental research.

3. Laboratory animals commonly used in functional experiments

(1) Amphibians

1) Frog

① **Genetic background:** Frogs belong to the amphibians of the phylum chordata, vertebrata, amphibia, lissamphibia, anura, ranidae, pelophylax, and amphibians of the black-spotted frog.

② **Biological characteristics:** Frogs have an inconspicuous neck and no ribs. The ulna and radius of the forelimb are united, and the tibia and fibula of the hindlimb are united, so the claws cannot rotate flexibly, but the limbs are muscular. The reproductive characteristics of frogs are dioecious, fertilized in water, hatching into tadpoles, breathing with gills, after mutation, adults mainly breathe with lungs, and also use the skin, which belongs to oviparous. The heart can still beat rhythmically for a long time in vitro.

2) Toad

① **Genetic background:** Toads belong to the class of amphibia, lissamphibia, anura, bufonidae, and bufo. Toad frog species of amphibians, its body surface has many bumps; there are poison glands. In China, it is divided into two species: bufo gargarigans and black orbit toad. The adult toad is a commonly used animal in medical experiments.

② **Biological characteristics:** Toads have a wide, short and sturdy body, and its skin is extremely rough, the back of the body is covered with scrofula of various sizes, which can secrete bufonin. The ventral surface is not smooth and creamy yellow, with brown or black fine spotted, the skin color of the back changes with the season, and is different between the females and males. During the breeding season, female toads are lighter and males are black green.

(2) Rodents

1) Mouse

① **Genetic background:** Mice belong to the mouse species of rodentia, mammalia, vertebrata, containing 20 pairs of chromosomes. At present, mouse is a laboratory animal with the largest dosage, the widest use, the most varieties (lines) and the most sufficient research in the world.

② **Biological characteristics:** The tail length of mice is about the same as the body length, and no more than 15.5 cm. The tail is covered with short hair and circular horny scales. The esophagus lacks mucus secreting glands and has a thick layer of keratinized squamous epithelium on the inner wall, which is conducive to gavage operation. The mouse has a gastric which is the small volume (1.0~1.5 mL) and poor function, and intolerance to hunger. Compared with guinea pig and experimental rabbit herbivores, its intestine is short, the cecum is underdeveloped, and the gallbladder and pancreas are scattered in the duodenum, gastric fundus and splenic hilum, light red and irregular, like adipose tissue; the lymphatic system is very developed, without palate or pharyngeal tonsils. External stimulation can proliferate the lymphatic system and be prone to lymphatic diseases; the mouse has no sweat glands and four obvious blood vessels in the tail, one vein on the back and abdomen and one artery on both sides. The body temperature of the mouse is about 38 (37~39) ℃, the heart rate is 600 (328~780) beats / min, the respiratory rate is 163 (84~230) time / min, the systolic blood pressure is 113 (95~125) mmHg, the diastolic blood pressure is 81 (67~90) mmHg, and the blood volume accounts for 8.4% of body weight.

2) Rat

① **Genetic background:** Rats belong to the rat species of rodentia, mammalia, vertebrata, with 21 pairs of chromosomes. The experimental rats are the offspring of wild brown rats, which originated in Asia and spread to Europe in the 14th to 18th century. In the middle of the 18th century, wild rats and albino mutant rats were used for the experiment for the first time.

② **Biological characteristics:** The appearance is similar to that of mice. The adult weight is more than 10 times that of mice. The sweat glands of rats are extremely underdeveloped. The tail is a heat dissipation organ, covered with short hair and circular horny scales. Rats can't vomit, so they can't be used for emetic experiment. The intestine is short, the cecum is large and the function is underdeveloped. It is intolerant of hunger. The pancreas is scattered and located at the curvature of duodenum and stomach. There is no gallbladder, and bile directly enters the duodenum through the common bile duct; The sphincter of common bile duct is relaxed and does not have the function of concentrating bile and storing bile. Basic physiological parameters of rats: the body temperature of rats is 39 (38.5~39.5) ℃, the heart rate is 475 (370~580) beats / min, the respiratory rate is 85.5 (66~114) times / min, the systolic blood pressure during anesthesia is 116 (88~138) mmHg, the diastolic blood pressure is 91 (58~145) mmHg, the blood volume account for 7.4% of body weight.

3) Guinea pig

① **Genetic background:** Guinea pigs belong to the guinea pig species of the vertebrata, mammalia, the rodent guinea pig family, with a total of 32 pairs of chromosomes. In 1780, Laviser used guinea pigs for the first pyrogen test. As guinea pigs are easy to be raised in the laboratory and used for experimental operations and are suitable for medical and biological research, guinea pigs gradually occupied a prominent position in the animals for scientific research, in the 19th and early 20th centuries.

② **Biological characteristics:** Guinea pigs have developed cochlear ducts, sensitive hearing, and a much larger hearing range. They are often used in hearing experiments. Their digestive system has typical herbivorous animal characteristics: developed mouth muscles, thin stomach wall with fold-like mucosa, and big stomach with the 20~30 mL capacity; the intestinal tube is longer, about 10 times the body length, the cecum is well developed, accounting for about 1/3 of the abdominal cavity volume, and when it is full, it accounts for about 15% of body weight. Guinea pig is large appetite, and strong ability to digest crude fiber. The digestibility reaches 38.2%. It cannot synthesize vitamin C by itself, because of L-glucose lactone oxidase lacked. It is sensitive to antibiotic treatment, especially penicillin, as well as bacitracin, erythromycin, chlortetracycline, etc., which can cause enteritis in some cases, and death in severe cases. It is extremely sensitive to histamine and other substances, and is often used in asthma models and anti-allergic experiments.

(3) Mammals

1) Rabbit

① **Genetic background:** Rabbits belong to the chordata, vertebrata, belong to the class mammalia, lagomorpha, leptoridae, and the oryctolagus cuniculus rallit. The rabbits used in biomedical research are domesticated from wild rabbits, and most of them are the offspring of European rabbits, with chromosomes 2n=44.

② **Biological characteristics:** Rabbits have large auricle and clear blood vessels, which are convenient for vascular injection and blood collection. Rabbits have large eyeballs, suitable for ophthalmological research. Rabbits have a single stomach with a very large fundus, and the total length of the small and large intestines is 10 times of the body length. The cecum is well developed, accounting for 1/3 of the abdominal cavity. In the ileocecal area, there is a unique round small sac, the wall of which is rich in lymphoid follicles, and its mucosa constantly secretes alkaline fluid, which can neutralize various organic acids produced by the decomposition of cellulose by microorganisms in the cecum, which is conducive to digestion and absorption. The depressor nerves in the cervical neurovascular bundle are easy to be separated, and their endings are distributed in the vessels of the aortic arch, which belong to afferent nerves.

2) Dog

① **Genetic background:** Dogs belong to the chordata, vertebrata, belongs to the mammalia, carnivora, canidae, canis, dog breeds, with 39 pairs of chromosome. Beagles are commonly used in animal experiments.

② **Biological characteristics:** Dogs are red-green color blind, so red-green conditioned stimuli cannot be used for conditioned reflex experiments. Dogs have a well-developed blood circulation and nervous system, their internal organs and proportions are similar to humans. The intestines are short, about 5 times of the body length. Its liver is large, and the pancreas is divided into left and right lobes, the islets are small and numerous. Skin sweat glands are extremely underdeveloped, with a few sweat glands on the toe pads. Male dogs have no seminal vesicles and bulbourethral glands, and have a penile bone. Female dogs have 4~5 pairs of nipples.

Section 2 Basic Operating Techniques of Medical Functional Animal Experiment

Mastering the correct basic animal operation could effectively prevent the experimenter from being bitten or scratched by the animal, as well as stabbed by sharp tools. Meanwhile, it can also reduce the stress and maintain the normal physiological state of the laboratory animals, which ensure the welfare of laboratory animals and guarantee the animal experiments go smoothly.

1. Basic operating techniques of amphibians experiment

(1) Handling and restraint

Frog is relatively easy to handle and generally do not hurt people. Hold the frog with the left hand, and then give drug administration with the right hand. When handling and restraint the frog, the operator use the index finger and middle finger of the left hand to clamps the left forelimb of the frog while use left thumb to hold the right forelimb of the frog, then use right hand to straightens the lower limbs of the frog and lastly use the ring finger and the little finger of left hand to clamp them. When performing complex techniques such as marrow destruction or surgery on frogs and toads, the operator could choose to fix them back upward, with thumb pressed on their back, index finger pressed on the front of the head to bend it forward, middle finger against their chest to protrude the connection between the head and the spine bulge (Figure 2-1A). When conducting anatomical or other physiological experiments, the operator could also choose an anatomical table or fixed plate to fix the animal body position according to the needs of the experiment, and use thumbtacks or needles to fix the limbs on the frog fixed plate . Because the venom glands protruding from the two ears of toad can spray highly toxic venom, when handling and restraint the toads, do not squeeze this location to avoid the venom from spurting into the eyes.

(2) Marrow destruction

Fix the frog according to the method in Figure 2-1A and find the foramen magnum. The operator uses the right hand with needle and pierces the probe vertically through the foramen magnum, and then pierces forward into the cranial cavity, and swings the probe left and right to destroy the brain tissue. The tip of the probe is then turned back and inserted into the spinal canal parallel to the spine, while rotates to destroy the marrow (Figure 2-1B~D).

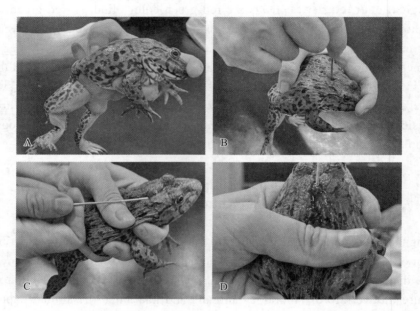

Figure 2-1   Handling, restraint and marrow destruction for frog and toad

(3) Drug administration (lymphatic sac injection)

Due to the poor elasticity of frog skin, the skin is not easy to heal after puncturing. Therefore the needle should pass through a diaphragm and then enter the subcutaneous lymphatic sac during injection. During the administration of the abdominal lymphatic sac, the needle was inserted from the upper thigh and then passed through the thigh muscle layer into the abdominal wall muscle layer, and lastly entered the abdominal subcutaneous lymphatic sac. The injection volume is 0.25~1 mL per animal.

2. Basic operating techniques of rodents experiment

(1) Handling and restraint

1) **Mouse handling and restraint:** two-handed method, single-handed method and mechanical restraint.

Two-handed method (Figure 2-2A~C): Grab the tail base of the mouse with one hand and lift it up. Place it on the cage lid or rough table, gently pull the mouse tail back. As the mouse crawls forward, grasp the skin surrounds the ear base and neck with the thumb and index finger of the other hand. Turn up the hand palm with the mouse and straighten its hind legs, so that the mouse body is in a straight line. Press the mouse tail with the ring finger and press the hind leg with the little finger to restraint the mouse. Pay attention to the right amount of skin to be pinched, if pinched too tight the mouse will suffocate, whereas too loose the mouse could turn back and bite the handler.

Single-handed method (Figure 2-2D~F): Use the thumb and index finger of one hand (usually the left hand) to pinch the tip of the mouse tail. Use the ring finger and little finger to press the tail base of the mouse on the palm of the hand. After that release the thumb and index finger and use the thumb and index finger to grasp the skin surrounds the ear base and neck in order to fix it and turn it over. The method is suitable for personnel who are proficient, or where one hand already holds instruments, articles or to avoids pollution.

Mechanical restraint (Figure 2-2G~I): When needed such as tail vein injection or blood collection, the mouse could be loaded into a mouse mechanical restrainer. Grab the mouse tail and make it move approach the restrainer, and then fix its position after the mouse drill into the restrainer, so that the tail is left outside for operation.

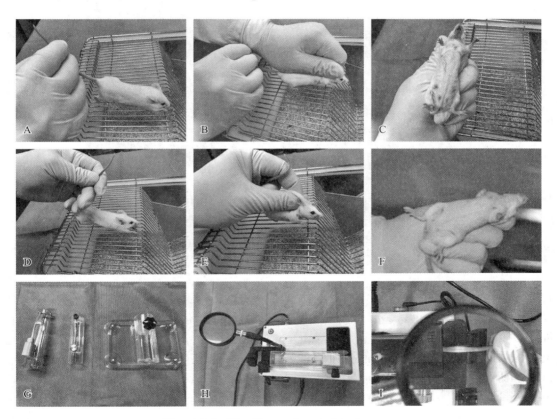

Figure 2-2　Handling and restraint of mouse
(refer to color picture on color pages)

2) Rat handling and restraint: The methods of handling and restraint of rat are basically the same as those of mice. When the rat be quiet and still, pinch the root of the rat tail and lift it up. Don't allow to grab the tip of the tail or hang in the air for too long. For those high-weight rats, the operator should hold the front part of the rat's body with the other hand. As the rat crawls forward, grasp the skin around both ears and neck with the other thumb and index finger, and the next three fingers grasped the skin of the back of the rat, and turn it over into a supine position, so that the body of the rat is in a straight line. Lastly, use the right hand to fix the hindlimb and the tail (Figure 2-3A~C). When drug is administrated, use thumb and index finger of the left hand to grasp the skin of its neck and back, and use the other three fingers to grab its back and fix the hindlimb. The other way is that the thumb and index finger are fastened to the neck of the rat, so that its head cannot be rotated at will, its forelimbs are fixed in T-rex grip or forelimb cross method, and the other three fingers fix its body trunk on the hand palm, which can be used for general operation (Figure 2-3D). When carrying out some special operations, the rat mechanical restraints can also be used. Rats are prone to bite when they are frightened or irritated. During handling and restraint of rat, it should be noted that beginners should wear canvas bite-proof gloves.

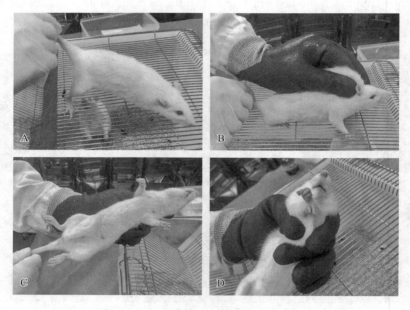

Figure 2-3   Handling and restraint of rat

3) Guinea pig handling and restraint: Guinea pigs have gentle temperament and generally do not bite people. When handling and restraining the young guinea pigs, they could be directed held up with both hands. For grasping of mature guinea pigs, firstly the operator quickly buckles their back with one palm to grasp the top of its shoulder blades, and then grasps their neck with the thumb and indexes finger, and lastly gently buckles the chest with middle and ring fingers. The other way is to grasp the skin among both ears and neck like rats, and hold the hip with the other hand. Those with lower body weight can be caught with one hand, while those with higher body weight should be caught with both hands.

(2) Drug administration

1) Gavage: It is suitable for acute toxicity experiment and the dosage is accurate.

In gavage administration of mice (Figure 2-4A): After attach the specialized smooth-tipped gavage needle to the syringe and inhale the administrated liquid, the operator grab and restraint the mouse with one hand with the mouse in position of high head and low tail (high head position), and then gently straighten the gavage needle and slowly insert it into the esophagus along the wall of the oral cavity and the posterior wall of the pharynx. The gavage needle should be inserted without resistance. If you feel resistance or the animal struggles, you should stop the administration or pull out the needle immediately to avoid damaging or breaking the esophagus or even entering the trachea by mistake. After the injection, gently withdraw the gavage needle. The movement should be gentle to avoid damaging the esophagus and diaphragm. Generally, when the gavage needle is inserted into the mouse for 3~4 cm, the drug can be administrated when there is succus gastricus visible after withdrawal the needle. The gavage dose shall not exceed 1% of body weight, and the commonly used gavage dose for mice is 0.2~1 mL. The method of gavage in rats (Figure 2~4B) is basically the same as that in mice. The depth of gavage needle is about 4~6 cm. In order to prevent insertion into the trachea, the needle bolt of the syringe can be withdrawn first. If there is no air extraction, it indicates that the needle is not in the trachea, and then the medicine could be injected. The dosage of each gavage of rat injection is about 1~4 mL. The gavage method of guinea pigs is basically the same as that of rats and mice, and the dosage of each gavage is about 1~5 mL.

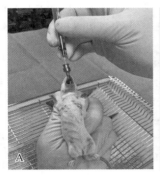 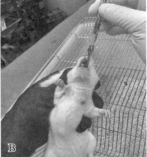

Figure 2-4   Gavage in mouse and rat

2) Injection

① **Subcutaneous injection:** During subcutaneous injection, the drug is pushed into the subcutaneous connective tissue and absorbed into the blood circulation through capillaries and lymphatic vessels. Mice are usually injected subcutaneously on the back. The specific method is that after local disinfection, the operator pinches the skin with the thumb and middle finger of the left hand, and presses the apex with the index finger to form a triangular fossa, then uses the right hand to hold the syringe perpendicular to the subcutaneous fossa, after that

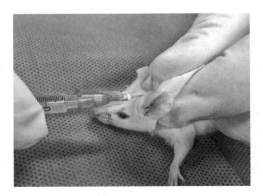

Figure 2-5   Subcutaneous injection of mouse

quickly pierces into the skin and releases the left hand after piercing (Figure 2-5). If there is no blood return to the tube when withdraw the syringe, the liquid could be injected. The subcutaneous injection site of rats can be either subcutaneously on the back or lateral hindlimb. During rat subcutaneous operation, the operator gently lifts the skin of the injection site and inserts the injection needle into the subcutaneous, and then pushes in the liquid medicine. The subcutaneous injection site of guinea pigs can be selected with less subcutaneous fat, such as the inner side of limbs, back and shoulder. Usually the operator injects the needle into the subcutaneous skin at a 45° between the needle and the skin on the inner thigh to make sure that the needle is under the skin, then injects the liquid medicine. After pulling out the needle, use thumb gently press the injection site. When correctly inserted under the skin, the needle can swing freely. If the injection dose is large, it can be injected at different sites. After the needle is pulled out, gently pinch the skin with your left hand at the acupuncture site for a moment to prevent the liquid medicine from flowing out.

② **Intradermal injection:** Intradermal injection is to inject the liquid medicine into the skin between the epidermis and dermis. It is mostly used for vaccination or allergy test. The hair of injection site is removal before injection. The operator pinches the skin into a fold with the left hand, and then holds the syringe with the right hand to make the needle pierce into the skin at an angle of 30° with the skin. A small papular bulge shows at the injection site indicates the correct injection. If the pushing resistance of intradermal injection is small, it indicates that the needle is injected subcutaneously, and the needle should be reinjected. Do not press hard after injection to avoid the outflow of liquid medicine.

③ **Intraperitoneal injection:** Owing to the strong absorption capacity and large injection dose, intraperitoneal injection is commonly used in animal experiments. When the mice were injected intraperitoneally (Figure 2-6), the operator grasps the animal with left hand and turns over the animal with the position of abdomen upward, head in low position and tail in high position, then disinfects the skin against the hair growth direction. Holding the syringe in the right hand to pierce the skin in the site of lower abdominal quadrant just off of midline, and push the needle forward to 0.5 cm and then pass through the abdominal muscle at an oblique angle of 45°. At this time, there is a sense of loss of resistance. After that, the operator fixes the needle and draws back with no liquid, and then injects the liquid slowly. The amount that can be injected at one time is 0.1~0.2 mL/10 g · BW. Do not

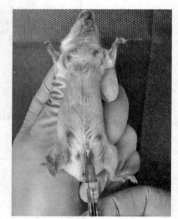

Figure 2-6　Intraperitoneal injection of mouse

inject the needle upward during intraperitoneal injection, so as not to stab the internal organs. The intraperitoneal injection of rats and guinea pigs can refer to the intraperitoneal injection of mice.

④ **Intramuscular injection:** For intramuscular injection in mice (Figure 2-7), after the animal is restraint, the operator uses one hand straightens one hindlimb of the mice, and uses the other hand to hold syringe pierces into the muscle lateral the thigh of the hindlimb to inject liquid. The single injection amount of mice shall not exceed 0.1 mL per mice. Intramuscular injection of rats and guinea pig is basically the same as that of mice. The single injection dose of rats and guinea pigs shall not exceed 0.5 mL per animal.

⑤ **Intravenous injection:** Intravenous injection of tail vein is often used in mice and rats. Generally, two lateral left and right vein are selected, and the injection is started from the thin skin of the distal end of the tail (1/3 from the tail tip), which is easy to puncture. First fix the mouse in the retainer and leave the tail outside. Before injection, flick the tail with the right index finger, or immerse the tail in warm water at 40~50 ℃, or wipe with alcohol to dilate the blood vessels and soften the cuticle of the epidermis. Then clamp the root of the tail with your fingers to block the blood flow of the tail vein and fill it. After that, one hand hold up the tail from the bottom, and the other hand hold

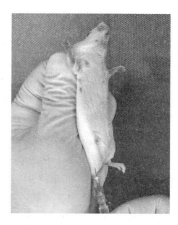

Figure 2-7   Intramuscular injection of mouse

the syringe parallel to the tail at a certain angle (15° ~30°) insert into the vein (Figure 2-8A). If there is blood return and there is no resistance to the injection of liquid medicine, a white line can be seen along the vein indicating that it is in the blood vessel. At this time, the injection should be stopped immediately and the injection should be carried out at the replacement position close to the tail root. The single injection volume was 0.05~0.1 mL /10 g · BW. For black mice whose tail blood vessels are not easy to be seen in the deep skin color, the tail vein injection instrument with light can be used to help confirm the blood vessels and improve the success rate (Figure 2-8B). Insulin syringe can be used for injection in mice with younger age or small body size. The operation method of intravenous injection in rats is basically the same as that in mice. However there are thick scales on the surface of rats tail skin, so it is difficult to puncture. The needle can be inserted at the thin skin between 1/4 and 1/3 from the tail tip.

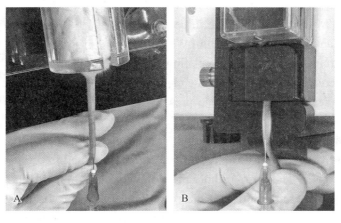

Figure 2-8   Intravenous injection
(refer to color picture on color pages)

(3) Blood collection

The blood collection methods of rats and mice are basically universal, and the appropriate blood collection method can be selected according to the blood collection volume, blood collection frequency, blood type and detection purpose.

1) Tail cutting and blood collection: This method is suitable for taking a small amount of blood samples, such as blood cell count. Before collecting blood, the mouse or rat tail vessel should be congested. After soaked in 50℃ warm water, dried and disinfected, the operator cut off the tail tip for 1~2 mm to collect blood. Massage from the tail root to the tail tip, and the blood will flow out of the tail tip. Cotton ball compression hemostasis and 6% liquid collodion applied to the wound to stop bleeding. The maximum amount of blood collected each time is 0.1 mL.

2) Tail-cut blood collection: A sharp blade is used to cut the vessel of the tail, and the blood flows out of the incision, which can be cut alternately and start from the tip of the tail. After the completion of blood collection, cotton ball compression can be used to stop bleeding.

3) Blood collection of posterior orbital venous plexus: This method is suitable for repeated blood collection in a short period of time. Mice can collect blood volume of 0.2~0.3 mL at a time and rats with volume of 0.5~1.0 mL. First of all, prepare the glass capillary and break it into 1~1.5 cm long before use, and immerse it in the anticoagulant as needed, and then take it out for drying. After the mouse was anesthetized, the operator uses left thumb and index finger grasps the skin on the back and neck to fix mouse head, then gently compresses both sides of the neck so as to hinder the venous reflux and makes the eyeball fully protruding and the orbital venous plexus congested. The operator holes the capillary tip in the right hand between the inner corner of the eye, and gently moves it to the bottom of the eye, and then rotates the capillary to cut the venous plexus and maintain the horizontal position of the capillary. The mice pierce into it for 2~3 mm, and the rats for 4~5 mm. When the resistance, stop piercing and the blood feel flows out (Figure 2-9). After collect blood, pull out the capillary tube immediately, release the left hand and press with a cotton ball to stop bleeding. This method can be used to collect blood from mice, rats and guinea pigs.

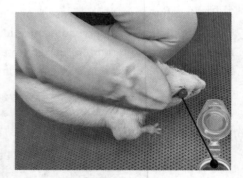

Figure 2-9　Mouse blood collection of posterior orbital venous plexus

4) Cardiac blood collection: The animals were anesthetized and fixed on supine position, and then disinfected routinely. The operator hold the syringe with right hand, and inserted the needle vertically at the place where the left 3~4 intercostal apical impulse was most obvious to extract blood (Figure 2-10A). The needle can also be inserted into the ventricle through the diaphragm from the upper abdomen to collect blood, and all the action procedure should be gentle (Figure 2-10B). Both mouse and rat can collect blood in this way.

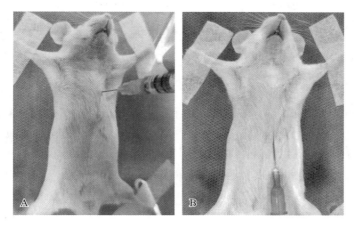

Figure 2-10   Cardiac blood collection of mouse

5) Eyeball extraction and blood collection: After the mouse was anesthetized, the operator uses left hand to grasp the back and neck skin of mouse, in order to make the eyeball protrude, then places the mouse in the lateral position (Figure 2-11). Then use right hand hold ophthalmic curved forceps to remove the eyeball quickly and the blood flows out of the orbit. Generally, the blood volume equivalent to 4%~5% of animal body weight can be obtained. The animal dies immediately after use, and it is only suitable for one-time blood collection.

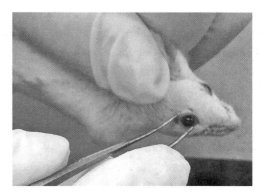

Figure 2-11   Eyeball extraction and blood collection of mouse

3. Basic operating techniques of mammals experiment

(1) Handling and restraint

1) Hand restraint method: The operator lifts it together with the fur on the back of the rabbit's neck as well as the ear, and then holds its hip with the other hand so that the weight of the rabbit mainly falls on this hand (Figure 2-12A). Rabbits generally do not bite people, however their claws are sharp. When they are caught and struggling, it is very easy to cause scratches to operators, so they should avoid the movement of their limbs. In addition, only grasp the rabbit's ears, hind legs, waist, and back fur were not allowed, so as to avoid damage to the rabbit's ears, kidney and cervical spine or subcutaneous hemorrhage.

2) Fixator restraint method: The restraint of anesthetized rabbits generally adopts box or desktop restraint fixator (Figure 2-12B). It is suitable for surgical experiments such as blood collection, injection, blood pressure measurement and so on.

(2) Drug administration

1) Gavage: It is suitable fot acute toxicity experiment and the dosage is accurate.

When giving gavage administration to rabbits, dogs and other animals, mouth openers should

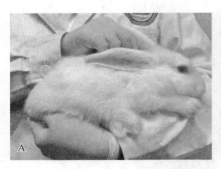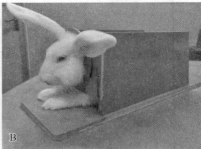

Figure 2-12　Handling and restraint of rabbit

be used to avoid animal molars and canine teeth, so as not to bite the gastric tube. The rabbit was fixed with a rabbit restraint fixator, the operator placed the opener horizontally in the rabbit mouth, and pressed the rabbit tongue under the opener, then inserted the gastric tube through the central hole of the opener, and slowly inserted the catheter along the upper palatal wall of the rabbit mouth into esophagus for about 15~18 cm. After intubation, put the outer end of the gastric catheter tube into the water. If bubble is observed from the catheter tube, it means that the catheter is not in the esophagus but in the trachea. The catheter should be pulled out and re-inserted. If there is no bubble observed, the drug can be pushed in. The amount of liquid injected each time can reach 80~120 mL. After gavage administration, the gastric catheter tube can be rinsed with a small amount of water, and then pulled out. When pulling out the gastric tube, the operator should hold the open end of the catheter and draw it out slowly. When approaching the throat, speed up the movement and pass quickly to prevent residual liquid from entering the throat and trachea.

2) Oral method: Suitable for chronic experiments and solid forms drugs.

Oral method is to mix drugs into feed or drinking water so that animals can take them freely. The advantage of this method is its simplicity and convenience, however the disadvantage is that the dose cannot be accurately quantified, and there are great differences among individual animals. When administered to large animals, if the drug is in solid dosage form, the drug can be directly put into the mouth of laboratory animals with tweezers or fingers and try to allow them swallow it orally.

3) Injection

① **Intravenous injection of rabbit marginal auricular vein:** The blood vessels in the rabbit ear are clearly distributed, with an artery in the center of the ear and a vein at the outer edge. Owing to the inner marginal vein is deep and difficult to fix, it is less used, while the outer marginal vein is shallow and easy to fix, so it is more commonly used. The marginal auricular vein walks along the back edge of the ear. After remove the hair on the surface skin and disinfected the part with alcohol, the blood vessel appears. Before injection, gently flick, rub the tip of the ear, or gently press the root of the ear to make the ear marginal vein congested. Insert the needle from the distal end as far as possible. The operator clamp the proximal end of the vein with the left index finger and middle finger while pad the ring finger and little finger under the ear, and then use syringe pierce the skin first and enter the vein, with the needle go deep 0.5~1 cm along the parallel direction of the blood vessel. After that loosen the index finger and index finger, move the left thumb and index finger to the puncture position of the needle and press it, fix the needle with the rabbit ear and push it into the liquid (Figure 2-13). If there is great resistance or local swelling during injection, it indicates that the needle has not pierced into the vein. The needle should be pulled out immediately and re-injected in the proximal segment of the original injection point.

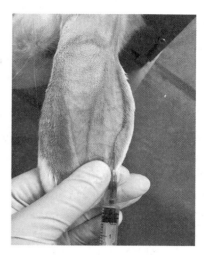

Figure 2-13　Intravenous injection of rabbit marginal auricular vein

After the injection, pull out the needle and press the iodine tincture cotton ball on the needle pinhole to stop bleeding. If multiple intravenous administrations are reguired during the experiment, the scalp needle can be substituted and an artery clamp used for fix the rabbit ear.

② **Intraperitoneal injection of rabbits:** When the rabbit is injected intraperitoneally, the experimental assistant needs to hold the rabbit in the supine position with its abdomen facing upward, and remove the hair at the injection site of the lower abdomen. The injection position is located at 1 cm on both sides of the white line of the lower abdomen and punctured at an angle of 45° . When the needle passes through the abdominal muscle and feels lost, it shows that the needle has entered the abdominal cavity. Fix the needle and if there is no liquid after withdraw the syringe, it can be injected.

③ **Rabbit subcutaneous injection:** The subcutaneous injection method of rabbits resembles that in the subcutaneous injection method of mice and rats. Subcutaneous injection was performed at the site of loose tissue, mostly in the neck and shoulder (Figure 2-14).

④ **Rabbit intramuscular injection:** The injection is usually carried out in the muscles of the hind legs. After the rabbit is restrained, the hair is sterilized with alcohol. After alcohol disinfection, the operator uses left hand fingers to tighten the skin of the injection site, right hand to hold the syringe at an angle of 60° with the skin and quickly stab into the muscle (Figure 2-15). If there is no blood return, the injection can be carried out. The amount of injection volume at one time should not exceed 2 mL.

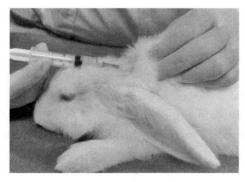

Figure 2-14　Rabbit subcutaneous injection

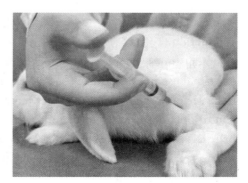

Figure 2-15　Rabbit intramuscular injection

⑤ **Rabbit intradermal injection:** First, remove the hair from the intradermal injection area, and then depilate with depilatory agent. Intradermal injection could be carried out after an interval of 1 day. The injection method is the same as that of mice and rats. The amount of injection volume at one time is about 0.1 mL.

(3) Blood collection

1) Rabbit marginal auricular vein blood collection: The operation method is the same as that of intravenous injection of marginal auricular vein. Local hair removal can dilate blood vessels, and blood can be drawn after successful puncture with syringe (Figure 2-13). You can also use only the needle without connecting the syringe to let the blood drop directly into the container with anticoagulant. You can also cut the marginal auricular vein with a blade to let the blood flow out naturally and drip into a container with anticoagulant. After blood collection, compress with gauze or cotton ball to stop bleeding. The blood collection volume is 5~10 mL each time.

2) Rabbit central auricular artery blood collection: There is a thick, bright red central artery in the middle of the rabbit ear. The method of blood collection is similar to that of rabbit marginal auricular vein. As the central auricular artery of the rabbit is prone to spasm, the rabbit ear must be fully congested and move gently before blood drawing. Too thin needle used for blood collection or low indoor temperature are not suitable for blood collection.

3) Rabbit cardiac blood collection: The rabbits are fixed in supine position after anesthesia, and the hair is removed and disinfected at the needle entry area. At the 3 rd~4 th intercostal space on the left, or the most obvious touched place where the heart beat is touched by the left index finger, is the needle entry point. The blood sampling needle is vertically inserted into the chest cavity, and the needle entry depth is about 3 cm. When there is a sense of loss, the needle tip can be felt to beat rhythmically with the heart, which means that the needle has been inserted into the heart and blood has entered the syringe. When there is no blood flowing into the syringe, the needle can be drawn while withdrawing the needle (or entering the needle). Once the blood is drawn, the needle shall be fixed immediately. The needle can only move up and down vertically, and are not allowed to swing left to right in the chest to avoid puncturing the heart.

Section 3　Welfare of Laboratory Animals and Ethics of Animal Experiment

1. Introduction

From ancient times, people have endeavored to understand the workings of nature and the universe. Animal use in science dates back to Eristratus and Herophilus in the third century BC. and Galen in the second century AD. All use of animals for human benefit creates a dilemma. There is a spectrum of opinion on whether there is justification for using animals for our own ends.Some people believe that animals have rights and it is wrong to use them, whether for food, in research, as servitude, as pets or to kill them as vermin. Another group believes it is acceptable for humans to use animals in any way we think fit. Most people fall somewhere in between these two extremes.

The debate about animal experiment has never gone away, whereas some aspects of the debate are essentially unchanged from those used a century ago. An important factual point is whether or not animal experiment has been essential in the development of important medical advances. Some groups claim that animal research has never resulted in any medical benefits, that it has misled scientists, or that it is unnecessary because we have alternative non-animal techniques. Most scientists agree that animal research has played a major role in medical advances in the past and will continue to do so.

There is no doubt that it was cruel, before the advent of modern anaesthetic and analgesic drugs. But today things are very different: advances in veterinary science have made painless surgery possible, and everyone involved in animal research is very much aware of the need to maintain animal welfare.

2. The welfare of laboratory animals

The Five Freedoms were originally developed for farm animals, but application of these principles has been extended to almost all captive species of animals, including those kept in laboratories. Because of the broad acceptance of the tenets of the Five Freedoms, they have come to be used as stand-alone, specific assessment criteria.

The revised Five Freedoms include:

① Freedom from thirst and hunger—by ready access to fresh water and a diet to maintain full health and vigor.

② Freedom from discomfort—by providing an appropriate environment including shelter and a comfortable resting area.

③ Freedom from pain, injury, and disease—by prevention or rapid diagnosis and treatment.

④ Freedom from fear and distress—by ensuring conditions and treatment that avoid mental suffering.

⑤ Freedom to express normal behavior—by providing sufficient space, proper facilities, and company of the animal's own kind.

Laboratory animal welfare is not a one-sided protection of animals, but considers the welfare of animals while using animals, and opposes the use of extreme means and methods. The Hasting Center report on Animal Research Ethics states "animal welfare is concerned with assuring humane treatment of animals: maintaining good health, minimizing negative states such as pain, enhancing positive states, and giving animals freedom to behave in ways that are natural to that species". Good animal welfare requires disease prevention and veterinary treatment, appropriate shelter, management, nutrition, humane handling and humane slaughter/killing.

3. Principles of 3R in animal experiment

"3R" proposed by Russell and Burch (1959) are: Replacement, the use of in vitro or computer methods; Reduction, using the minimum number of animals to obtain valid results; Refinement, minimizing pain/distress and/or increasing animal well-being.

In vitro methods can replace animals in some circumstances and also be important in characterizing potentially effective compounds prior to preclinical research on animals. When animals cannot be replaced, proper planning of experiments is required in order to produce reliable data with the fewest and most suitable animals. Examples of how animal numbers can be reduced include: experimental design with standardization and control of variation, high levels of control of dose administration; and appropriate combinations of safety testing. Refinement can improve welfare by acting on both direct and contingent suffering. The search for refinement must be continual to take advantage of technological advances.

In 1993, the "International Foundation for the Study of Ethicalization" in Chicago, USA added "Responsibility" as the 4th principle on the basis of "3R" . Strengthen ethical concepts in animal experiments, and call on experimenters to have a sense of responsibility towards humans and animals. Advocating animal welfare does not mean that you cannot use animals and conduct animal experiments, but how to use animals rationally and humanely to achieve a balance between scientific research needs and animal welfare.

4. The ethical review of animal experiment

Ethical review is an essential part of any systems regulating animal use in research and testing. It provides a framework for deciding whether animal use can be justified within each scientific project, taking into account animal welfare, scientific and ethical issues.

The review principles include: the principle of necessity, the principle of protection, the principle of welfare, the principle of ethics, the principle of the balance of interests, the principle of fairness, the principle of legality, the principle of taking account of national constraints. The content of the review includes the purpose, necessity, significance and experimental design of the experiment, the information on the animals to be used (including the reasons for selecting the type and number of experimental animals), the expected damage to the animals and the prevention and control measures (including anesthesia, analgesia, etc.) , merciful endpoints and euthanasia, etc.), animal replacement, reduction of animal dosage, reduction of animal pain and injury, the main measures and benefit analysis, etc.

The ethical review of animal experiments has attracted more and more attention from scientific and technological workers and scientific research management units during the application and implementation of scientific research projects. Each province and each user unit has established a strict review mechanism; and the ethical review of experimental animals for teaching has not been Pay attention to the fact that users of teaching experimental animals are all practitioners of future scientific research, and their ethical reviews should be paid more attention to. Jinan University's application for experimental animal ethics in teaching experiments is submitted to the university's experimental animal ethics committee at the beginning of each semester to apply for experimental ethics review, and continuously optimize experimental programs and operating methods.

Section 4   Introduction to BL-420 Biological Data Acquisition and Analysis Systems

1. Overview of BL-420 system

BL-420 biological data acquisition and analysis system (hereinafter as BL-420 system) is a 4 channels system configured on the computer for biological signal acquisition, amplification, displaying, recording and processing. It can be applied to physiological, pharmacological, toxicology and pathological experiments, and is one of the main equipment and means to study biological function activities. It is composed of the following three major parts: personal computer, BL-420 system hardware, BL-420F biological signal display and processing software (hereinafter as BL-420F software), as shown in Figure 2-16.

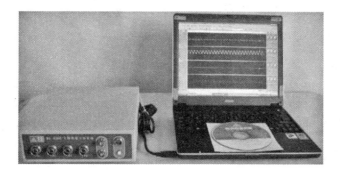

Figure 2-16 BL-420 biological data acquisition and analysis system

2. Principle of BL-420 system

In the detection of biological electrical signals or biological non-electrical signals introduced through sensors, because the signal is often very weak (such as depressor nerve discharge, the signal is a microvolt level signal), and many interfering signals including acoustic, light, electrical signals, etc. are mixed in the biological signals, such as 50/60 Hz signal from the electric network. The amplitude of these interfering signals is always greater than bioelectrical signals themselves. If these interfering signals are not filtered, it may cause that the useful biological signals themselves can not be observed because interfering signals are too strong. The working principle of the BL-420 system(Figure 2-17) is to first amplify and filter the original biological function signals and then digitize the processed signals through analog-to-digital conversion and transmit the digitized biological function signal to the computer through the special BL-420 software. After that, it will process the signals received in real time, i.e., display the biological function wave and save the biological function signal. In addition, it is possible to process and analysis the specified data according to users' command, such as the smooth filtering, differential and integral calculus and spectrum analysis, etc.

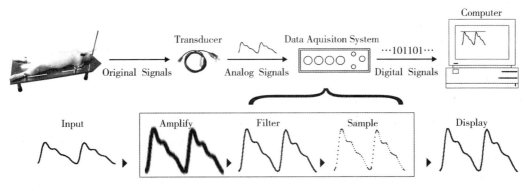

Figure 2-17   Schematic diagram of BL-420 system

3. Introduction to BL-420F software tool bar

At first we will make a brief introduction to the whole tool bar. See Figure 2-18.

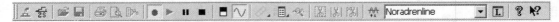

Figure 2-18   Tool bar of BL-420F software

Tool bar is used to directly display some commonly used commands in convenient and visualized mode (in form of graphs). Each graph button on the tool bar is called tool bar button. Each tool bar button corresponds to a command. When it is displayed in emboss form (in gray), it indicates that this tool bar button is currently not available. At this moment, it has no response to user's input.

There are total 23 tool bar buttons and a label edit and selection group box on main tool bar of BL-420F software, of which two tool bar buttons are pull-down type. The detailed description of the important toolbar button commands is as below.

(1) System reset

System reset command is used to reset all hardware and software parameters of BL-420 system. That is to say, these parameters will be reset to default ones.This command works when the system is in non-real-time experiment status and in replay state.

(2) Zero-rate sampling

Zero-rate sampling command is similar to pause command. The execution of this command in real-time status will stop the movement of the wave, and stop any data saving. However, the change in wave will be displayed at the screen where new data appear. The up-to-date measured point data values will also be displayed at the upper-right corner of the hardware parameter adjusting area. This command is mainly used to observe the change in extremely slow-speed signals. For example, this function can be used to observe signals in which change occurs after 1 h. This command only works when the system is in real-time sampling status.

(3) Open

This command opens a previously logged data file that has an extension name of bmp (.tme type). By default, the BL-420F software uses the "temp. tme" to name the files recording the original data waveform data.

(4) Save as

Select this command to pop the save as dialog, as shown in Figure 2-19. The save as command works only during the data display, allowing storing the data file with a different name, or save it in a different directory.

(5) Print

Print is used to print the wave displayed on the current screen. When you select this command, a "custom print" dialog box will pop up. See Figure 2-20.

When "print whole file" parameter is set, the whole replay data file will be printed. Generally you are better not set this parameter, because it will cause much waste of print paper if the file contains many invalid data. It is preferable to use the print whole file function after you have established a smaller data file through data edit function.

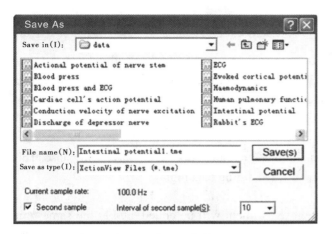

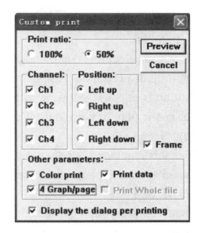

Figure 2-19   "Save as" dialog box

Figure 2-20   "Custom print" dialog box

(6) Print preview

When you select this command, a "custom print" dialog box (Figure 2-20) will pop up. When you press "preview" command button after the print parameters have been selected in this dialog box, you may enter the print preview status. Wave displayed by means of print preview is consistent with the printed one. See Figure 2-21.

Note: Print and print preview functions are associated with the channel display window. If you want to use print or print preview function during data replay or real-time experiment, you should set the channel display window to activated status, otherwise these two function buttons will be not available (in gray). If the two buttons are in gray when you perform printing operation, you only need to click left mouse button on any channel display window to activate these two buttons.

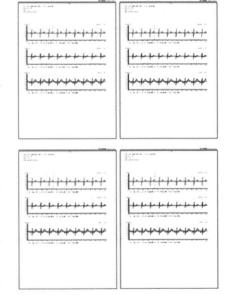

Figure 2-21   Print preview of wave (4 Copies/Group)

(7) Last experiment config

When an experiment is over, each item of parameter that has been set for this experiment will be saved in configuration file config.las. If you want to repeat the last experiment without repeating the setting operation, you can realize it just by selecting "open last experiment config" command. The computer will automatically set the experimental parameters to the same as those in last experiment.

(8) Record data

"Record data" command is a two-state command. It means that each time when this command is executed, the status that it represents will change once. When red solid circular label of the record command button is in pressed state, it indicates that the system is now in recording state, otherwise the system is only in observation state, in which the observed data will not be recorded.

(9) ▶ Start

When you select this command, data acquisition will be started, and the acquired experimental data will be displayed on computer screen. When you select this command in the event that data acquisition is in pause status, it will continue to start wave display. This command is used to start the automatic play of wave during data replay.

(10) ▮▮ Pause

After this command is selected, data acquisition and dynamic display of wave will pause. This command is used to pause the automatic play of wave during data replay.

(11) ▪ Stop

When you select this command, the current experiment will be ended, and at the same time "system reset" command will be sent, which makes the whole system return to the default status at the moment of start-up. But this command will not reset the screen parameters that you have set, such as channel background color, baseline display switch, etc. During the course of replay, this command is used to stop data replay.

(12) ▦ Switch background color

When you select this command, the background color of the displayed channel will be switched between black and white. No matter what background color of the channel you have set before, this command will unconditionally set the background to black or white.

(13) ∿ Grid line display

This is a two-state command, which is used to show or hide background grid line.

(14) Measurement

Measurement button is a pull-down tool button. That is, when you press and hold left mouse button on this button, a pull-down sub-tool bar will pop up(Figure 2-22). This sub-tool bar contains 4 commands associated with measurement, which are respectively section measurement, two-point measurement, frequency measurement and cardiac functional parameter measurement.

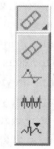

Figure 2-22 The sub-toolbar of measurement

1) Section measurement: is used to measure the parameters such as time difference, frequency, maximum value, minimum value, mean value, peak-to-peak value, area, maximum elevating speed, maximum lowering speed, etc. of the selected wave segment in any channel wave. The measurement results will be displayed in general information display area. If Excel worksheet is opened during the course of measurement, the measured data will also enter Excel worksheet.

Procedures for section measurement:

① Click section measurement command button, at this moment wave scanning will pause.

② Move your mouse cursor to the starting point of the wave segment in any channel that you want to perform section measurement. Then click left mouse button to determine the starting point. At this moment, a vertical line will appear, which represents the starting point that you have selected for section measurement.

③ When you move your mouse cursor, another vertical line will appear and move along with your mouse. This straight line is used to determine the end point of the wave segment for section measurement. When this straight line moves, time difference between two vertical lines will be displayed dynamically at the upper-right corner of the channel display window. After the end point is selected, click left mouse button to confirm the end point.

④ At this moment, a horizontal straight line will appear within the interval between two vertical lines(Figure 2-23), used to determine the baseline for frequency counting (if you are conducting section measurement for electrocardiosignal, the horizontal baseline that you have selected will not act as the frequency counting line, because template analysis method is adopted for heart rate analysis, which is in dependent of frequency counting line). This horizontal baseline will move along with your mouse cursor up and down. The value at the position that the horizontal straight line locates will be displayed at the upper-right corner of the channel. You can click left mouse button to confirm the position of this baseline to complete the section measurement.

⑤ Repeat the above procedures ② ~ ④ to perform section measurement for different wave segments in different channels.

⑥ Click right mouse button in any channel to end this section measurement.

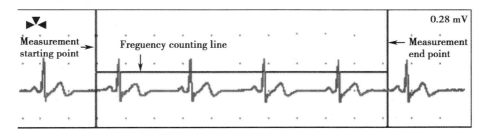

Figure 2-23   Schematic diagram of section measurement

2) ．Two-point measurement: is used to measure the maximum value, minimum value, mean value and peak-to-peak value of certain wave segment in any channel, time difference between two points, change ratio and change rate of the signal. All the information will be displayed in general information display area. The change rate and change ratio of the signal are two different concepts. The former refers to the variance relative to time, i.e. it is worked out by the result that is obtained by subtracting the value of the first point from that of the second point, and then divided by time difference between these two points. The unit is mV/ms; the latter refers to the variance relative to the value of the first point, i.e. it is worked out by the result that is obtained by subtracting the value of the first point from that of the second point, and then divided by the value of the first point. The unit is %.

Procedures for two-point measurement:

① Click two-point measurement command button, at this moment the wave scanning will pause (if the wave scanning has been started). .

② Click left mouse button at the starting point of the wave segment that you want to measure to determine the position of the first point. At this moment, a red straight line will appear, with one end fixed on the first point that you have just confirmed, and the other end moving along with your mouse cursor. This line is used to determine the second point for two-point measurement.

③ Click left mouse button when you have determined the position of the second point. This red straight line will be fixed. The two-point measurement is completed. See Figure 2-24.

④ Repeat the above procedures ② and ③ to perform two-point measurement for different wave segments in different channels.

⑤ Click right mouse button in any channel to end this two-point measurement.

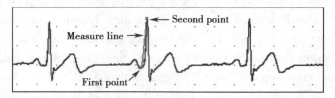

Figure 2-24   Schematic diagram of two-point measurement
(refer to color picture on color pages)

3) ᴧᴧ **Frequency measurement:** is used to manually measure the frequency of certain wave.

As wave curves recorded by BL-420F software are diverse, for example, gastrointestinal electricity is extremely slow, while the depressor nerve charge is extremely fast; cardiac electricity is regular, while the rule of brain electricity is ambiguous. Although the displayed graphs are different, it is not reflected by the computer, which always use a few limited frequency algorithms to calculate the wave frequency. Therefore, in the event of the great variation in wave or dominant wave mixed with secondary wave, the computer can not work out correct wave frequency. As the complementation for accurate measurement of frequency for these extremely special waves, the manual measurement method can be adopted. That is to say, this frequency measurement command and measurement results are displayed at the heart rate area of the general information display area of the software.

Procedures for frequency measurement:

① Click frequency measurement command button.

② Select the position of the first dominant wave, and click left mouse button.

③ Select the position of the second dominant wave, and click left mouse button.

④ Select the position of the third dominant wave, and click left mouse button to complete the measurement. See Figure 2-25.

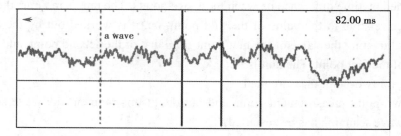

Figure 2-25   Schematic diagram of frequency measurement

⑤ Repeat the above procedures ② ~ ④ to conduct frequency measurement for different wave segments in different channels.

⑥ Click right mouse button in any channel to end this frequency measurement operation.

4) ⚡**Cardiac functional parameter measurement:** is used to manually measure various parameters on an electrocardiaogram (ECG), including 13 parameters such as heart rate, R wave amplitude, ST interval, etc. This is a switching command. The measurement is available only when this command is opened.

There are two kinds of measurement methods for cardiac functional parameters: One is overall measurement, and the other is local measurement. Overall measurement can measure all 13 parameters of the selected cardiac electricity in single operation, while local measurement can measure 1 parameter in single operation. If Excel worksheet has been opened using the "open Excel" command button on the tool bar during the course of measurement, the measured data will directly enter the Excel worksheet.

Overall measurement method uses area selection function to select a complete ECG. Attention shall be paid to that in overall measurement mode, time width of wave segment that you have selected is used to calculate heart rate, therefore you should try to select an ECG with a complete cycle, otherwise the measured heart rate will be inaccurate. When you click right mouse button after the selection, a cardiac functional parameter measurement shortcut menu will pop up. You may select "overall measurement" command in this menu to complete overall measurement. See Figure 2-26 and Figure 2-27.

In local measurement mode, a datum will be measured in single operation. Datum to be measured can be either a time difference value, or an amplitude difference value. Therefore you must use mark to complete the measurement. For example, for measurement of PR interval,   the starting point and end point should be determined, first, then determine a point with mark, and move cursor to determine another point. After confirmation, click right mouse button, a shortcut menu will pop up. Then select "PR interval" command to complete the measurement. See Figure 2-26 and Figure 2-27

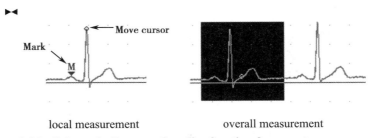

local measurement   overall measurement

Figure 2-26   Schematic diagram of cardiac functional parameter measurement

(15) 🖼️ Cut bitmap window

Cut bitmap window button is a pull-down tool button. See Figure 2-28.

When you click this pull-down tool button, a Sub-tool Bar relating to Window will pop up. This sub-tool bar contains 5 commands, which are cut bitmap window, X-Y input window, parameter set window, display window of section measurement result and Excel open window. cut bitmap window can be exited only when you have selected the cut bitmap exit command button 🔲 on the tool bar.

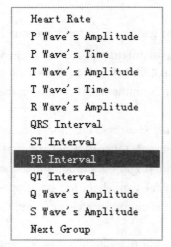

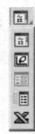

Figure 2-27   Shortcut menu of   Figure 2-28   The sub-toolbar
cardiac functional parameter   of cut bitmap window
measurement

1) 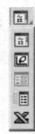 **Cut bitmap window:** It is divided into two parts: cut bitmap page and cut bitmap tool bar. See Figure 2-29.

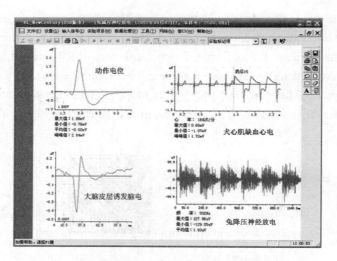

Figure 2-29   Cut bitmap window

Cut bitmap page is at the left side of the cut bitmap window, which takes up most space thereof. Cut bitmap page is used to piece together and modify the wave graphs cut from raw data channel. The graphs cut can only move within the white area of the cut page.

Cut bitmap tool bar is at the right side of the cut bitmap Window, which contains 12 command buttons relating to cut bitmap. These buttons are: open, save, print, print preview, copy, paste, undo, refresh, select, erase, write and exit.

2) 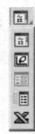 **X-Y input window:** When you select this function, X-Y vector graph display window will appear. See Figure 2-30.

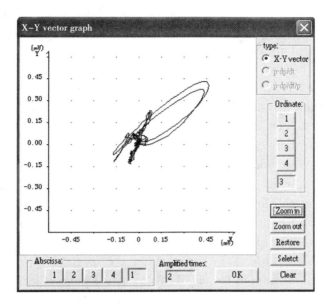

Figure 2-30   X-Y vector graph dialog box

The "type" parameter in X-Y vector graph dialog box is used to set the type of the plotted X-Y vector graph. 3 types are optional: electrocardial vector (X-Y vector), p-dp/dt and p-dp/dt/p, among which, the latter two types are available only when user has completed the differential for experimental data of certain channel, because dp/dt refers to differential, otherwise the latter two options will be ineffective (the color will change to gray).

"Abscissa" refers to the input channel selected in X-axis direction in X-Y vector graph, which may be any one of the four channels; "Ordinate" refers to the input channel selected in Y-axis direction in X-Y vector graph.

X-Y vector graph display window contains 5 function buttons, respectively "Zoom-in", "Zoom-out", "Restore", "Select" and "Clear". "Zoom-in" button is used to double the size of the original X-Y vector graph; "Zoom-out" button is opposed to the function of "Zoom-in". "Restore" button is used to restore the graph that has been zoomed in or out to its original size; "Select" button is used to select a wave segment to complete X-Y vector graph of the input channel on X-Axis. The wave segment selection method is just the same as that during section measurement; "Clear" button is used to clear the unwanted or unsatisfied X-Y vector graph.

3) 🔲 **Set parameter window:** It is designed to change the initial parameter setting of certain experiment model with optional parameter setting during the course of experiment.

4) 🔲 **Section measurement result display window:** BL-420F software has a dual view display system. The measured data in the two sets of display systems can be displayed in general information display area. In real-time experiment, raw data are obtained from the right view for calculation, and the measurement results in general display area will be automatically refreshed. If you want to analyze the data in left view, the measurement results can not be displayed.

When you select this command, the section measurement result display window will be opened(Figure 2-31), which is used to display the measured results in left view. Of course it can also be used to display the measured results in right view.

5) ✖ Open Excel: This command is used to open Excel worksheet If you want to directly write some measurement results of BL-420F software in Excel, such as section measurement results, hemodynamic measurement results or cardiac functional parameter measurement results, you must open Excel worksheet, and establish a write-in relationship between BL-420F software and Excel worksheet application. When you use this function, Excel worksheet will be opened. What is more important is that a communication relationship has been established between BL-420F software and Excel. Therefore, if you want to write data directly in Excel, you must use this command to open Excel worksheet application.

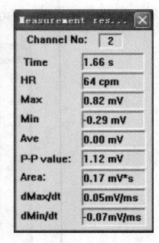

Figure 2-31   Measurement result window

(16) ᴬᴬ Selected wave zoom-in

This function is used to zoom in the detail of very small wave to facilitate observation and analysis. After you have selected a detail of a wave segment using area selection function, this function becomes available. When you select this command, a "wave zoom-in" window will pop up. See Figure 2-32. In this window, we can further zoom in or zoom out the wave

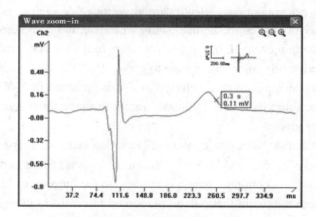

Figure 2-32   "Wave zoom-in" window

(17) ▥ Cut bitmap

Cut bitmap means that the segment of wave that you have selected in channel display window together with the data measured in this segment of wave are sent into a common data area of windows operating system in graphical form. Thereafter you can paste this graph that you have selected into cut window of BL-420F software or any windows application that can display graphs, such as Word, Excel or Paint. You can easily complete it by selecting "Paste" command in "Edit" menu of these applications.

The operational procedures for cut bitmap are as follows:

① During the course of real-time experiment or data replay, press "Pause" button to suspend the experiment. At this moment cut bitmap button 🔳 on the tool bar is in activated state. When you press this button, the system will be in cut bitmap status.

② Conduct area selection for the segment of wave that you are interested in. You can only select one-channel graph or select multi-channel graphs simultaneously. See Figure 2-33 and Figure 2-34.

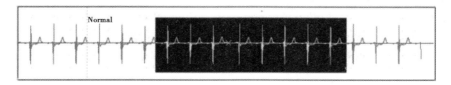

Figure 2-33   Area selection in one-channel display window

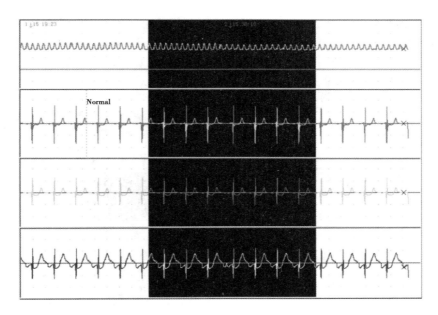

Figure 2-34   Area selection in multi-channel display window

③ When area selection is completed, cut bitmap window will appear. The graph that you selected last time will automatically be pasted into the cut bitmap window.

④ Select "Exit" button 🔳 on the tool bar at the right side of the cut bitmap window to exit the cut bitmap window.

⑤ Repeat the procedures of ① to ④ to continue the graphic cut for other segments of the waves, and then piece them together to form a complete graph. Now you can print or save this graph, or copy it into other applications, such as Word and Excel.

(18) ✂ *Cut data*

Cut data means to extract the selected one or more segments of original sampled data of inverse wave in BL-420 data format, and save them in your designated BL-420 format file named by you. As BL-420 data format is adopted for the extracted data using cut data command, such data can be read by software of BL-420 biological data acquisition and analysis system, and can be further analyzed and extracted. This command is available only when area selection for experimental data of certain channel has been completed. The operational procedures of cut data are as follows:

① Search the segment of wave that you want to cut in the whole recorded data.

② Use area selection function to select a segment of wave that you want to cut. Multi-screen data can be selected simultaneously.

③ Press cut data command button on the Tool Bar, or select "cut data" function in the pop-up shortcut menu when you click right mouse button on the selected area. Then, cut data for a segment of wave is completed. Data segment that has been cut will be displayed in gray. See Figure 2-35.

④ Repeat the above 3 procedures to conduct data cut operation for different segments of waves.

⑤ When you stop replay, a data cut file with the name of "cut.tme" will be generated automatically. You may rename it according to your own need, whereas the file name shall not be the same as the opened replay file. The file that has been cut is saved under \data subdirectory, with an extension file name of "tme".

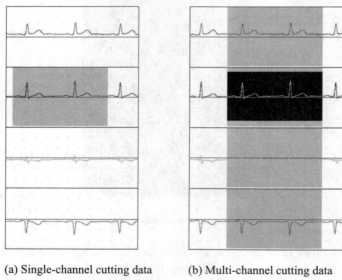

(a) Single-channel cutting data   (b) Multi-channel cutting data

Figure 2-35   Cut data

(19) Data deletion

Data deletion is to delete the useless data in raw data so that the rest ones are useful, which can form a new file. This function is useful only when the file has a small number of invalid data. Attention shall be paid to that data cut and data deletion can not be used simultaneously. If you have at first used cut data on a file, data deletion function will be disabled, and vice versa.

(20) Sign

When you click this command during the course of real-time experiment, a sign in the shape of a downward arrow will be added at the top of the wave display window. Before the arrow is the No. of this label. The serial number starts from 1, such as "20 ↓ " . After the arrow the time that indicates when this label is added. During single experiment, you can add 200 general experimental labels at most.

(21) 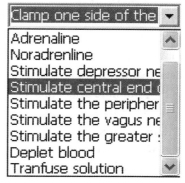 *Label edit and selection group box*

In fact label edit and selection group box is not a toolbar button. It is placed on toolbar in order to facilitate operation.

Relevant label groups have been preset in some experiment models of BL-420F software, such as in depressor nerve discharge experiment model. But these labels are not preset in most models.

If label group has been preset in certain experiment model itself, when you select this experiment model, all preset label in this experiment model will be listed in the label edit and selection group box(Figure 2-36). If in the list there are no labels you need, you may directly edit them in edit box. After the edit is completed, press "Enter" button to confirm it. At this moment, the edited labels may directly be added on the real-time wave, and at the same time they will be automatically saved into corresponding label groups.

If label group is not preset in certain experiment, you can also directly input new labels in edit group box. After the input,

Figure 2-36　Label list

a new label may be directly added onto the wave displayed in real time, whereas it can not be saved. You should use the label edit dialog box to add new label group.

In real-time experiment, the method to add a Label is very simple. You can select or edit a label in label edit and selection group box, and then click left mouse button at the position on the wave where you want to add the Label. See Figure 2-37. Attention shall be paid to that the selected label can only be added once. If you want to add the same label for the second time, you should re-select this label in the group box .

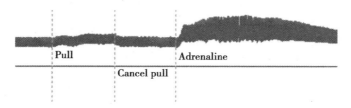

Figure 2-37　Add a label

After the label is added, you may also move (relocate), edit or delete the label that you have added. The method is very simple. Use your mouse cursor to point at the name of the label. Then click and hold left mouse button to move the label.

This command is only applicable to data replay. It is used to add a label to the specified location of the replay wave.

When you select this command by clicking right mouse button at the blank place of a waveform display channel, "Edit label" dialog box will pop up for you to input the content of the label. See Figure 2-38. Then you can press "OK" button, the label will be added to the place where you click right mouse button. If you press "Cancel" button, such operation will be ineffective. Attention shall be paid to that the label to be added shall not exceed 30 Chinese characters or 60 English letters.

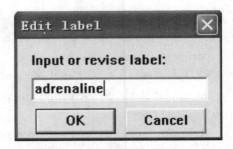

Figure 2-38   Edit label dialog box

(22) L _Open label dialog box_

When you click this command, "Edit experimental label" dialog box will be opened. See Figure 2-39.You may select an edited label group in label dialog box, or establish a new label group by yourself, and then press "OK" button to select this label group.

1) Add: After you press "Add" button, a "New Label Group" option will appear at the lowest part of the label group list, at the same time a new label named "New Label" will be automatically added for this label group in label list, because at least one label is required in each label group. At this moment, "New Label Group" will also be displayed in label group edit area. You may change the name of the experiment group in the edit area, and then press modify button to make it become effective. See Figure 2-39.

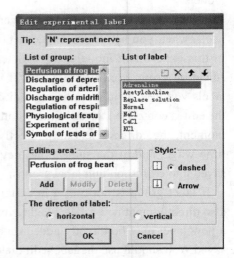

Figure 2-39   Edit experimental label
dialog box

2) Modify: This command is to make the modified name of the label group become effective.

3) Delete: This command is used to delete the whole label group that you have selected, including all labels inside it. Generally, you should use this command with care.

4) Edit label list : Label list box is a special list box, which not only have data list function like common list boxes, but also can add new list data, modify and delete list data in the list box, etc. It has a powerful function. There are 4 function buttons at the top of this list box, which are in turn "Add", "Delete", "Shift Up" and "Shift Down".

Add an internal label of the group: After you select Add button, a blank edit box will appear at the last line of the label list box, where a text edit cursor will flash, which indicates that you may edit this newly-added label now.

Delete button is to delete the currently selected label.

Shift Up button is to shift up the currently selected label by certain distance.

Shift Down button is to shift down the currently selected label by certain distance.

5) Label mode: Besides the literal description at the labeling place of label, there is a label point indicator. You may select the dotted line or arrow mode to complete labeling operation. See Figure 2-40.

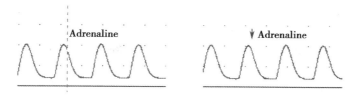

Figure 2-40 Label mode of label

6) Label text display direction: The text of label may either be horizontally or vertically displayed according to the requirement.

(23) *About*

This command contains the version of the BL-420F software, copyright information, and some configuration information of this computer.

(24) *Help*

This command can realize the context-dependent timely help function. After you have selected this tool bar command, the mouse pointer will become an arrow with a question label. At this moment you can use your mouse to point at different parts on the screen, and then click left mouse button. The help information about the specified part will pop up.

Section 5 Classical Animal Experiments in Medical Functional Experiment

Experiment 1 Sciatic-gastrocnemius preparation

1. Aims

1) To practice the method of brain pithing and spinal pithing of a toad or a frog.

2) To practice the method of making the sciatic-gastrocnemius preparation.

2. Principles

The physiological property of the tissue of frogs is similar to that of warmblood animal. It is easy to maintain the environment for their survival. Therefore,the sciatic-gastrocnemius preparation is often used in the laboratory to study the excitability, excitation process, some general rules of stimulation and the characteristics of skeletal muscle contraction.

The sciatic nerve runs down the leg between the large thigh muscles, i.e., between the semimembranosus and the lateral and medial femoral muscles. It branches several times and the peroneal branch is found deep between the two large calf muscles, i.e., the peroneus and gastrocnemius muscles.

3. Experimental materials

1) Animal: frogs.

2) Equipment: frog anatomy device (frog board, glass needle, bone scissors, tissue scissors, ophthalmic scissors, pin, dropper, petri dishes, zinc-copper arch) , probe, BL-420 system.

3) Reagents: Ringer's solution.

4. Procedures and observations

(1) Destroy the brain and the spinal cord

① The frog is held in the left hand with the dorsal side up and its head directed away from the experimenter (Figure 2-41A).

② Locate the position of the foramen magnum (It is in a concave fossa on the skull and you can feel it with the needle when move it down. Figure 2-41B).

③ Insert the pithing needle into the foramen magnum and push forward into the cranium. Move the point from side to side (Figure 2-41B).

④ Insert the pithing needle at the same point that it was inserted as step ①.Run it down through the neural canal to destroy the spinal cord (Figure 2-41C).

Sign: an extension of the hind legs is seen just before the reflexes are lost and then the legs relax.

(2) Removal of the upper trunk and the viscera

① Find the sacraliliac joint (Figure 2-41D). Make a section of the spinal column at the level 1~2 cm above the sacraliliac joint (Figure 2-41E).

② Cut off the part of the frog above the spinal cord where the sciatic nerves appear along the spinal cord. Remove and discard the viscera, the head and the chest and keep the remaining parts including hind legs, sacrum and spinal column (Figure 2-41F).

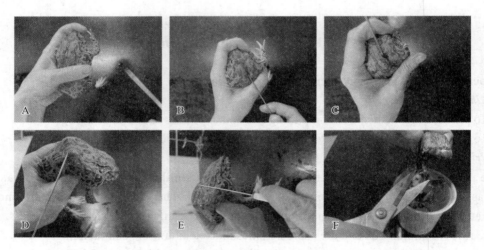

Figure 2-41   The procedures of pithing and removal of the viscera and upper trunk

(3) Skinning

① Tear off the skin. Place the specimen in a petri dishes containing Ringer's solution.

② Clean hands and instruments (apparatus) after skinning the frog.

(4) Division of the specimen

① Cut the spinal column into two halves along the midline with bone scissors (Figure 2-42A).

② Make an incision at the center of the symphysis pubis to have the two legs separated and place the legs into a petri dishes containing Ringer's solution (Figure 2-42B).

(5) The sciatic-gastrocnemius preparation

① Fix the specimen on the frog board with its dorsal side (flip the frog over) upward by pins (Figure 2-42C).

② Free the sciatic nerve with a glass needle along the column to the hip joint (Figure 2-42D).

③ Free the nerve till the hip joint and connect this part to the part of column (Figure 2-42E).

④ Dissect the Achilles tendon and tie it with a thread (Figure 2-42F).

⑤ Connect the spinal segment with the thigh segment, with upper part of sciatic nerve connected to a small piece of spine (Figure 2-42G)

⑥ Cut the tendon and free the muscle upward to the knee joint (Figure 2-42H).

⑦ Cut the femur and all the muscles around the knee joint (Figure 2-42I).

⑧ Complete the sciatic-gastrocnemius preparation (Figure 2-42J).

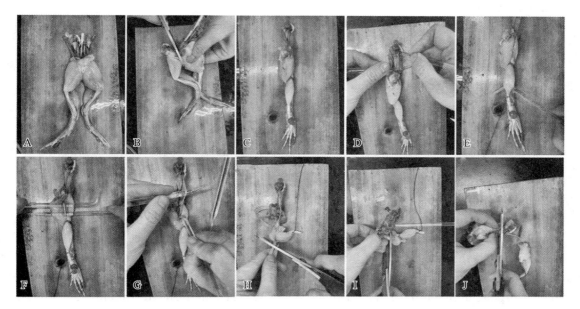

Figure 2-42   The procedures of making a sciatic-gastrocnemius preparation

(refer to color picture on color pages)

(6) Test on the excitability of the preparation

The preparation consists of a little piece of spinal column, sciatic nerve and gastrocnemius muscle (Figure 2-43A).Test the excitability of the preparation by stimulating the nerve with a zinc-copper arch (Figure 2-43B).

5. *Cautions*

1) Do not overstretch the nerve during the separation.

2) Don't touch the tested portion of specimen with sharp instrument or hands.

3) Moisten constantly the specimen with Ringer's solution during the whole experiment.

4) Free the sciatic nerve from the surrounding tissue by cutting the surrounding tissue parallel to the nerve.

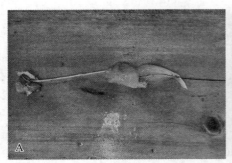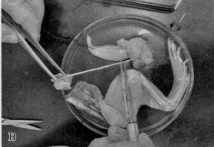

Figure 2-43　Sciatic-gastrocnemius preparation and excitability test

(refer to color picture on color pages)

6. Questions

1) Who is the first person to use the zinc-copper arch to test the excitability of nerve and muscles?

2) What is the mechanism underlying the function of zinc-copper arch?

3) How to use the zinc-copper arch correctly?

Experiment 2　The effects of stimulation intensity on muscle contraction

1. Aims

To observe the relationship between the intensity of stimulation and the strength of skeletal muscle contraction.

2. Principles

In neuroscience, the threshold potential is the critical membrane potential level at which the stimulus causes the membrane potential to depolarize and initiates the action potential, which determines whether the intensity of the stimulus is sufficient to produce the action potential (AP). The minimum stimulus that can cause the action potential is the threshold stimulus, and the corresponding intensity is the threshold intensity. The subthreshold stimulus refers to the stimulus with the intensity less than the threshold intensity. The subthreshold stimulus can produce local potentials, while the local potentials can be summated. Once the summation of the local potentials reaches the threshold, AP will burst. The value of the threshold potential can vary with many factors, such as changes in conductance of the sodium or potassium ion can cause a change in the threshold. Meanwhile, a decrease in the sample excitability may make it difficult to respond to the stimuli.

In one skeletal muscle cell, threshold stimulus is the stimulus with the smallest intensity, which just can cause the contraction of skeletal muscle cells with the highest excitability. Excitability of the skeletal cell can be evaluated by the threshold stimulus. The lower the threshold stimulus for causing the skeletal muscle contraction, the higher the excitability of this muscle cell. Subthreshold stimulus is the stimulus with the intensity lower than that of threshold stimulus, which cannot cause the contraction of any skeletal muscle cell. Supra-threshold stimulus is the stimulus with the intensity higher than that of threshold stimulus, which can cause the greater contraction strength of the skeletal muscle. Maximal stimulus is the stimulus with the lowest intensity, which just can excite all the cells in one skeletal muscle tissue to generate the maximum contraction strength. In one skeletal muscle tissue, each skeletal muscle cell has its own definite threshold stimulus. The contraction strength of one skeletal muscle depends on the numbers of the excited skeletal muscle cells involving in contraction. Therefore, the minimum stimulus intensity that causes the contraction of all muscle cells in a muscle is called maximal stimulus or optimal stimulus, which can cause the muscle to produce the maximum response. See Figure 2-44.

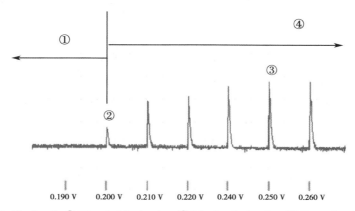

0.190 V   0.200 V   0.210 V   0.220 V   0.240 V   0.250 V   0.260 V

① Subthreshold stimuli; ② Threshold stimulus; ③ Maximal stimulus; ④ Suprathreshold stimuli.

Figure 2-44   The relationship between stimulation intensity and the strength of muscle contraction

3. Experimental materials

1) Animal: frogs.

2) Equipment: frog anatomy device, electronic stimulator, universal support stand, mechanical-electrical transducer, BL-420 system.

3) Reagents: Ringer's solution.

4. Procedures and observations

1) Making the sciatic-gastrocnemius preparation. Refer to experiment 1.

2) Connecting the muscle to the input of BL-420 system with a mechanical-electrical transducer.

3) Adjusting the stimulating electrodes and keep them to contact with the sciatic nerve closely.

4) Using BL-420 system to generate the stimulation to the sciatic nerve and record the contraction of the skeletal muscle.

① Stimulate the preparation with the weakest stimulus. There will be no contraction. This is the subthreshold stimulus.

② Increase the amplitude of stimulus step wisely till the muscle gives a slight twitch. This is the threshold stimulus.

③ Increase the amplitude of stimulus continuously, the increased amplitude of muscle contraction will reach a saturation point, there will be no further increase even increasing the stimulus intensity and the corresponding stimulus is called the maximal or optimal stimulus.

5. Cautions

1) Don't over stretch the nerve.

2) Keep the nerve wet with Ringer's solution during the whole experiment.

3) Don't touch the portion of specimen with sharp instrument or your hands.

4) A pause lasting about 30 seconds should be given between two stimuli.

5) Keep the experimental condition stable in the process of recording the curves, don't touch the specimen or related devices.

6. Questions

1) What is the "all or none" principle? Who is the first one to find it?

2) When we talk about the concepts of subthreshold, threshold and suprathreshold, do we mean the same thing as single nerve fiber and a bundle of nerve fibers?

3) The muscle contraction increases correspondingly with the increment of the stimulus intensity between the threshold and optimal stimulus, how to explain this phenomenon?

Experiment 3　The effects of stimulation frequency on muscle contraction

1. Aims

To observe the relationship between the stimulation frequency and the patterns of muscular contraction.

2. Principles

When an action potential travels along a motor nerve to a muscle cell, it causes a depolarization on the muscle cell membrane. The action potential generated on the muscle cell membrane travels to the centre of the muscle cell, which causes the sarcoplasmic reticulum to release calcium ions which initiate the contractile process. After the calcium level is restored by calcium ions pump, the contraction ceases. The whole process is called single muscle twitch.

Under a low frequency of stimulation, individual contraction occurs one after another, which is displayed on the left of Figure 2-45. Eventually as the frequency increases, new contraction will occur before the previous is over. As a result, the second contraction is partially added to the first one, and thus the contraction strength rises with the frequency. When the frequency continues to rise, it will reach a critical level that the successive contractions fuse together and the whole muscle contraction appears to be completely smooth and continuous as shown in the right side of Figure 2-45. This phenomenon is called complete tetanus, and the frequency before complete tetanus is given a name of incomplete tetanus. Tetany occurs when enough calcium ions are maintained in the muscle sarcoplasm, even between action potentials. Therefore, full contractile state is sustained without allowing any relaxation between the action potentials.

3. Experimental materials

1) Animal: frogs.

2) Equipment: frog anatomy device, electronic stimulator, universal support stand, mechanical-electrical transducer, BL-420 system.

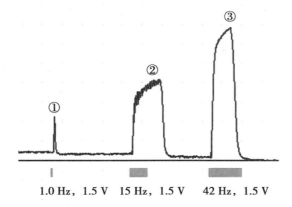

1.0 Hz，1.5 V   15 Hz，1.5 V   42 Hz，1.5 V

① Single twitch; ② Incomplete tetanus; ③ Complete tetanus.

Figure 2-45   The patterns of muscular contraction with increased stimulus frequency

3) Reagents: Ringer's solution.

4. Procedures and observations

1) Making the sciatic-gastrocnemius preparation as done before.

2) Connecting the muscle to the input of BL-420 system with a mechanical-electrical transducer.

3) Putting the stimulating electrodes on the sciatic nerve or muscle directly.

4) Using BL-420 system to generate the stimulation to the muscle tissue and record the contraction of the skeletal muscle.

5) Adjust the frequency of stimulation. When the frequency of stimulation is low, a series of simple muscle twitch occurs. Increase the frequency of stimulation and take the record of muscular contraction after each increase in frequency. Different patterns of incomplete tetanus and complete tetanus will be obtained in doing so.

5. Cautions

1) Don't overstretch the nerve.

2) Moisten the specimen constantly with Ringer's solution during the whole experiment.

3) Don't touch the portion of specimen with sharp instrument or your hand.

4) A pause lasting about 30~60 s should be given between two stimulations.

5) Keep the experimental condition stable in the process of recording the curves, and don't touch the specimen or related devices.

6. Questions

1) The muscle contraction can be summated, can the action potential that induces the muscle contraction also be summated? Why?

2) How does the stimulation frequency determine the patterns of muscle contraction?

3) Compare the amplitude of the single twitch, incomplete and complete tetanus and analyze the physiologic significance of the differences.

Experiment 4　Induction of the compound AP of nerve trunk

1. Aims

1) To learn the basic operation of sciatic nerve specimen.

2) To record and identify the waveform of the AP on the sciatic nerve: the diphasic and monophonic AP.

3) To observe the relationship between the intensity of stimulation and the amplitude of nerve trunk action potential.

2. Principles

In a nerve trunk, there are thousands of axons whose size, myelination and position are different, therefore, the recording we obtained is expression of a compound action potential (CAP). See Figure 2-46. This CAP is the algebraic summation of all the action potentials produced by all the fibers that were fired by that stimulus. An extracellular method can be used to record the CAP.

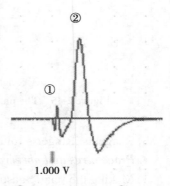

① Stimulus artifact; ② AP of nerve trunk.

Figure 2-46　The stimulus artifact and AP of nerve trunk

Each nerve fiber has its own threshold stimulus. Therefore, the amplitudes of AP of nerve trunk are determined by the numbers of the excited nerve fibers. The more the excited nerve fibers there are, the greater the AP of nerve trunk will be. The amplitude of AP will reach the maximal one as all the nerve fibers are excited by the maximal stimulus.

Stimulus artifact (Figure 2-46) is the sign of the start of stimulation, the size of artifact increase with the increment of stimulus intensity. Too large artifact will stimulus affect the waveform of the action potential.

The out membrane potential is lower than resting potential (RP) in exciting part. With the nerve impulse passing, the out membrane potential returns to RP. The process of membrane potential changing in nerve trunk is call AP of nerve trunk. If two leading electrodes are placed on the surface of a normal nerve trunk, two reverse potential deflection are induced which is called biphasic AP (Figure 2-47) when an excitation traverses two electrodes successively. If the nerve tissue between two leading electrodes are injured, the excitation only traverses the first leading electrodes, but it doesn't pass the second one. A unidirectional potential deflection is induced that is named a monophasic AP (Figure 2-47) in the situation.

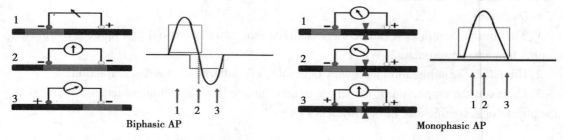

Biphasic AP　　　　　　　　　　　　　　　　Monophasic AP

Figure 2-47　The biphasic and monophasic AP of nerve trunk

3. Experimental materials

1) Animal: frogs.

2) Equipment: frog anatomy device, electronic stimulator, shielded nerve box, universal support stand, BL-420 system.

3) Reagents: Ringer's solution.

4. Procedures and observations

1) Refer to the step (1) to (4) of experiment 1.

2) Make a sciatic nerve specimen.

① Fix the specimen to the frog board with pins, dissect and separate the spinal and thigh segments of the sciatic nerve along the sciatic nerve groove carefully.

② Free the nerve upwards till the hip joint and then move down to the knee, the sciatic nerve extending into the knee is divided into two parts (Figure 2-48A). Cut the tendon which covers the nerve at the knee.

③ Free the nerve down the length of the calf to the ankle(Figure 2-48B and Figure 2-48C).

④ Free the sciatic nerve from surrounding tissue by cutting the surrounding tissue parallel to the nerve, be careful and do not cut the nerve.

⑤ Tie off the nerves at the ankle, leaving about 4~5 cm of thread for mounting (2-48D). Cut the nerves just beyond where it is tied.

⑥ Tie off the sciatic nerves at the backbone where it leaves the spinal cord, leaving about 4~5 cm of thread attached for manipulating the nerve. Cut the nerve between the knot of thread and the spinal cord.

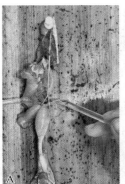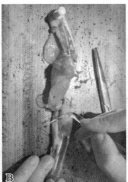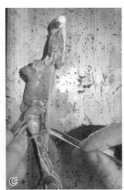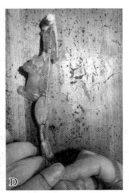

Figure 2-48   The isolation of the sciatic nerve

(refer to color picture on color pages)

3) Place the nerve on stimulating electrodes and recording electrodes properly which are embedded in the shielded nerve box. Please make sure that stimulating electrode is in contact with the proximal end of the nerve trunk and the recording electrode to the distal end. See Figure 2-49.

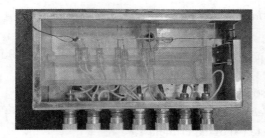

Figure 2-49   The placement of the sciatic nerve in shielded nerve box

4) Connect the shielded nerve box to BL-420 system (Figure 2-50), then stimulate the nerve trunk with an adequate stimulus to initiate a CAP from the most distal pair of recording electrodes. The recorded waveform consists of an early component that occurs within a fraction of a millisecond after the stimulus which is a Stimulus artifact and a later, diphasic component that occurs after a delay of a few milliseconds which is the real AP of nerve trunk.

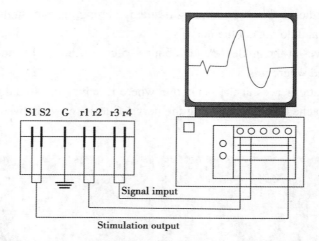

Figure 2-50   The assembly of the shielded nerve box and BL-420 system

① Start with a weak stimulus and gradually increase the level to determine the threshold current for the CAP for pulse, change the amplitude of the stimulus and see whether there is any change in the action potential. Observe the relationship between stimulation intensity and the amplitude of CAP. Find out the minimal stimulation intensity and maximal stimulation intensity that can cause the maximum CAP.

② Press and crush a small portion of the nerve midway between the two recording electrodes using forceps or a hemostat. On stimulation, a monophasic AP will be shown. Compare it with the biphasic AP before injury.

5. Cautions

1) Do not hurt the nerve during separation in order not to affect the results.

2) The sciatic nerve specimen should be as long as possible, 8 cm above is the best.

3) Wash it with Ringer's solution on times to keep its good excitability.

4) Keep the nerve trunk in touch with electrodes. The distance between two recording

electrodes should be as long as possible.

5) Avoid applying too much Ringer's solution to the nerve.

6) Avoid large currents which can damage the nerve.

6. Questions

1) The too large stimulus artifact will change the AP waveform, how can we decrease the amplitude of the stimulus artifact?

2) Does the CAP have "all-or-none" response?

3) Why is the amplitude of positive phase of AP lower than the negative phase of AP?

Experiment 5 Observation of the cardiac pacemaker of a frog

1. Aims

1) To locate and observe the cardiac pacemaker in amphibian.

2) To detect the autorhythmicity of cardiac muscle in various parts of the frog's heart.

2. Principles

The special conduction system of the heart has the automatic rhythm, but the autorhythmicity of each part is different. the venous sinus has the highest autorhythmicity in amphibian. Every excitement of the normal heart starts from the part of the highest autorhythmicity to the atrium and ventricle in turn, then cause the contraction of atrium and ventricular successively. The part with the highest autorhythmicity is called the pacemaker of the heart. When the normal pacemaker is affected, the activity of the atrium and ventricle also changes accordingly. If the impulses transmitted from the pacemaker are blocked, the activity of atrial and ventricular will temporarily stop, and then show their respective autorhythmicity.

The normal pacemaker of the amphibian is the sinus venosus, an enlarged region between the vena cava and the right atrium. Each region of the heart has its intrinsic rate of beating, for example sinus venosus 72 beats/min; atrium 60 beats/min; ventricle 25 beats/min. The cells that are depolarized fastest control the rate of contraction of all other cells, thus they act as the pacemaker of the heart. Only when the faster pacemaker region is blocked is it possible to observe the intrinsic rate of the slower regions. The heart of the frog has three chambers, one ventricle and two atria (Figure 2-51 and Figure 2-52). The frog's heart differs from the mammalian heart anatomically in that they are three-chambered rather than fourchambered. In this experiment, the frog's heart will be used because it functions well at the room temperature and will continue to beat even when excised from the body.

3. Experimental materials

1) Animal: frogs.

2) Equipment: frog anatomy device, timer, cotton thread.

3) Reagents: Ringer's solution.

4. Procedures and observations

1) Destroy the brain and spinal cord of the frog. Place it on a frog board in a supine position.

2) Cut the skin over the thorax along the midline and open the thorax with a pair of scissors. Slit the pericardium carefully to expose the heart.

3) Preset a piece of suture under the sinus groove and atrioventricular groove respectively.

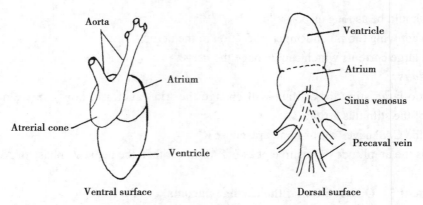

Figure 2-51   The structure of a frog heart

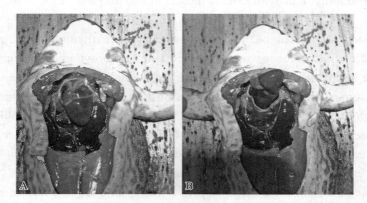

Figure 2-52   The ventral side (A) and dorsal side (B) of a frog heart

(refer to color picture on color pages)

4) Identify the sinus venosus, the atria and the ventricle, and then observe the sequence and contraction rate of each part of them.

5) Tie the heart between the sinus venosus and the atria with a piece of thread, and then observe the sequence and contraction rate of each part of the heart (the sinus venosus and the atria).

6) Tie the heart between the atria and ventricles with a piece of thread, and then observe the sequence and contraction rate of each part of the heart (the atria and the ventricle).

Table 2-1   Frequency of heart beating (times/min)

Observation item	Sinus venosus	Atrium	Ventricle
Control			
Tie the sinus groove			
Tie the atrioventricular groove			

5. Cautions

1) Moisten constantly the specimen with Ringer's solution.

2) Don't touch the portion of specimen with sharp instrument or your hand.

3) When tie the heart between the venous sinus and the atrium, make ligation as close to the atrium as possible.

6. Questions

1) How does the normal pacemaker control the beating rate of the whole heart?

2) What is the work mechanism underlying the clinical cardiac pacemaker? What should be paid attention to the use of heart pacemaker?

Experiment 6   Extrasystole and compensatory pause of the frog heart

1. Aims

To observe stimulate the extrasystole and compensatory pause of the frog heart.

2. Principles

Ventricular muscle cells have a very long refractory period lasting from the beginning of systole to the end of early stage of diastole (Figure 2-53). Any stimulus cannot induce a new contraction during the refractory period. After the refractory period, an extra effective stimulus before the normal impulse from the normal pacemaker arriving at the ventricle muscles can induce an extra ventricular contraction, called extrasystole (Figure 2-53). The cardiac muscle is also absolutely refractory in the contraction period of the extrasystole, if the closely following impulse coming from the normal pacemaker arrives at the refractory period of the extrasystole, it cannot induce a normal ventricular contraction, because the impulse arising normally from the sinus venosus drops in the absolute refractory is ineffective, so a long pause which is called compensatory pause will be resulted.

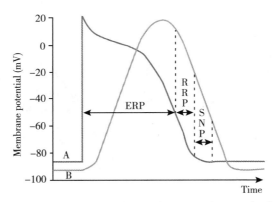

A. The graph of AP of cardiac muscle cell; B. The contraction graph of cardiac muscle;

ERP. Effective refractory period; RRP. Relative refractory period; SNP. Superanormal period.

Figure 2-53   The relationship between excitability during AP and contraction of ventricle muscle

The extrasystole is normally followed by a long period of diastole, which is called compensatory pause (Figure 2-54).

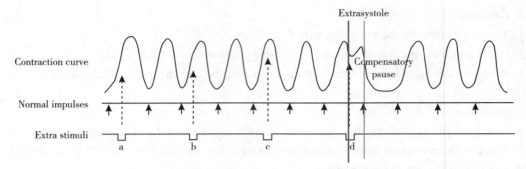

Figure 2-54   Extrasystole and compensatory pause of the frog heart

3. Experimental materials

1) Animal: frogs.

2) Equipment: frog anatomy device, electronic stimulator, universal support stand, BL-420 system.

3) Reagents: Ringer's solution.

4. Procedures and observations

1) Destroy the brain and spinal cord of the frog as before mentioned. Expose the heart.

2) Clip the apex of the heart during diastole(2 mm).

3) Set up the apparatuses as shown in Figure 2-55A.

4) Adjust the two poles of the stimulating electrode so that they are in close contact with the ventricle during systole as well as diastole, see Figure 2-55B.

5) Identify which part of the curve corresponds to ventricular systole and which part to diastole.

6) Take a record of several heartbeats. Stimulate the ventricle with a single impulse of moderate amplitude during systole and diastole respectively. When will extrasystole be initiated? Is there a compensatory pause in consequence?

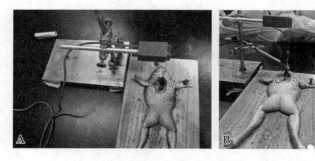

Figure 2-55   The settings of the frog heart

5. Cautions

1) Don't overstretch the nerve.

2) Moisten constantly the specimen with Ringer's solution.

3) Don't touch the portion of specimen with sharp instrument or your hands.

4) A pause lasting about 30 seconds should be given between two stimulations.

5) Keep the experimental conditions stable in the process of recording the curves, don't touch the specimen or related devices.

6. Questions

1) Were you able to demonstrate tetanus in the frog's heart? Why or why not?

2) Why do we say extrasystole is not always followed by compensatory pause?

Experiment 7   Regulation of respiration movement

1. Aims

1) To learn the basic technique of tracheal incubation/cannula.

2) To observe the effects of some factors on the respiration movement.

2. Principles

The main function of the lung is to obtain oxygen from the external environment to supply the oxygen to cells and to remove from the body the carbon dioxide produced by cellular metabolism. To realize this function, the respiratory movement should be under the control of the central nervous system.

The respiratory control system is very sensitive to alterations in the internal environment of the body. Changes in PCO_2, pH and PO_2 cause changes in alveolar ventilation designed to restore these variables to their normal values. Chemicals in the body such as oxygen, carbon dioxide, and hydrogen ion concentrations greatly influence respiration. There are two types of chemoreceptor, peripheral chemoreceptors (PCRs) and central chemoreceptors (CCRs). PCRs are located in the carotid arteries and the aortic arch and mainly sensitive to PO_2, but can also respond to CO_2, H^+ and pH. They cause an increase in breathing rapidly when stimulated and therefore called hypoxic receptors. CCRs are located in the medulla oblongata, they are separated from the blood by the extracellular fluid, cerebrospinal fluid (CSF) and the blood brain barrier (BBB). CCRs respond to CO_2, H^+ and pH but not to O_2. They respond more slowly but have a greater effect on breathing.

Besides chemical control, Hering-Breuer reflex can influence respiration. There are two types of reflex: inflation reflex and deflation reflex. Inflation reflex increased stretch due to overinflation of lungs causes activation of stretch receptors that send impulses to respiratory center via pathways to vagus which causes the inhalation to be inhibited. Deflation reflex which serves lung deflation causes activation of receptors in the lung walls (pleura) that send impulses to respiratory center via pathways to vagus which causes the exhalation to be inhibited. When one side of vagus is cut, breath becomes a little deeper and less frequently because the efficiency of Hering-Breuer reflex is reduced by half. After cutting both of vagus, breath becomes deeper and less frequently because Hering-Breuer reflex has been completely tampered.

3. Experimental materials

1) Animal: rabbit, 2.0~2.5 kg.

2) Equipment: mammalian surgical instruments (skin clamp, tissue scissors, hemostatic forceps, tissue tweezers, surgical blade, scalpel handle, ophthalmic scissors, opthalmic tweezers, sutures, suture needles, needle holders), dissecting table for rabbit, mechanical-electric transducer, electronic stimulator, tracheal tubing, syringes, rubber tubing of 50 cm in length, balloon filled with CO_2,

balloon filled with N₂, thread, gauze, universal support stand, double clamp, frog heart clip.

3) Reagents: 25% urethane solution, 3% lactic acid solution, saline solution.

4. Procedures and observations

1) Anesthetization and restraint of the rabbit.

① Anesthetization: inject 4 mL/kg 25% urethane solution via the marginal ear vein.

② Restraint: fix the anesthetized rabbit on the dissecting table in supine position.

2) Clear the hairs on the neck in front of the larynx.

3) Make a midline incision about 5~7 cm long just at the lower border of the thyroid cartilage.

4) Free the vagus nerve on both sides. See Figure 2-56.

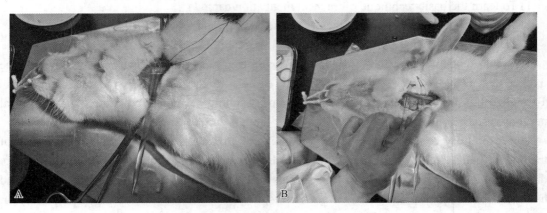

Figure 2-56　The isolation of vagus nerves
(refer to color picture on color pages)

5) Isolate the muscles covering the trachea and dissect the connective tissues on both sides of the trachea and between the trachea and esophagus with a pair of hemostat. After the trachea is freed, a piece of cotton thread is put under it.

6) Tracheal intubation (tracheotomy)

① Make a cross cut on the anterior wall between the two cartilage rings at the level about 2~3 cm below the distal margin of larynx with a scalpel. Make another longitudinal cut on the anterior wall at the proximal end of the trachea. A converse "T shape" incision is thus formed. See Figure 2-57A. Clean the secretion and/or blood from the wound with cotton ball.

② Insert the tracheal tubing into it. Pick up the cotton thread underneath the trachea with one hand and insert the tracheal tubing of appropriate diameter into the distal end of the trachea. See Figure 2-57B.

③ Fix the tracheal tubing tightly with the thread.

7) Observation

① Take a record of normal respiratory movement curve. Check its rhythm and frequency. Identify the relation of the inspiration and expiration with the upward stroke or downward stroke of the respiratory movement.

② Effect of CO_2: bring the balloon filled with CO_2 close to the opening of the tracheal tubing. Observe the changes of the respiratory movement. Take the balloon away and watch the recovery

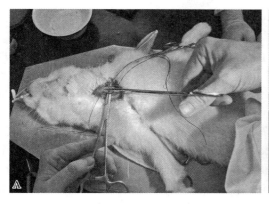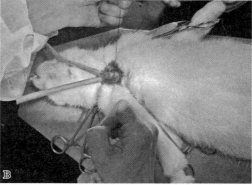

Figure 2-57   Tracheal intubation

(refer to color picture on color pages)

of the respiratory movement.

③ Effect of anoxia: close one of the branches of the tracheal tubing and connect the other branch to a balloon filled with N_2. While the animal is breathing through the balloon, what will be the result? Take the balloon away and open the branches of the tracheal tubing. Will the respiration resume to its original condition?

④ Effect of increases in dead space: connect a rubber tubing of 50 cm in length to the other branch of the tracheal tubing. What change will occur?

⑤ Effect of pH of blood: inject 2 mL of 3% lactic acid solution via the marginal ear vein. What is the result?

⑥ Effect of the vagus nerve on respiration movement: cut off the vagus nerve on one side. What is the result? Then cut another side. Observe the changes in respiratory frequency and depth of breath after severing bilateral vagus nerves.

5. Cautions

1) Notes to use anesthetics.

① There is individual variation in the tolerance of anesthetics. It is, therefore, necessary to manage the dosage of anesthetics by monitoring the condition of the animal to avoid overdosage.

② The degree of anesthesia can be determined by the depth and the rate of respiration, the character of corneal reflex, the tone of the muscles over the extremities and abdominal wall and the response to picking of skin. In case of the aforementioned response diminishes greatly or disappears, the infusion of anesthetics should be discontinued.

③ When intravenous infusion is used, it should be carried on slowly. A rapid infusion is liable to lead to sudden death of the animal.

2) Notes to isolation of nerve and blood vessels.

① Nerves and blood vessels are fragile and liable to be damaged. Care must be taken while isolating them from the surrounding tissues. Don't use the toothed forceps, lest damage structurally and /or functionally induces.

② While isolating a large nerve trunk or blood vessel, it is better to separate first the surrounding connective tissues with a pair of ophthalmic scissors or ordinary hemostat and then free them from the adhered connective tissues.

③ The normal anatomical relationship should be reserved while dissecting the twigs of nerve and blood vessel. A pair of glass needle is preferred for dissection in this case.

④ When the nerve or blood vessel is freed, put a piece or pieces of thread socked in saline under them for identification.

⑤ Cover the incision with a wet gauze pad or add a few mL of liquid paraffin of 37 ℃ to bathe the nerve.

6. Questions

1) What are the differences that the acting mechanism on the respiration movement caused by anoxia or excessive CO_2 in the blood? And compare their acting mechanism.

2) What is the function of the vagus nerve during rhythmic respiration movement?

3) Who found the peripheral chemoreceptors (PCRs)? How did he design experiments to identify the locations and functions of PCRs ?

Experiment 8　Regulation of cardiovascular system activities

1. Aims

1) To practice the basic technique of arterial cannulation.

2) To observe the effect of nerves and hormones on heart and blood vessels.

2. Principles

Cardiovascular activities are mainly controlled by nervous system and humoral agents. Taking blood pressure as an index of cardiovascular activities, the effects of various factors on cardiovascular system can be demonstrated.

(1) Effect of baroreceptors

There are baroreceptors presented in the arch of the aorta, and the carotid sinuses of the left and right internal carotid arteries. Baroreceptors serve for maintaining mean arterial blood pressure to allow tissues to receive the right amount of blood. Baroreceptors respond very quickly to maintain a stable blood pressure, but they only respond to short-term changes. Also, they work by detecting the amount of stretch. The more the baroreceptor walls are stretched, the more frequently they generate action potentials.

(2) Effect of vagus nerve

Parasympathetic innervation of the heart is mediated by the vagus nerve. The vagi innervate the sinoatrial node (SN) and predispose the heart to atrioventricular (AV) blocks. Vagus nerves secrete substances called acetylcholine which has effects on M receptors in heart. Acetylcholine causes SN cells to increase efflux of K^+ in phase 4 and decrease influx of Ca^{2+}. Therefore, the activation of the vagus nerve leads to a reduction in heart rate and blood pressure.

(3) Effect of adrenaline

Adrenaline or epinephrine plays a vital role in the short-term stress reaction. It is secreted by the adrenal medulla. When injected into the bloodstream, epinephrine binds to α, β_1 and β_2 receptors of smooth muscle in skeletal muscle arterioles. As binding to α receptors that cause the vasoconstriction, binding to β_1 receptors that cause the increase of cardiac activity and binding to β_2 receptors that cause vasodilatation, adrenaline increases heart rate and stroke volume. Increasing stroke volume can cause the increase of blood pressure.

(4) Effect of noradrenaline

Norepinephrine or noradrenaline is released from the medulla of the adrenal glands as a hormone into the blood, but it is also a neurotransmitter in the nervous system where it is released from noradrenergic neurons during synaptic transmission. When injected into the bloodstream, norepinephrine binds to α and β_2 receptors of smooth muscle in arterioles. Binding to α receptors causes vasoconstriction and binding to β_2 receptors causes vasodilatation. Noradrenaline has a much greater affinity for α than for β_2 receptor; therefore, it causes vasoconstriction rather than vasodilatation, so,activating the sympathetic nervous system directly increases the heart rate and blood pressure.

(5) Effect of acetylcholine

The chemical compound acetylcholine, often abbreviated as ACh, was the first neurotransmitter identified. It is a chemical transmitter in both the peripheral nervous system (PNS) and central nervous system (CNS). Acetylcholine is the neurotransmitter in all autonomic ganglia.

When acetylcholine binds to M receptors of heart, it causes sinus node cells to increase efflux of K^+ in phase 4 and decrease influx of Ca^{2+}.Therefore, injection of acetylcholine induces decreased contraction in cardiac muscle fibers. So, there are decreases in heart rate and blood pressure.

3. Experimental materials

1) Animal: rabbits, 2.0~2.5 kg.

2) Equipment: mammalian surgical instruments, dissecting table for rabbits, mechanical-electric transducer, electronic stimulator, shielded electrodes, polyethylene tubing, tracheal tubing, syringes, 3 way stopcock, suture thread, gauze, universal support stand, double clamp, arterial clip.

3) Reagents: liquid paraffin, heparin (1:1000 unit/mL), 25% urethane solution, 3% lactic acid solution , saline solution, 0.01% adrenaline solution, 0.01% noradrenaline solution, 0.01% acetylcholine solution.

4. Procedures and observations

1) Anesthetization of the rabbit: inject the rabbit with 25% urethane solution at 4 mL/kg via the marginal ear vein.

2) Restraint of the rabbit: fix the anesthetized rabbit on the dissecting table in supine position.

① Restraint of the extremities: place the rabbit in a supine position. Tie the hindlimb at the level just above the ankle joint with one end of a piece of cotton thread. Tie the forelegs at the level just above the elbow joints. Fix them to both sides of the dissecting table.

② Restraint of the head: tie the two upper incisors of the animal with one end of a piece of cotton thread and tie the other end to an iron rod fixed on the dissection table.

3) Dissection: isolate the common carotid artery, vagus nerve, aortic depressor nerve and sympathetic nerve.

① Make a midline incision about 5~7 cm long on the neck just at the lower of the thyroid cartilage. Using a pair of hemostat to separate the subcutaneous tissue and muscle by blunt dissection.

② Locate the trachea and separate the muscle lying over it with the hemostat. The left and right common carotid arteries will be seen lying laterally to the trachea on both sides. Several nerves are running parallel to the common carotid artery; they are, namely, vagus nerve (the thickest one), sympathetic nerve and aortic depressor nerve (as fine as a hair).

③ Isolate sections of about 2~3 cm of the artery and nerves (Figure 2-58A). Put threads of different colors under each of them for identification. Two pieces of thread should be placed around the left common carotid artery for further double ligation.

4) Cannulation of the carotid artery.

① Tie the distal end of the left common carotid artery with one thread and clamp the proximal end with a bulldog (arterial clip). The distance between these two ties is approximately 3 cm. See Figure 2-58B.

② Pick up the thread at the distal end and make a "V" shape incision on the arterial wall close to the knot with a pair of fine sharp scissors. The cut edge should have an angle of 45 degree in relation to the long axis of the artery. Be careful not to section it. See Figure 2-58B.

③ Insert the tip of an arterial cannula that has been filled with heparin sodium solution into the artery against the direction of blood flow. See Figure 2-58C.

④ Fix the tip of the cannula tightly with the other piece of thread.See Figure 2-58D.

⑤ Check the closure of 3 way stopcock, and then open the arterial clip, letting the blood enters the transducer through the arterial cannula.

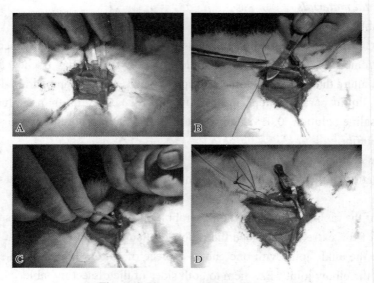

Figure 2-58   Arterial cannulation
(refer to color picture on color pages)

5) Observations.

① Record the normal blood pressure curve. Observe the systolic and diastolic change.

② Occlude the right common carotid artery for 15 seconds. How will the blood pressure and heart rate change?

③ Stimulate the whole right aortic depressor nerve with medium intensity via a pair of shielded stimulating. Then stimulate the peripheral and proximal ends of it respectively.

④ Make a ligature on the right vagus nerve. Cut the nerve cephalad to the ligature. Then stimulate the peripheral and proximal ends of the right vagus nerve respectively.

⑤ Inject 0.3 mL of 0.01% adrenaline solution into the marginal ear vein.

⑥ Inject 0.3 mL of 0.01% noradrenaline solution into the marginal ear vein.

⑦ Inject 0.3 mL of 0.01% acetylcholine solution to the marginal ear vein.

5. Cautions

Same as experiment 7.

6. Questions

1) Analyze the different effects of noradrenaline and adrenaline on the heart and blood vessels; and how are they applied in clinical practice?

2) Who is the first one to find acetylcholine, and how? What is the significance?

3) Both the anoxia and excessive CO_2 in the blood can increase the cardiovascular activities. Please compare their acting mechanisms.

4) How was noradrenaline first identified and what is the significance?

Experiment 9   Physiological properties of smooth muscle of digestive tract

1. Aims

1) To practice the method of in vitro perfusion of intestine.

2) To investigate the physiological properties of smooth muscle of digestive tract by observing the effects of some chemicals on smooth muscle movement of digestive tract.

2. Principles

The gastrointestinal tract has its own nervous system called the enteric nervous system (ENS), which lies entirely in the wall of the tract. This system functions to control the gastrointestinal movement and secretion. Although the ENS can function independently of the peripheral nerves, stimulation by the parasympathetic and sympathetic systems can greatly enhance or inhibit gastrointestinal functions. The autonomic nerve fibers innervate smooth muscle, and the vesicles of the autonomic nerve fiber endings contain acetylcholine in some fibers and norepinephrine in others, and occasionally other substances as well.

The smooth muscle is highly contractile, because there are many sodium or calcium channel on the membrane of smooth muscle. When stimulated by nerve or other chemical factors, influx of sodium or calcium either initiates action potential, which induces sarcoplasmic reticulum to release calcium ions; or allows extracellular calcium ions enters the cell. The calcium ions activate calmodulin, which binds to myosin light chain kinase. This kinase activates the regulatory chain of the myosin in smooth muscle, which allows the attachment-detachment cycling of the myosin head. Hence, the contraction of the smooth muscle is greatly dependent on calcium ions rather than action potentials.

Smooth muscle as a whole are easily stretched and possess different degrees of tonus and autorhythmicity. On the basis of the resting membrane potential, automatic depolarization and repolarization produce the slow waves whose amplitude and frequency are small (about 10~15 mV) and slow (lasting for several seconds). When a slow wave reaching to certain level (more positive than −40 mV), it can initiate AP and contraction of smooth muscles. The mechanical stretch, temperature and chemicals of the food in the tract are the sensitive stimuli of the gastrointestinal smooth muscle.

3. Experimental materials

1) Specimen: segments of small intestine (2~3 cm) of rabbit.

2) Equipments: thermostat water bath, thermostatic bath, curved needle and threads, mechanical-electric transducer, BL-420 system.

3) Reagents: Tyrode's solution, 25% urethane solution, 0.01% adrenaline solution, 0.01% acetylcholine solution, 0.01% atropine sulphate solution, 1 mol/L HCl solution, 1 mol/L NaOH solution.

4. Procedures and observations

1) Preparation.

① Set up the thermostatic bath and fill it with Tyrode's solution of 38℃.

② Inject the rabbit with 25% urethane solution at 4 mL/kg via the marginal ear vein.

③ Open the abdominal cavity and isolate a segment of intestine of 2~3 cm in length and take it out. Tie the two cut ends with cotton threads. Fix one end to the tip of the L-shaped glass tubing and the other end to the lever via the thread.

④ Assemble the recording device and record the contractions of the intestine through the transducer. See Figure 2-59.

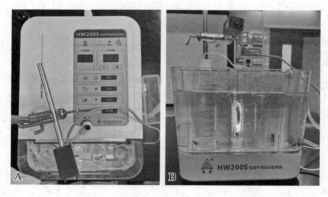

Figure 2-59   The connection of intestine to the transducer

2) Observations.

① Normal contraction curve.

② Add 1~2 drops of 0.01% adrenaline solution to the bath. After the observations, wash the specimen three times.

③ Add 1~2 drops of 0.01% acetylcholine solution to the bath. After the observations, wash the specimen three times.

④ Add 1~ 2 drops of 0.01% atropine sulfate solution. After the observations, go directly to the next step.

⑤ Add 1~ 2 drops of 0.01% acetylcholine solution to the bath. After the observations, wash the specimen three times.

⑥ Add 1~ 2 drops of 1 mol/L HCl solution to the bath. After the observations, wash the specimen three times.

⑦ Add 1~ 2 drops of 1 mol/L NaOH solution to the bath. After the observations, wash the specimen three times.

⑧ Decrease the temperature from 38℃ to room tempreture.

5. Cautions

1) Care must be taken to avoid overstretching of the specimen when connecting the segment between the level to the transducer.

2) Ligate the mesenteric vessels before cutting out that segment.

3) Before the next item, wash several times with 38℃ Tyrode's solution and wait till the last effect is subsided.

4) Check the temperature and the oxygen flow in the Magnus bath regularly, and complete the experiment as soon as possible.

6. Questions

1) Can 1 mol/L HCl solution induce the same effects on the tonus and frequency of the intestinal contraction as 1 mol/L NaOH solution do? Why or why not?

2) What will be the changes of the intestinal contraction when the 0.01% atropine sulfate solution is added to the thermostatic bath before and after the addition of acetylcholine?

3) How to prove the important action of the calcium ions on the smooth muscle contraction of the small intestine?

Experiment 10　Factors affecting urine formation

1. Aims

1) To practice the abdominal operation.

2) To learn the basic techniques of ureters intubation.

3) To observe the influences of some factors on urine formation.

2. Principles

As the key organ in the urinary system, kidneys serve various vital functions in regulating homeostasis. The most familiar one is to rid the body of waste materials that are either ingested or produced by metabolism. These wastes include urea, creatinine, uric acid, etc., which must be eliminated from the body as rapidly as they are produced. The kidneys also eliminate most toxins and other foreign substances that are either produced by the body or ingested, such as pesticides, drugs, and food additives. The second function is to regulate water and electrolyte balances. For the maintenance of homeostasis, excretion of water and electrolyte must precisely match its intake, which stabilizes the body fluid osmolarity and electrolyte concentrations; regulate acid-base balance; and in turn stabilizes the arterial blood pressure by controlling total blood volume. This regulatory function of the kidneys maintains the stable internal environment which is necessary for the cells to perform their various activities. The kidneys perform their most important functions by filtering the plasma and removing substances from the filtrate at variable rates, depending on the needs of the body. Ultimately, the kidneys "clear" unwanted substances from the filtrate by excreting them in the urine while returning substances that are needed back to the blood.

In summary, urinary formation is the main function of the kidney, which includes the processes of glomerular filtration, tubular reabsorption and secretion. Any factor that acts on these processes will result in the alteration of the quality and quantity of the urine.

3. Experimental materials

1) Animal: rabbits, 2.0~2.5 kg.

2) Equipment: mammalian surgical instruments, dissecting table for rabbits, drop meter, shielded electrodes, polyethylene tubing, 3 way stopcock, gauze, syringes, testing paper for glucose, BL-420 system.

3) Reagents: 25% urethane solution, saline solution, 20% glucose, 0.01% noradrenaline, furosemide, antidiuretic hormone.

4. Procedures and observations

1) Anesthetization: inject 4 mL/kg 25% urethane solution via the marginal ear vein.

2) Restraint: fix the anesthetized rabbit on the dissecting table in supine position.

3) Isolate the right vagus nerve; place a thread around it for later use.

4) Isolate the cervical shallow vein and place a thread under it, tie the cephalic end and make a "V" shape incision on the wall of it, and insert a polyethylene tubing that has been filled with saline and connected the other end with a 3 way stopcock for injection of the drugs and tie it with the thread tightly.

5) Ureters intubation (Figure 2-60).

① Clear the hair over the skin of lower abdomen. Make a middle incision of 5~7 cm long at the level 2 cm above the symphysis pubis.

② Cut through the abdominal muscles along the linear alba. Slit the peritoneum, and open the abdominal cavity.

③ Locate the urinary bladder and ureters on both sides near the base of it. Free the ureters by blunt dissection.

④ Put a piece of thread under one ureter at the level of 2~3 cm above the tie, and then make a ligation (tie a knot) near the bladder.

⑤ Make a "V" shape incision on the wall of the ureter, insert a polyethylene tubing filled with saline into the ureter, and fix it firmly. The urine is now draining through the tubing. Connect the tubule with a drop-meter, and record the drops of urine with BL-420 system.

⑥ After this operation, cover the opening of abdomen with a piece of gauze sucked in warm saline.

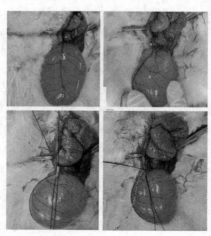

Figure 2-60   Ureter intubation
(refer to color picture on color pages)

6) Observations.

① Record the amount of urine as a control.

② Inject intravenously 20 mL of saline of 38℃. Record the change of urine volume and continue the next item after the urine volume returns to normal level.

③ Inject intravenously 0.5 mL of 0.01% noradrenaline. Record the change of urine volume and continue the next item after the urine volume returns to normal level.

④ Inject intravenously 5 mL 20% glucose of 38℃. Make a qualitative test of urine sugar before injection and repeat the test at the peak of increase in urine after injection.

⑤ Stimulate the peripheral end of the right vagus nerve. Record the change of urine volume and continue the next item after the urine volume returns to normal level.

⑥ Inject intravenously furosemide 5 mg/kg. Record the change of urine volume and continue the next item after the urine volume returns to normal level.

⑦ Inject intravenously 2 unit of pitressin.

⑧ Fill the results into Table 2-2, and you can also design your own table to record results.

Table 2-2 Influences of some factors on urine formation

Observations	Urine volume (drops/min)	Urine glucose (+/−)
Normal		
Saline		
Noradrenaline		
20% glucose		
Stimulate the right vagus nerve		
Furosemide		
ADH		

5. Cautions

1) Before and after each item, the drops of urine should be recorded as controls (the drop of urine before each item can be expressed by the normal drop of urine).

2) Proceed on the next item only when the effect of the last factor has subsided.

3) The vein of the outer ear edge should be protected for multiple injections. It is necessary to inject from the distal end firstly, and gradually move closer to the root.

4) Abdominal surgery should be done before the artery cannulation, lest the struggle of the rabbit makes the arterial cannula fall off or break the carotid artery wall, which causes the blood loss and even death of the rabbit.

6. Questions

1) How to avoid blood clotting which blocks the polyethylene tubing and affects the urine collection.

2) Will the urine volume increase greatly after the injection of hypertonic glucose? And why?

3) What is the mechanism of furosemide-induced diuresis? How to use furosemide in clinical situations?

Experiment 11　The analysis of reflex arc

1. Aims

To understand the relationship between the integrity of reflex arc and the performance of reflex action through analyzing the components of a reflex arc.

2. Principles

The structural basis of all kinds of reflexes is the reflex arc which includes five parts, namely, the receptors, the afferent fibers, the centers, the efferent fibers and the effectors. Flexor reflex happens when harmful stimulation to the skin produces contraction of the flexor of the limb in the stimulated side. This reflex can be realized by the spinal animal in which the spinal cord has been separated from the higher centers. And spinal animal means the animal in which the portion of the central nervous system other than the spinal cord is damaged by the experimenter.

In summary, reflex arc consists of a sense organ, an afferent neuron, the central nervous system, an efferent neuron, and an effector. Structural and functional integrity is the prerequisite of practicing reflex action. (Spinal animal means an animal in which the portion of the central nervous system other than the spinal cord are damaged by the experimenter)

3. Experimental materials

1) Animal: frogs.

2) Equipments: frog anatomy device, pithing needles, universal support stand, test tube holder, gauze, porcelain plate, beaker.

3) Reagents: Ringer's solution, 0.5% H_2SO_4 solution.

4. Procedures and observations

1) Preparation of a spinal frog. Make brain pithing only and keep the spinal intact. Clip the lower jaw with the test tube holder mounted on the support stand.

2) Place a few mL of 0.5% H_2SO_4 solution (sulfuric acid) into a petri dish.

3) Drop the frog's toe of the left or right hindlimb into the 0.5% H_2SO_4 solution (Figure 2-48A). See whether there is a flex or reflex. Wash the 0.5% H_2SO_4 left on the skin with tap water in the beaker. Dry the skin.

4) Make an incision of the skin at the lower part of the left or right hindlimb and take off the skin thoroughly. Repeat step 3) (Figure 2-48B).

5) Drop the frog's toe of the right hindlimb into the 0.5% H_2SO_4 solution. See whether there is a flex or reflex. Wash the 0.5% H_2SO_4 left on the skin with tap water in the beaker. Dry the skin.

6) Free the right sciatic nerve and make a double ligation on the nerve. Cut it between two ligatures (Figure 2-48C).

7) Repeat step 5) to see whether there is a flex or reflex (Figure 2-48D).

8) Stimulate the central and peripheral ends of the nerve, what will happen (Figure 2-48E)?

9) Take another frog and destroy its brain and spinal cord, repeat steps 3) or 5) to see whether the flexor reflex will happen.

5. Cautions

Each time after applying the sulfuric acid, the portion of the stimulated skin should be cleaned with tap water and wiped with a piece of gauze.

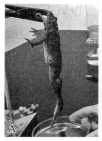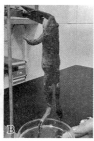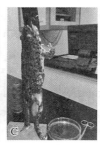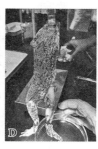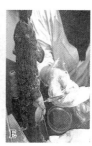

Figure 2-61   Analysis of flexor reflex arc on a frog

6. Questions

1) Who is the first person to propose the concept of spinal animal? Why do we need to make a spinal animal?

2) What reflex will be observed on the basis of flexor reflex if we increase the concentration of sulfuric acid?

3) What is the physiological significance of flexor reflex? What else manifestation will occur if we induce the flexor reflex in the intact body?

Experiment 12   Preparation and observation of hypoxia model

1. Aims

1) To establish the animal model of hypotonic hypoxia and hemic hypoxia.

2) To compare the changes in respiration, blood color and the pathogenesis of different types of hypoxia in mice.

2. Principles

Oxygen in the atmosphere enters the alveoli through respiration, diffuses into the blood and combines with hemoglobin, and then is transported to the whole body by blood circulation, and then used by tissues and cells. Hypoxia is a pathological process in which tissue oxygen supply is reduced or oxygen cannot be fully utilized, resulting in abnormal changes in tissue metabolism, function and morphological structure. According to the causes of hypoxia and the characteristics of blood oxygen changes, hypoxia can be divided into four types: hypotonic hypoxia, hemic hypoxia, circulating hypoxia and tissue hypoxia. Only hypotonic hypoxia and hemic hypoxia are replicated in this experiment.

1) Hypotonic hypoxia: There are 2 main causes of hypotonic hypoxia: hypoventilation and low pressure of O_2 (PO_2) in inspired air. The characters of hypotonic hypoxia are that the arterial blood PO_2 is below the normal range. As a result, the oxygen content and the hemoglobin O_2 saturation also fall down. During the experiment, the mouse is placed in an airtight flask with soda lime. Oxygen in the flask is consumed by the mouse while the carbon dioxide (CO_2) exhaled is absorbed by soda lime. Thus the PO_2 in the flask decreases gradually, while the concentration of CO_2 in the flask does not increase. This model is usually referred to as hypotonic hypoxia.

2) Hemic hypoxia: Hemic hypoxia is mainly caused by the low oxygen capacity of blood owing to the reduction of the amount of hemoglobin (Hb) or its ability to combine oxygen.

① **Carbon monoxide (CO) poisoning:** CO can combine with hemoglobin (Hb) to form carboxyhemoglobin (HbCO) and loses the oxygen carrying capacity. The affinity of HbCO is 210 times stronger than that of oxygen. A mouse is placed in a bottle linked to the CO generator. CO rapidly binds to hemoglobin to form carboxyhemoglobin that is unable to carry oxygen, leading to hemic hypoxia.

② **Nitrite poisoning:** The iron in hemoglobin is normally in ferrous state (Fe^{2+}). As a powerful oxidant, sodium Nitrite ($NaNO_2$) oxidizes the iron in hemoglobin to ferric state (Fe^{3+}), forming a methemoglobin (Hb-Fe^{3+}OH) that has lost the ability to carry oxygen. Via an intra-abdominal injection of sodium nitrite to the mouse in the experiment, the model of nitrite poisoning is established. Methylene blue is a reductant, which reduces the iron from Fe^{3+} to Fe^{2+} and the oxygen-carrying capacity of hemoglobin returns to normal when the mouse is injected with proper dose of methylene blue immediately after injection of $NaNO_2$.

$$\text{Hb-Fe}^{2+} \xrightarrow{\quad NaNO_2 \quad} \text{Hb-Fe}^{3+}$$

$$\text{Hb-Fe}^{3+} \xrightarrow{\quad \text{Methylene blue} \quad} \text{Hb-Fe}^{2+}$$

3. Experimental materials

1) Animal: adult mouse, 22~25 g, male or female.

2) Equipments: mouse hypoxia device (Figure 2-62), CO generator (Figure 2-62), scissors, tweezers, 1 mL syringes, 1 mL pipettes.

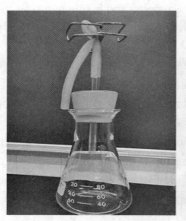 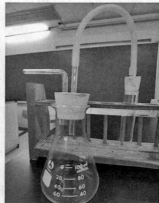

Figure 2-62   Mouse hypoxia device (left) and CO generator (right)

3) Reagents: soda lime (NaOH•CaO), formic acid, sulfuric acid, normal saline, 5% sodium nitrite solution, 1% methylene blue.

4. Procedures and observations

1) Hypotonic hypoxia (A): take one mouse and place it in a flask with sodium lime (5 g). Tighten the flask, clamp the rubber tube and seal the flask with water. Observe its general condition, respiratory rate, skin and mucous membrane color until death.

2) Blood hypoxia

① Carbon monoxide poisoning hypoxia (B): set up a CO generator according to Figure 2-62. Place a mouse in the bottle, observe its respiratory rate, color of skin and mucous membrane, and record its respiratory rate. Pour 4 mL formic acid into the test tube of the CO generator. Then add 2 mL of sulfuric acid slowly so that carbon monoxide is generated. Connect the bottle containing a mouse to the CO generator (refer to Appendix 4), measure the parameters as mentioned above.

② Nitrite poisoning hypoxia: select 2 mice (C and D), then treat the mice as follows.

C is intraperitoneally injected with 0.3 mL of saline immediately after intraperitoneal injection of 0.3 mL sodium nitrite (5%). Observe the changes in the general conditions, respiratory rate, color of skin and mucous membrane.

D is injected with 0.3 mL methylene blue (1%) immediately after the injection of 0.3 mL sodium nitrite (5%). Observe the changes in the general conditions, respiratory rate, color of skin and mucous membrane.

3) Control group (E): take one normal mouse as the control group and observe its general condition, respiratory rate, skin and mucous membrane color. Kill it after all other experiments are finished.

4) Open the abdominal cavity of the mouse A, B, C, D and E, and then compare the differences in color of the liver.

5) Fill the table 2-3 based on what you have observed and measured.

Table 2-3　Results

Mouse	Model	General activity	Respiratory rate	Skin and mucous membrane color	Liver color
A	Hypotonic hypoxia				
B	CO poisoning				
C	Nitrite poisoning				
D	Methylene blue treatment				
E	Control				

5. Cautions

1) The flask used to induce hypotonic hypoxia must be kept airtight by applying water to the interspace between the flask and rubber stopper, and between the glass tube and the rubber stopper.

2) In order to exclude the influence of age, the weight of mice in each group should be close.

3) Make the intraperitoneal injection accurately on the low left quadrant of abdomen to avoid the liver or bladder injury.

4) In the CO poisoning test, formic acid should be added first and then sulfuric acid. The spent acid must be collected in a special container after experiment.

5) Connect the bottle with CO generator immediately after the CO is produced. Do not seal up the tube exposed to atmosphere.

6. Questions

1) What are the differences in blood color in different type of hypoxia? Why?

2) What are the differences in respiratory patterns associated with different type of hypoxia? Why?

3) What is the key characteristic change in blood gas related to different type of hypoxia? What is the mechanism?

Experiment 13　Factors affecting hypoxic tolerance

1. Aims

1) To establish the mouse hypotonic hypoxia model.

2) To observe the effects of ambient temperature, nervous system activity and metabolic state on hypoxia tolerance in mice.

2. Principles

The tolerance to hypoxia is not only affected by the degree and speed of hypoxia, but also related to many other factors. Metabolic oxygen consumption rate is an important factor affecting the body's tolerance to hypoxia. When the basic metabolic rate is high, such as the increase of ambient temperature, hyperthyroidism, nervous system excitation, the metabolic oxygen consumption rate increases, and the body's tolerance to hypoxia decreases. However, when the ambient temperature decreases and the nervous system is inhibited, the metabolic oxygen consumption rate decreases and the body's tolerance to hypoxia increases. During this experiment, changing the ambient temperature, central stimulant (isoproterenol + coramine) and inhibitor (pentobarbital sodium) are used and the oxygen consumption and survival time of mice are observed to clarify factors affecting hypoxia tolerance.

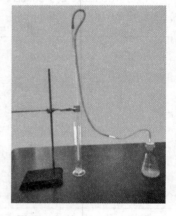

Figure 2-63　Apparatus for measuring oxygen consumption

3. Experimental materials

1) Animal: adult mouse, 22~25 g, male or female.

2) Equipments: mouse hypoxia device, scales (Figure 2-62), apparatus for measuring oxygen consumption (Figure 2-63), syringes, thermostatic bath.

3) Reagents: sodium lime (NaOH • CaO), normal saline, 0.5% sodium pentobarbital, isoprenaline (4 mg/100 mL) + nikethamide (1 g/100 mL) mixture.

4. Procedures and observations

1) Hypoxia tolerance affected by different ambient temperatures

① Place 5 g soda lime into each of the 3 flasks.

② Select 3 mice with similar body weight, put them into the 3 flasks respectively and label the flasks as A, B and C. Flask A is placed at room temperature, flask B is immersed in ice water and flask C is immersed in warm water (42 ℃). After adapted the mice in the specific temperatures for 5 min under the condition of flask A, B and C respectively, tighten each flask and clamp up the rubber tube to induce hypoxia.

③ Observe the activities, breathing pattern and skin color of the mice in the flasks and record the survival time. Remove the flask from ice or warm water as soon as the mouse is dead. After equilibrated at room temperature for 15 min, the flask is connected to an apparatus for measuring the oxygen consumption of the mouse (refer to Appendix 5).

④ Calculate the oxygen consumption rate (R) according to the following equation, where W is the weight of the mouse, T is the survival time, and A is the total volume of oxygen consumption.

$$R\,[\text{mL/(g}\cdot\text{min)}] = \frac{A\,(\text{mL})}{W\,(\text{g})\cdot T\,(\text{min})}$$

2) Hypoxia tolerance affected by different state of body metabolism

① Place 5 g soda lime into each of the 3 flasks.

② Select 3 mice with similar body weight. The animals are injected intraperitoneally with 0.1 mL/10 g · BW of normal saline (D), 0.1 mL/10 g · BW of 0.5% pentobarbital solution (E) and 0.1 mL/10 g · BW of isoprenaline + nikethamide mixture (F), respectively.

③ 5 min after injection, place the mice into the airtight flasks respectively, and clamp up the rubber tubes to induce hypoxia.

④ Observe the activities, breathing pattern and skin color of the mice in the bottles until the animals die, record the survival time.

⑤ Measure the volume of oxygen consumption and calculate the oxygen consumption rate of each mouse.

⑥ Fill in the data to Table 2-4.

Table 2-4   Results

Animal	Treatment	Weight W (g)	Survival time T (min)	Oxygen consumption A (mL)	Rate of oxygen consumption R [mL/(g · min)]
A	Room temperature				
B	0 ℃				
C	42 ℃				
D	Normal saline				
E	Pentobarbital sodium				
F	Isoprenaline+Nikethamide				

5. Cautions

1) Make the intraperitoneal injection accurately at the low left side of the abdomen.

2) All flasks must be kept airtight by applying water to the interspace between the bottle and rubber stopper, and between the glass tube and the rubber stopper.

3) Determine the oxygen consumption by reading the falling level of water in graduated cylinder of the measuring apparatus.

6. Questions

1) What is the cause of death in mice during the experiment?

2) State the factors affecting the tolerance to hypoxia, and explain how they work?

Experiment 14　Hyperkalemia and its rescue

1. Aims

1) To establish the animal model of hyperkalemia.

2) To observe the toxic effect of potassium on the heart and the characteristic of electrocardiogram in hyperkalemia.

3) To understand the principles of therapeutic strategy for hyperkalemia.

2. Principles

The normal potassium concentration in serum is 3.5~5.5 mmol/L. Hyperkalemia refers to a serum potassium concentration higher than 5.5 mmol/L. Hyperkalemia happens when potassium intake is increased, potassium excretion is decreased, or potassium shift from the intracellular fluid to the extracellular fluid. Hyperkalemia has a toxic effect on myocardium, such as fatal ventricular fibrillation and cardiac arrest. The irritability increases in the mild hyperkalemia and decreases in the severe hyperkalemia. The autonomy and conductivity of myocardium are reduced and contractility is weakened in the hyperkalemia. The above effects of hyperkalemia on cardiac action are usually manifested by changes in the electrocardiogram (ECG), including a sharp T wave, a lower P wave, a lower and wide QRS complex wave, as well as a prolonged P-R interval. During this experiment, 1% KCl is injected from the marginal ear vein to establish the animal model of hyperkalemia and the ECG is continuously monitored at the same time. The therapeutic measurements for rescuing arrhythmia (even cardiac arrest) induced by hyperkalemia are also performed with this animal model.

3. Experimental materials

1) Animal: rabbit, 2.0~2.5 kg, male or female.

2) Equipments: mammalian surgical instruments, dissecting table for rabbit, electrocardiograph (ECG), centrifuge, Na^+-K^+ analyzer, intravenous infusion device, syringe, scalp needle, 5 mL anticoagulant tube.

3) Reagents: 25% urethane solution, 0.3% heparin sodium solution, 1% potassium chloride (KCl), 4% sodium bicarbonate, 10% calcium chloride, 50% glucose solution, insulin, normal saline.

4. Procedures and observations

1) Operation preparation: The rabbit is weighted and anesthetized with 25% urethane solution (4 mL/kg) intravenously in the marginal ear vein. Fix a rabbit in supine position on the rabbit holder. Clean the surgical field in the cervical region by removing the fur with scissors.

2) The carotid artery cannula (Appendix 6): Make a 4~5 cm long longitudinal incision along the middle of the neck, separate the subcutaneous tissue and muscle layer by layer, and burst the trachea. Find the carotid artery sheath on the dorsolateral side of the trachea and carefully separate one side of the carotid artery (about 3 cm long). Ligate the distal end with a suture and clamp the proximal end with an artery clamp. The arterial catheter filled with 0.3% heparin sodium solution or 22G venous indwelling needle is inserted to the artery and fixed.

3) Blood collection and serum preparation: 1 mL blood is collected from the carotid artery and put into the anticoagulant tube. The blood is mixed up and down and centrifuged at 1000 *g* for 15 min, and then the supernatant is taken to detect the normal blood potassium concentration.

4) Stick the needle electrodes subcutaneously into the ankles of the corresponding limbs and make the correct settings as follows: RED-right forelimb, YELLOW-left forelimb, BLACK-right hindlimb and GREEN - left hindlimb.

5) Turn on the electrocardiograph, select Lead II or avF to record the normal electrocardiogram (ECG) for control.

6) Connect the infusion needle to the apparatus of intravenous transfusion. Get rid of all air bubbles in the tub. Insert the infusion needle into the marginal ear vein of the rabbit and fix it on the pinna of the ear securely with sticky tape. Begin at low dose, speed up the transfusion rate of 1% KCl to 60 ~80 drops/min according to the physical state of the rabbit.

7) Record the ECG every 2 min until the typical ECG of hyperkalemia is observed (a sharp T wave, a lower P wave, a lower and wide QRS complex, and a prolonged P-R interval). The serum samples are collected and the potassium concentration is measured again.

8) One of the following methods is used for rescue the hyperkalemic rabbit and record the ECG. The serum samples are collected and the potassium concentration is measured again.

① Intravenously inject 6~10 mL of 4% sodium bicarbonate slowly.

② Intravenously inject 1~2 mL of 10% calcium chloride slowly.

③ Intravenously inject 20 mL of 50% glucose solution containing 4 U of insulin slowly. Observe the change of electrocardiogram during injection.

9) Maintain the transfusion of KCl and record the ECG until the rabbit dies. Pay close attention to the change of ECG during the transfusion.

10) Dissect the rabbit, open the thorax and observe the situation of cardiac arrest.

11) Fill table 2-5 with what you have observed and measured.

Table 2-5   Results

Treatment	ECG	K^+ (mmol/L)
Control		
1% KCl		
4%NaHCO$_3$		
10%CaCl$_2$		
50% glucose + insulin		

5. Cautions

1) Inject urethane slowly and a fast injection may induce respiratory inhibition and sudden death of the animal. Add a small dose of urethane intravenously or 1% procaine as local infiltration anesthesia if the animal still has pain reaction during the experiment.

2) Some animals may need higher dose of KCl than others to induce abnormal changes in the ECG because of the different tolerance to hyperkalemia.

3) The electrocardiograph should be connected to the ground to avoid interference. Clean the

needle electrodes to keep them in good condition after use.

4) Control the speed of intravenous injection of KCl solution to prevent tachycardia. The speed of calcium injection to rescue hyperkalemia should be slow; otherwise it is easy to cause hyperkalemia and animal death.

6. Questions

1) What are the toxic effects of hyperkalemia on myocardium?

2) What are the ECG changes during hyperkalemia? Try to explain its possible mechanisms.

3) Is it in the state of diastole or systole when the cardiac arrest?

4) What are the principles of hyperkalemia rescue?

Experiment 15   Ischemia reperfusion injury in intestines

1. Aims

1) To establish an animal model of ischemia reperfusion injury in intestine.

2) To observe the pathological effects of intestinal ischemia/reperfusion on the blood pressure, small intestinal mesenteric microcirculation during intestinal ischemia-reperfusion injury. and discuss the possible mechanism of ischemia/reperfusion injury.

2. Principles

The restoration of blood flow after transient tissue ischemia, it not only fails to restore the organ function, but also associates with further irreversible cell damage, which is called ischemia-reperfusion injury. The mechanisms of ischemia-reperfusion injury have not been fully clarified. It is considered that the role of free radicals, intracellular calcium overload and leukocyte activation are important pathogenesis of ischemia-reperfusion injury. By clamping the superior mesenteric artery for a period of time, acute ischemia and structural injury on the barrier of intestinal mucous membrane in the intestine are developed, including extensive separation of epithelium and villi, epithelial necrosis, massive neutrophil infiltration, destruction of lamina propria, bleeding and ulcer formation. At this time, reopening the superior mesenteric artery and returning the blood flow into intestinal tissue may not recover the functions of the barrier of the intestinal mucous membrane. On the contrary, the intestinal mucosal injury and intestinal wall capillary permeability are even higher. As a result, severe damage of the intestines occurs, more toxic materials in the enteric cavity are absorbed into the systemic circulation and the toxemia results in hypotension.

3. Experimental materials

1) Animal: rabbit, 2.0~2.5 kg, male or female.

2) Equipments: mammalian surgical instruments, dissecting table for rabbit, BL-420 system, microcirculation perfusion device, dynamic microcirculation image analysis system, pressure transducer, arterial clamp, suture, syringe, 100 mL beaker, arterial catheter, three-way valve, gauze.

3) Reagents: 25% urethane, 1% procaine, 0.3% heparin sodium solution, normal saline.

4. Procedures and observations

1) Operation preparation: The rabbit is weighted and anesthetized with 25% urethane (4 mL/kg) intravenously in the marginal ear vein. Fix a rabbit in supine position on the dissecting table for rabbit. Clean the surgical field in the cervical region by removing the fur with scissors.

2) Separation of superior mesenteric artery: At 5 cm below the xiphoid, make a 5~10 cm long midline incision. Follow the Linea Alba in the upper abdominal wall, open the peritoneal cavity. Push the intestines to the left side to expose the right kidney. Locate and isolate the root of the superior mesenteric artery below the right hilum, threading a suture as a marker for further use.

3) Observation of mesenteric microcirculation: Find the ileocecal junction at the right lower abdomen, and remove a section of ileum connected with the appendix through fascia where the mesentery is long and convenient for observation. Lay the mesentery on the stage in the perfusion box, select the appropriate position (containing arteries, veins, arteriovenous anastomotic branches and capillaries in the view) to observe. Observe the normal mesenteric microcirculation with an anatomical microscope (flow pattern, flow rate and caliber).

Flow pattern is divided according to the morphology of blood flow in capillary vessels.

Grade 0 (line): the blood flow can be observed clearly but not the shape of blood cells.

Grade I (granular): the morphology of blood cells can be observed clearly.

Grade II (stasis): the blood cells stop moving or swing back and forth.

Flow rate: the flow rate can be read using the software.

Caliber: a proper position with clear vascular edge is selected and the diameters are measured using the software.

4) Inject 1 mL heparin sodium solution intravenously for anti-coagulation.

5) The carotid artery cannula (Appendix 6): Make a 4~5 cm long longitudinal incision along the middle of the neck, separate the subcutaneous tissue and muscle layer by layer, and burst the trachea. Find the carotid artery sheath on the dorsolateral side of the trachea and carefully separate one side of the carotid artery (about 3 cm long). Ligate the distal end with a suture and clamp the proximal end with an artery clamp. The arterial catheter filled with 0.3% heparin sodium solution or 22G venous indwelling needle is inserted to the artery. After ligation and restraint, it is connected with BL-420 system through the pressure transducer, and the normal arterial blood pressure curve is recorded (systolic pressure, diastolic pressure and mean arterial pressure).

6) Establish animal model of the ischemia/reperfusion injury in intestine: Clamp the superior mesenteric artery with artery clamp for 30~60 min. Put the intestinal back into the abdominal cavity and clamp the intestinal wall with two forceps. Cover the abdominal incision with saline gauze. The arterial blood pressure and mesenteric microcirculation are observed during superior mesenteric artery occlusion.

Release the artery clamp to recover the blood perfusion of the intestines and touch the distal end of the superior mesenteric artery with your finger. It indicates that the blood flow of the small intestine is restored an arterial pulse can be feel. The arterial blood pressure and mesenteric microcirculation are recorded at 0 min, 5 min, 15 min and 30 min after ligation separately.

7) Animal euthanasia: Double dose of urethan is injected intravenously to euthanize the animal after finishing the experiment.

5. Cautions

1) Inject urethane slowly and a fast injection may induce respiratory inhibition and sudden death of the animal. A small amount of 1% procaine can be used as local infiltration anesthesia if

the animal still has pain reaction during the experiment.

2) Turn the intestines gently to avoid hypotension caused by excessive pulling of the intestines.

3) Do not use sharp instruments to separate superior mesenteric artery avoid of vessel damage.

4) Release of the artery clamp may not recover the blood perfusion in the intestines sometimes because the arterial wall may be sticky together by clumping. Using your fingers to massage the artery softly will help to restore the blood perfusion.

6. Questions

1) What is the change in mean arterial pressure during the experiment? Describe the possible mechanisms.

2) What is the change of mesenteric microcirculation before and after reperfusion? Discuss the possible causes and mechanisms.

Experiment 16　Hemorrhagic shock

1. Aims

1) To establish the model of hemorrhagic shock in rabbit.

2) To observe the changes of mean arterial pressure, microcirculation and hemodynamics before and after shock treatment. and explore the pathogenesis, pathophysiological process and treatment principles of hemorrhagic shock.

2. Principles

Shock is a pathological process in which the effective circulating blood volume decreases sharply and the tissue perfusion is seriously insufficient under the pathogenic factors such as severe blood loss, infection and trauma, resulting in widespread impairment of cellular metabolism. The blood pressure and tissue perfusion can be maintained basically by compensation when the blood is lost less than $10\% \sim 15\%$ of the total blood volume within $15\sim20$ minutes. However, the hemorrhagic shock will happen when the blood is lost more than 20% of the total blood volume within 15 minutes. During this experiment, the blood pressure of rabbits is maintained at 40% of normal blood pressure for a long time by femoral artery bleeding in order to induce the hemorrhagic shock model, and different therapeutic measures, such as blood infusion and vasoactive drugs, are also applied in this experiment.

3. Experimental materials

1) Animal: rabbit, 2.0~2.5 kg, male or female.

2) Equipments: mammalian surgical instruments, dissecting table for rabbit, BL-420 system, pressure transducer, arterial clamp, artery catheter, suture, three-way valve, syringe, scalp needle.

3) Reagents: 25% urethane solution, 1% procaine solution, 0.3% heparin sodium solution, normal saline, norepinephrine, anisodamine (654-2).

4. Procedures and observations

1) Operation preparation: The rabbit is weighted and anesthetized with 25% urethane (4 mL/kg) intravenously in the marginal ear vein. Fix a rabbit in supine position on the dissecting table for rabbit. Clean the surgical field in the cervical ,stomach, and groin regions by removing the fur with scissors.

2) The carotid artery and femoral artery cannula (Appendix 6).

① Isolate the carotid artery and femoral artery in the neck and groin.

② Inject l mL heparin sodium solution intravenously for anti-coagulation.

③ Ligate the artery at the end far from the heart and place a suture under the artery at the end near to the heart.

④ Insert the artery catheter filled with heparin sodium solution into the femoral artery and connect it to a 50 mL syringe containing 20 mL of 0.3% heparin sodium solution for releasing blood.

⑤ Insert the artery catheter filled with heparin sodium solution into the carotid artery and connect it to the BL-420 system through a pressure transducer for monitoring blood pressure (BP).

3) Observation of mesenteric microcirculation: find the ileocecal junction at the right lower abdomen, and remove a section of ileum connected with the appendix through fascia where the mesentery is long and convenient for observation. Lay the mesentery on the stage in the perfusion box, select the appropriate position (containing arteries, veins, arteriovenous anastomotic branches and capillaries in the view) to observe. Observe the normal mesenteric microcirculation with an anatomical microscope (flow pattern, flow rate and caliber).

Flow pattern: is divided according to the morphology of blood flow in capillary vessels.

Grade 0(line): the blood flow can be observed clearly but not the shape of blood cells.

Grade I (granular): the morphology of blood cells can be observed clearly.

Grade II (stasis): the blood cells stop moving or swing back and forth.

Flow rate: the flow rate can be read using the software.

Caliber: a proper position with clear vascular edge is selected and the diameters are measured using the software.

4) Establish of shock model.

① After the blood pressure is stable, release blood from the femoral artery via the 50 mL syringe containing 20 mL of 0.3% heparin sodium solution. When the blood pressure drops to 3/4 of the baseline value, stop releasing blood and observe the compensatory responses of the rabbit (the changes of BP) for 10 min.

② Continuously release blood from the femoral artery via the 50 mL syringe to 40% of the baseline value and maintain this level for 30 min. Observe the mesenteric microcirculation (flow pattern, flow velocity and caliber).

5) Treatments: the following ① or ② treatment can be selected respectively and observe the blood pressure as well as mesenteric microcirculation (flow pattern, flow velocity and caliber) after treatment.

① Blood transfusion: make the blood transfusion by inputting back all arterial blood released from the femoral artery and observe the changes of blood pressure. 654-2 (10 mg/animal) is injected intravenously through the ear margin vein before and after blood transfusion, and the changes of blood pressure are observed.

② Vasoactive drug use: inject 2 mL norepinephrine (75 μg/mL) through the ear margin and observe the changes of blood pressure. When the blood pressure drops back to the level before injection, give the second injection of 2 mL norepinephrine through the ear margin vein. The third injection of 2 mL norepinephrine will be made when the blood pressure drops back to the level before injection again. Compare the blood pressure responses of the 3 injections.

6) Animal euthanasia: Double dose of urethan is injected intravenously to euthanize the animal after finishing the experiment.

5. Cautions

1) Inject the urethane slowly. A fast injection may induce respiratory inhibition and sudden death of the animal. A small amount of 1% procaine can be used as local infiltration anesthesia if the animal still has pain reaction during the experiment.

2) Pay attention to distinguish between arteries and veins. The arteries are thin with light red or bright red and pulsation.

3) The artery catheter should be filled up with 0.3% heparin sodium solution before use. 20 mL of 0.3% heparin sodium solution must be left in the 50 mL syringe to prevent the blood from coagulation.

4) The ileocecal loop should be used to observe the mesenteric microcirculation because of its long mesentery and less fat. Turn the intestines gently and keep the intestine warm to avoid hypotension caused by excessive pulling of the intestines.

6. Questions

1) How can you make a correct judgment on the occurrence of shock? What symptoms and signs can help you to make the diagnosis in this experiment?

2) Describe the changes of mean arterial blood pressure during the experiment and try to discuss the pathophysiological mechanism.

3) What are the characteristics of the microcirculation before and after shock treatment. Discuss the pathogenesis and compensatory responses of the microcirculatory changes.

4) Why the blood pressure cannot be maintained stably by injection of norepinephrine only in shock rabbit? What are the differences of the blood pressure responses in the three injections of norepinephrine?

5) What is the difference of the blood pressure responses between the two injections of anisodamine in the experiment? What are the principles of using vasodilator?

Experiment 17　Acute right heart failure

1. Aims

1) To establish a model of acute right heart failure, and observe the main changes of hemodynamics in acute right heart failure.

2) To explore the etiology and pathogenesis of acute right heart failure.

2. Principles

Heart failure is the pathophysiological process in which the systolic and/or diastolic function of the heart is impaired, and as a result, cardiac output decreases and is unable to meet the metabolic demands of the body. The underlying causes include primary myocardial diastolic and systolic dysfunction and overload of myocardium, including pressure overload (afterload) and volume load (preload). In this experiment, pulmonary arteriole embolism (intravenous injection of liquid paraffin) and excessive transfusion will be used to increase the afterload and preload of the right heart. The mean arterial blood pressure and central venous pressure are observed to indicate the pathogenesis of heart failure.

3. Experimental materials

1) Animal: rabbit, 2.0~2.5 kg, male or female.

2) Equipments: mammalian surgical instruments, dissecting table for rabbit, BL-420 system, pressure transducer, arterial clamp,suture, syringe, scalp needle, three-way valve, arterial catheter (or 22G venous indwelling needle), intravenous transfusion device, central venous pressure determinator (Figure 2-64).

3) Reagents: 25% urethane solution, 1% procaine solution, 0.3% heparin sodium solution, normal saline, liquid paraffin.

4. Procedures and observations

1) Operation preparation: The rabbit is weighted and anesthetized with 25% urethane (4 mL/kg) intravenously in the marginal ear vein. Fix a rabbit in supine position on the dissecting table for rabbit. Clean the surgical field in the cervical region by removing the fur with scissors.

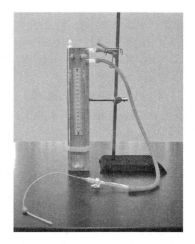

Figure 2-64   Central venous pressure determinator

2) Isolation of carotid artery and jugular vein: Make a 4~5 cm long longitudinal incision along the middle of the neck, separate the subcutaneous tissue and muscle layer by layer, and burst the trachea Isolate one side of the carotid artery and two sides of the jugular veins.

3) Inject 1 mL heparin sodium solution intravenously for anti-coagulation.

4) The carotid artery cannula (Appendix 6): Ligate the distal end with a suture and clamp the proximal end with an artery clamp. The arterial catheter filled with 0.3% heparin sodium solution or a 22G venous indwelling needle is inserted to the artery. After ligation and fixation, it is connected with BL-420 system through the pressure transducer, and the normal arterial blood pressure curve is recorded (systolic pressure, diastolic pressure and mean arterial pressure).

5) The jugular vein cannula (Appendix 6).

① Adjust the "0" position of the central venous pressure determinator to the altitude of the midaxillary line.

② Insert one catheter, which is connected to the central venous pressure determinator, into the right side of jugular vein. During the cannula, the liquid level of the central venous pressure determinator falls continuously. When the tube is inserted in about 5~6 cm, the liquid level stops dropping and fluctuates with the breathing movement. Fix the artery catheter securely and record the normal center vein pressure (CVP).

③ Insert another catheter into the left side of jugular vein. Link it to the normal saline transfusion apparatus at a speed of less than 10 drops/min.

6) Establishment of rabbit model of acute right heart failure.

① Make venipuncture at the marginal ear vein of the rabbit with an infusion needle, slowly inject 38℃ liquid paraffin at speed of 0.1 mL/min with a 2 mL syringe and closely observe the changes of BP and CVP. Stop injection when arterial BP decreases by 10~20 mmHg or CVP increases by 20~30 mmH$_2$O (the total dose of liquid paraffin is no more than 1 mL/kg).

② Speed up the normal saline transfusion to 80~100 drops/min intravenously until the rabbit dies. The changes of BP and CVP are observed.

7) Open the chest and abdominal cavity and observe the appearance of the lung, heart, mesenteric vessels, intestinal wall and liver. Make sure whether there is pleural effusion and ascites.

5. Cautions

1) Inject the urethane slowly. A fast injection may induce respiratory inhibition and sudden death of the animal. A small amount of 1% procaine can be used as local infiltration anesthesia if the animal still has pain reaction during the experiment.

2) Fill the central venous pressure determinator and the artery catheters with 0.3% heparin sodium solution to avoid clotting.

3) Control the volume and injection speed of liquid paraffin and the changes of BP and CVP should be observed at any time. When one of the indicators changes sharply, the injection speed should be slowed down.

4) Try to add a little more liquid paraffin if the transfusion volume of normal saline is over 200 mL/kg and heart failure is still not induced.

6. Questions

1) What symptoms and physical signs can help you to judge the development of acute right heart failure? Why?

2) What are the factors affecting central venous pressure? Try to describe the mechanisms of elevated central venous pressure in right heart failure.

3) What are the main pathophysiological changes in right heart failure?

4) What is the clinical significance of central venous pressure in the diagnosis and treatment of heart failure?

Experiment 18　Respiratory failure

1. Aims

1) To establish different animal models of respiratory failure (suffocation, pneumothorax and pulmonary edema), and observe the changes of blood gas and respiration curve in different types of respiratory failure.

2) To understand the mechanisms of pulmonary ventilation and ventilation dysfunction in respiratory failure.

2. Principles

Respiratory failure is a pathological process in which the external respiratory dysfunction leads to an abnormal decrease of arterial partial pressure of oxygen (PaO_2) with or without carbon dioxide retention. According to the characteristics of blood gas, it is divided into type I respiratory failure (hypoxic respiratory failure, $PaO_2 < 60$ mmHg) and type II respiratory failure (hypercapnic respiratory failure, $PaO_2 < 60$ mmHg and $PaCO_2 > 50$ mmHg). The main causes of respiratory failure are ventilation disorder (restrictive and obstructive hypoventilation) and gas exchange disorder (diffusion impairment, ventilation-perfusion imbalance, anatomical shunt). In this experiment, the type II respiratory failure model is established by suffocation and type I respiratory failure model is establish by intratracheal instillation of 20% glucose. Furthermore, pneumothorax is artificially induced in rabbit to establish acute respiratory dysfunction caused by restrictive hypoventilation and ventilation-perfusion imbalance.

3. Experimental materials

1) Animal: rabbit, 2.0~2.5 kg, male or female.

2) Equipments: mammalian surgical instruments, dissecting table for rabbit, BL-420 system, respiratory sensor, arterial catheter, Y-shape tracheal cannula, suture, syringe, arterial clamp, needle (18-0), clamp, three-way valve, blood gas analyzer.

3) Reagents: 25% urethane solution, 1% procaine solution, 20% glucose solution.

4. Procedures and observations

1) Operation preparation: The rabbit is weighted and anesthetized with 25% urethane (4 mL/kg) intravenously in the marginal ear vein. Fix a rabbit in supine position on the dissecting table for rabbit. Clean the surgical field in the cervical region by removing the fur with scissors.

2) The carotid artery cannula (Appendix 6): make a cervical median incision and isolate the carotid artery and trachea. Inject an arterial catheter into the carotid artery and 0.5 mL of blood is taken from the carotid artery for blood gas analysis.

3) The trachea cannual (Appendix 6): Make a T-shaped incision 0.5~1 cm below the thyroid cartilage of the trachea and insert a Y-shape tracheal cannula toward the lung. Fix it firmly with a suture. Connect the BL-420 system through the respiratory sensor to record the respiratory frequency and depth. Record the respiratory frequency and depth.

4) Establish the model of suffocation: Clamp up the rubber tube connected to the Y-shape tracheal cannula with clamp for 30 s and Record the breathing curves. Release the clamp and let the animal recover from suffocation until the breathing waves return to normal. Take 0.5 mL arterial blood for blood gas analysis after clamping for about 25 s.

5) Establish the model of pneumothorax: Locate the 4th or 5th intercostal space on the right side of midaxillary line. Make a small cut to open the skin under local anesthesia with procaine. Insert a needle (18-0) connected to a 50 mL syringe via a three-way stopcock into the thoracic cavity (a sense of sudden disappearance of resistance will be experienced when the needle gets properly into the pleural cavity). Inject 30 mL air slowly into the pleural cavity. Collect the blood sample when the rabbit has obvious changes in respiration curve and cyanosis of oral and lip mucosa. If the changes are not obvious, continue to inject air (30 mL/injection) until the changes can be observed. Drain off all the air from the pleural cavity with the 50 mL syringe and remove the needle rapidly. Wait for 10~20 min until the respiration of the rabbit returns to normal.

6) Establish the model of pulmonary edema: Elevate the head side of the dissecting table for rabbit about 5 cm. Inject 20% glucose 2 mL slowly (drop by drop) into the trachea through one branch of the Y-shape tracheal cannula. Observe the changes in breathing frequency and depth. Record the breathing curves until the bubbles show up from the trachea. If the bubbles do not show up 20 min after injection, add 1~2 mL glucose as described above.

7) Animal euthanasia: Double dose of urethan is injected intravenously to kill the rabbit.

8) Open the chest and observe the pathologic changes of the lungs. Carve up the lungs and observe whether bubble-like exudate effuses or not.

5. Cautions

1) Drain off all the air from the pleural cavity after the pneumothorax is established as soon

as possible.

2) Inject glucose solution into the Y-shape tracheal cannula slowly (drop by drop). A fast injection will cause suffocation.

6. Questions

1) What are the characteristics of blood gas changes in different types of respiratory failure models? Try to explain the possible mechanisms.

2) What type of respiratory failure is established in this experiment by suffocation, pulmonary edema or pneumothorax?

3) What pathological changes of the lung can be observed? Try to give the explanations.

Experiment 19   The role of ammonia in the pathogenesis of hepatic encephalopathy

1. Aims

1) To establish an animal model of acute hepatic dysfunction.

2) To discuss the role of elevated blood ammonia in the pathogenesis of hepatic encephalopathy.

2. Principles

Hepatic encephalopathy (HE) is a complex, potentially reversible disturbance in central nervous system that occurs as a consequence of severe liver disease. The mechanisms responsible for HE are undefined. The following hypotheses are generally recognized to explain the pathogenesis of HE, such as ammonia intoxication, false neurotransmitters, amino acid imbalance, and the γ-aminobutyric acid hypothesis, etc. In this experiment, the acute hepatic insufficiency resulting from ligation of most liver lobes combined with injection of ammonium chloride solution will result in the rapid increase in blood ammonia, thus the animal will show some symptoms similar to hepatic encephalopathy, such as convulsions, coma and spasm. This demonstrates the pathogenesis of ammonia intoxication in hepatic encephalopathy. Another animal is injected with normal saline instead of ammonium chloride solution after most of the liver lobes are ligated, in order to demonstrate that "acute hepatic insufficiency" itself is not enough to cause hepatic encephalopathy during the experiment under the same condition without injection of ammonium chloride solution. The third animal, without ligation of the liver lobes, is injected with the same amount of ammonium chloride solution as the first one, and it usually does not present any symptom. This demonstrates that the liver has detoxifying functions for ammonia.

3. Experimental materials

1) Animal: rabbit, 2.0~2.5 kg, male or female.

2) Equipments: mammalian surgical instruments, dissecting table for rabbit, syringe, urinary catheter, cotton thread.

3) Reagents: 1% procaine solution, 2.5% compound ammonium chloride solution (25 g ammonium chloride, 15 g sodium bicarbonate, dissolved in 1000 mL 5% glucose solution), 2.5% compound sodium chloride solution (25 g sodium chloride, 15 g sodium bicarbonate, dissolved in 1000 mL 5% glucose solution).

4. Procedures and observations

1) Operation preparation: Three rabbits with similar weight are weighed and fixed in supine

position on the dissecting table for rabbit. Clean the surgical field in the upper abdominal wall by removing the fur with scissors. Inject 1% procaine solution (5~10 mL/ region) subcutaneously in the incision site to make a local anesthesia.

2) Ligation of liver lobes: Make a 6~8 cm long midline incision on the upper abdominal wall below the xiphoid. Follow the linea alba abdominis in the upper abdominal wall, open the peritoneal cavity and expose the liver located in the right upper abdomen. Press the liver down on both sides of the sickle ligament with the index and middle fingers of the left hand, and cut the falciform ligament between the liver and the diaphragm with scissor. Turn the liver lobe up, and separate the liver and hepatogastric ligament to dissociate the liver. Ligate the left outer lobe, left middle lobe, right middle lobe and quadrate lobe of the liver at the root firmly by a cotton thread. Leave the caudate lobe and the right outer lobe free.

3) Intestinal cannula: Make a purse-string suture on the duodenum. Snip a small incision and insert a urinary catheter (or plastic tube) about 4 cm depth into the duodenum and fix it. Suture the incision of the abdominal wall. Fix the outer end of the urinary catheter on the rabbit's ear.

4) Release the animal from the dissecting table for rabbit, observe the reactions of the rabbit, such as respiration, pupil size, corneal reflex, limb muscle tension and response to pain stimulation.

5) Experimental groups:

Group A (Model group). Do the experiment following the steps 2) ~ 4). Inject 5 mL of NH_4Cl via the urinary catheter in every 5 min until onset of spasm, convulsion and ankylosis (angular tension). At the same time, record the time and dose used and calculate the dosage per kg body weight of the rabbit.

Group B (Sham group). Do the experiment as group A, but do not ligate the lobes of the liver.

Group C (Control group). Do the experiment as group A, but inject the same dose of 2.5% compound sodium chloride solution instead of NH_4Cl.

Record the dosage of drug in table 2-6.

Table 2-6   Results

Group	Ligation of liver lobes	Drug	Dose	Total dose
A	Yes	NH_4Cl	5 mL/5 min	
B	No	NH_4Cl	5 mL/5 min	
C	Yes	NaCl	5 mL/5 min	

5. Cautions

1) In order to eliminate the influence of anesthetics on animal nervous system, 1% procaine was injected subcutaneously for local infiltration anesthesia.

2) Move the liver out smoothly to expose the liver lobes. Make sure that the thread is on the root of the liver avoid damaging the liver lobes and bleeding.

3) Pay attention to avoid injuring the diaphragm when cutting the falciform ligament.

4) Select the position to make purse-string suturing on the duodenum wall where the blood

vessels are sparse. Fix the urinary catheter onto the duodenum securely to prevent the compound ammonium chloride solution from leaking out of the duodenum into the peritoneal cavity.

6. Questions

1) Describe the basic viewpoint of ammonia intoxication hypothesis in the pathogenesis of hepatic encephalopathy according the results.

2) Describe the causes of hepatic encephalopathy according to the composition of compound ammonium chloride solution and discuss how to prevent hepatic encephalopathy.

3) What are the clinical manifestations and laboratory tests of patients with hepatic encephalopathy?

Experiment 20   Influence of administration route on drug action

1. Aim

To observe the influence of administration route on pharmacological action of magnesium sulfate.

2. Principle

Different administration routes do not only affect the onset, strength and sustainability of drug action, they also lead to "quantitative difference" (i.e. different action intensity with the same effect) and "qualitative difference" (i.e. different pharmacological effects).In some occasions, the nature of the drug action results in different pharmacological effects. Magnesium sulfate, when taken orally, it can not be systemically absorbed but acts as a osmotic laxatives for constipation. However, when is injected and enter the blood circulation, magnesium sulfate produces systemic action and therefore it is often used for the treatment of eclampsia by injection in clinic.

3. Experimental materials

1) Animal: 4 mice, 18~22 g.

2) Equipments: syringe,mouse gastric lavage needle, mouse cage.

3) Reagents: 4% magnesium sulfate solution.

4. Procedures and observations

1) Four mice are weighed and labelled. Four mice are received 4% magnesium sulfate solution at a dose of 0.2 mL /10 g · BW, two by i.p. (intraperitoneal) while the other two via gastric gavage.

2) Observe the symptoms and record them in table 2-7 accordingly.

Table 2-7   The Influence of administration routes on drug action

Mouse number	Weight (g)	Drug/ Dosage	Route of administration	Before giving drug		After giving drug		Stool
				Tension of muscle	Breath	Tension of muscle	Breath	
1								
2								
3								
4								

5. Cautions

1) Pay attention not to put the gastric perfusion needle into the trachea, so as to avoid suffocation of animals; If the mouse given drug by orally, presents any signs of suppression or even respiratory paralysis and death, it must be due to technical errors.

2) During intraperitoneal injection, the position and angle (30° ~45°) of the injection site (middle and lower abdomen) should be mastered to avoid injury to internal organs.

3) If obvious muscle relaxation and severe respiratory depression are found after administration, 0.2 mL calcium chloride can be injected intraperitoneally for rescue treatment.

6. Questions

1) Why do animals have different drug effects when the same dose of the same drug is administered in different ways?

2) Can you discuss the pharmacological mechanism and clinical application of magnesium sulfate? How to rescue when excessive magnesium sulfate poisoning?

Experiment 21   Dose-effect relationship of drugs

1. Aim

The dose-effect relationship of acetylcholine (ACh) was studied with rabbit isolated intestine as the experimental observation object.

2. Principle

In vitro intestinal experiment can be used to observe the effects of drugs on the relaxation and contraction function of small intestinal smooth muscle. ACh can activate the M-receptor on rabbit small intestine and make it contract, and its contractility increases regularly with the increase of ACh concentration. The pharmacological effect is dose-dependent. So, it can be used to quantitatively analyze the relevant pharmacodynamic parameters, such as E_{max} (maximum effect) and EC_{50} (half-maximum effect concentration, produce 50% maximum effect at this concentration).

3. Experimental materials

1) Animal: rabbit, 2.0~2.5 kg.

2) Equipments: mammalian surgical instruments, dissecting table for rabbit, thermostatic smooth muscle bath, tension transducer, BL-420 system，1 mL sampler, syringe, beaker, petri dishes, oxygen cylinders, etc.

3) Reagents: acetylcholine chloride solution (10^{-7} mol/L, 10^{-6} mol/L, 10^{-5} mol/L, 10^{-4} mol/L, 10^{-3} mol/L, 10^{-2} mol/L, 10^{-1} mol/L), Tyrode's solution, 25% urethane solution.

4. Procedures and observations

1) Animals are fasted for 12 h before the experiment.

2) Adjust the constant temperature smooth muscle bath 3 h before the experiment by adding water in the bath and keep the water temperature at 37℃.

3) Preparation of intestinal tube: After injecting 25% urethane (4 mL/kg) intravenously into the ear margin to anesthetize the rabbit, open the abdominal cavity quickly to find the junction of gastric pylorus and duodenum as the starting point, then cut and take out about 20 cm long intestinal tube by cutting off the mesentery connected with this segment of intestinal tube along

the intestinal margin, quickly put the intestinal tube in the Tyrode's solution at about 4℃, and rinse the contents of intestinal cavity with Tyrode's solution, Separate the intestine into 2~3 cm long segments and put them in Tyrode's solution at about 4℃ for future use; The rest part of intestine which is placed in a refrigerator at 4℃ can be used within 12 h.

4) Hanging the specimen: Add 20 mL of Tyrode's solution into the bath tube and adjust the air inlet to let 1~2 bubbles in per second. Fix both ends of the intestinal segment with suture. One end is tied to the L-shaped hook and put into the bath tube. The other end is connected to the tension transducer with thread, and then connected to the BL-420F biological function system. When the intestinal tube is completely relaxed, the muscle tension size (X g) is recorded by the system, then the tightness of the line is adjusted by setting the tension degree at the value larger than that measured at the complete relaxation status (X+2~3 g). After adjusting the appropriate muscle tension, the intestinal segment was placed in the specimen slot and stabilized for 10 min, and then the next step will be continued.

5) Open BL-420 system, click the pharmacological experiment module (effect of drugs on isolated intestine) and start to record the contraction curve.

6) Dosing: Record a section of pre dosing curve as a control. Add ACh of different concentrations according to the following table. Each time, when the contraction curve does not rise, rinse it with Tyrode's solution for three times, then stabilize it for 5~10 min, and then add ACh of the next concentration in sequence, and so on.

7) Figure drawing: Measure the maximum tension of small intestine (g), that is, the maximum amplitude of rise of contraction curve, and fill in the following table. Draw the dose-effect curve with E as Y and LG (d) as X, and input the data into the prepared Excel table to generate the corresponding dose-effect curve.

Table 2-8   Experimental data

Drug sequence	ACh concentration (mol/L)	ACh volume (mL)	ACh concentration in the bath tube (mol/L)	X (g)	Amplitude of contraction (g)
1	10^{-7}	0.2	10^{-9}		
2	10^{-6}	0.2	10^{-8}		
3	10^{-5}	0.2	10^{-7}		
4	10^{-4}	0.2	10^{-6}		
5	10^{-3}	0.2	10^{-5}		
6	10^{-2}	0.2	10^{-4}		
7	10^{-1}	0.2	10^{-3}		

5. Cautions

1) Avoid injury when preparing intestinal segments. Try to operate in Tyrode's solution and do not expose them to air for too long.

2) Keep the intestine in appropriate tension , the thread and intestinal segment should not be

close to the pipe wall.

3) The dosage must be accurate and ACh should be added on the liquid level, but not on the intestinal segment directly.

4) Once the experiment starts, the transducer and various parameters shall not be adjusted to keep stable until the experiment is over..

6. Question

What are the characteristic parameters of dose-effect curve and what is the significance of these parameters?

Experiment 22　Influence of hepatic function on the hypnotic effect of pentobarbital sodium

1. Aim

To observe the influence of impaired liver function on drug actions.

2. Principle

Pentobarbital sodium is predominantly cleared and deactivated by the liver. The state of liver function directly affects its metabolic process, such as blood drug concentration and duration, so as to affect the strength and duration of its pharmacological action, and finally affect the pharmacological action of pentobarbital sodium, i.e. sleep time and sleep duration. Carbon tetrachloride is a colorless, toxic and volatile liquid with a slightly sweet smell of chloroform. It can dissolve many substances such as fat and paint; It has a serious toxic effect on hepatocytes. It is a common tool drug to establish an animal model of toxic liver damage. (if pentobarbital sodium cannot be obtained, 3% urethane can be used instead for the experiment)

3. Experimental materials

1) Animal: 4 mice,18~22 g.

2) Equipments: syringe,mouse gastric lavage needle, mouse cage.

3) Reagents: 5% carbon tetrachloride solution, 0.3% pentobarbital sodium solution, normal saline, picric acid.

4. Procedures and observations

1) Take 4 healthy mice, male or female, and number them as A1, A2 and B1, B2 after weighing.

2) 48 hours before the formal experiment, the mice in group A were injected subcutaneously (subcutaneously, intraperitoneally or by gavage) 0.1 mL/10 g·BW of 5% carbon tetrachloride oil solution to make models, and the mice in group B were subcutaneously injected with normal saline 0.1 mL/10 g·BW as comparison.

3) During the formal experiment, mice in groups A and B were intraperitoneally injected with 0.3% sodium pentobarbital 0.15 mL/10 g·BW.

4) Observe the reaction of the mice after administration, record the time of falling asleep (from administration to disappearance of righting reflex) and sleep duration (disappearance of righting reflex to recovery), and fill in the results in Table 2-9, The results of each group in the whole room were combined for the between-group t-test.

Table 2-9　The influence of liver function on drug actions

Mouse number	Weight (g)	Liver function	Drug/Dosage	Given time	Sleeping time	Sleep duration	Liver appearance
A1		CCl_4					
A2		CCl_4					
B1		saline					
B2		saline					

5. Cautions

1) If the room temperature is lower than 20℃, keep the mice warm, otherwise the animals will not wake up easily due to the decrease of body temperature and slow metabolism.

2) Carbon tetrachloride can be prepared with vegetable oil or glycerol.

6. Question

1) Why does the pharmacological effect of pentobarbital sodium prolong after injection in mice with liver damage?

2) Please discuss the relationship between liver function status and clinical application of drug by clinical examples.

3) What is the pathological difference between the liver of mice poisoned by carbon tetrachloride and that of normal mice, and why?

Experiment 23　Effect of drugs affecting the autonomic nervous system on blood pressure

1. Aim

On the basis of mastering the method of direct measurement of blood pressure in animals, the effects of efferent nerve drugs on animal blood pressure were observed, the understanding of the interaction between these drugs was deepened, and the mechanism of action was preliminarily analyzed according to the receptor theory.

2. Principle

The potency of a cardiovascular drugs depends on the direct effects at the cellular level by combining the corresponding receptors on heart and vascular smooth muscle cells and also depends on the response of the cardiovascular control mechanisms. The experiment is designed to evaluate cardiovascular drugs on pressure effects in anesthesia rabbit. Blood pressure is affected by cardiac output, arterial tension and blood volume. Adrenergic drugs can act on the heart and blood vessels α、β receptors affect cardiac output and arterial tension, and then regulate blood pressure. Adrenaline is α、β receptor agonists have effects on heart and blood vessels, with obvious pressure rise; Norepinephrine is mainly strong α receptor agonists, weak β receptor activation mainly has a great impact on vascular tension, obvious enhancement of peripheral resistance, very significant pressure rise and strong and fast effect; Isoproterenol is mainly β receptor agonists have a great impact on vascular tension and weaken peripheral resistance, but at the same time, they enhance cardiac contractility and cardiac output. The two effects offset each other. Therefore, the pressor effect is not obvious, and there may be a slight depressor effect.

3. Experimental materials

1) Animal: rabbits, 2.0~2.5 kg.

2) Equipments: physiological pressure transducer, artery catheter, artery clamp, BL-420F recording & analyzing software.

3) Reagents: 25% urethane solution, 0.003% epinephrine hydrochlaride, 0.125% noradrenaline bitartrate, 0.005% isoprenaline, 1% phentolamine, 1% propranolol hydrochloride, heparin sodium solution (50 U/mL, 1000 U/mL).

4. Procedures and observations

1) Anesthesia: weigh the rabbit and administer 25% urethane solution 4 mL/kg via marginal ear vein and fix it on the operation table.

2) Trachea catheterization: cut off the neck fur and open the skin along midline, dissect the connective tissue and free the trachea. Insert a reverse "T" shape cannula and fix it tightly.

3) Heparinization: administer 1000 U/mL heparin sodium solution 1 mL/kg from marginal ear vein.

4) Carotid catheterization: isolate either lateral carotid artery, ligate the heart-distal terminal with thread tightly, clamp the heart-proximal terminal by artery forceps, and then make a "V" shape incision near to ligating point and insert an arterial cannula filled with heparin sodium solution connect to the force-displacement transducer linking the physiological pressure detector. After the pressure detector is well regulated, open the artery forceps and record normal blood pressure.

5) Recording methods: before administering the drugs, trace normal blood pressure. Then inject the following drugs in turn. After administration, infuse 2 mL normal saline through infusion tube immediately to make the drug enter the blood circulation entirely. observe and record the alteration in blood pressure. Don't give the next drug until the physiological condition is back to the normal or stable level.

6) Observe the blood pressure changes after the injection of the following drugs in sequence, and consider the principles of the blood alterations.

① To exam the effects of epinephrine-mimic drugs.

- IV epinephrine hydrochlaride 0.2 mL/kg via marginal ear vein, when the effects of epinephrine hydrochlaride disappear, do the next step as following.
- IV isoprenaline 0.2 mL/kg, when the effects of isoprenaline disappear, do the next step as following.
- IV noradrenaline bitartrate 0.2 mL/kg, when the effects of noradrenaline bitartrate disappear, do the next step as following.

② To exam the effects of epinephrine-mimic drugs after applying α -receptor antagonists on blood pressure.

- IV phentolamine 0.5 mL/kg, conduct the following steps after 15 min.
- IV epinephrine hydrochlaride 0.2 mL/kg via marginal ear vein, when the effects of epinephrine hydrochlaride disappear, do the next step as following.
- IV noradrenaline bitartrate 0.2 mL/kg, when the effects of noradrenaline bitartrate disappear, do the next step as following.

- IV isoprenaline 0.2 mL/kg, when the effects of isoprenaline disappear, do the next step as following.

③ To exam the effects of epinephrine-mimic drugs after applying β-receptor antagonists on blood pressure.

- IV propranolol hydrochloride 0.5 mL/kg, conduct the following steps after 15 min.
- IV isoprenaline 0.2 mL/kg, when the effects of isoprenaline disappear, do the next step as following.
- IV epinephrine hydrochlaride 0.2 mL/kg via marginal ear vein, when the effects of epinephrine hydrochlaride disappear, do the next step as following.
- IV noradrenaline bitartrate 0.2 mL/kg, observe the effects of noradrenaline bitartrate.

7) Print blood pressure curve, analyze the experiment results and give a correct conclusion.

5. Cautions

1) This experiment was carried out in rabbits. Because rabbits have poor tolerance, some results may not be very typical.

2) The dose in the experiment is calculated according to the general situation, and can be increased or decreased appropriately according to the specific situation if necessary.

3) In order to avoid thrombosis, normal saline should be continuously and slowly injected into the established venous channel without administration.

4) The administration speed of agonists should be fast, and the administration speed of two blocking drugs should be slow.

5) Mark each administration.

6) Keep warm after anesthesia.

6. Question

What are the effects of adrenergic drugs and antiadrenergic drugs on blood pressure? What is the interaction between them? What is the mechanism?

Experiment 24　The effect of diazepam on convulsion induced by central stimulants

1. Aim

To observe the effect of antiepileptic drugs against convulsions induced by pentylenetetrazol, and to see the behavior characteristics of convulsion mouse and the method of making the model.

2. Principle

Pentylenetetrazol is a central stimulant drug, which can cause excitation of brain and spinal cord, so it appears strong clonic convulsions, and gradually appear rigidity convulsion. The convulsive area may be located in brain stem and cerebrum. The pathological mechanism concerns the increase of brain nervous cell's permeability to K^+ and enhance the concentration of extracellular K^+, resulting in cell membrane depolarization and increasing neuron excitement and facilitation of stimulant synapse. When the dose is too large, it can over excite the brain and spinal cord and cause convulsive reaction. It is characterized by strong involuntary contraction of skeletal muscles of the whole body, causing clonic convulsions. Its convulsive action site is in the brain. The mechanism may be to increase the concentration of K^+ outside the nerve cell membrane, depolarize the cell membrane, reduce the threshold of excitation, and improve the excitability. Because gamma-amino butyric acid (GABA) is a central inhibitory neurotransmitter, pentetrazol may inhibit the release of GABA, pentetrazol enhance the excitability by reducing central inhibition. Diazepam can promote the combination of central GABA and GABA receptor, promote Cl^- influx, hyperpolarize nerve cells and inhibit nerve excitation, so it has anticonvulsant effect.

3. Experimental materials

1) Animals: mouse (or rat), 18~22 g.

2) Equipments: syringe and so on.

3) Reagents: 0.02% diazepam, 0.5% pentylenetetrazol, normal saline.

4. Procedures and observations

(1) Four mice are divided into 2 groups randomly (each group has 2 mice), and then the mice of group A is administered with diazepam 0.1 mL/10 g · BW, group B treat with normal saline by ip. After 30 min, all animals are treated with 0.5% pentylenetetrazol (0.3 mL/10 g · BW) by ip and the number of convulsion and dead in 30 minutes are recorded, and then calculating the rate of convulsion and dead. The standard appearance of mice's maximal seizure convulsion: clonus convulsion after 5~15 min or excitability jump, then forelimb flection, hindlimb rigidity as convulsive indications.

(2) Fill the experimental data in table 2-10 and figure out the rate of convulsion.

Table 2-10   Experimental data

group	Number of animals	Number of convulsion	Rate of convulsion (%)	Number of dead	Rate of dead (%)
Normal saline					
Diazepam					

5. Cautions

1) The intraperitoneal injection dose must be accurate, and the injection position must be confirmed in the intraperitoneal cavity.

2) The occurrence and frequency of convulsions in animals are judged by the occurrence of tonic convulsion contracture, and slight tremor is not used as the calculation index of convulsion.

6. Question

How about the anticonvulsant mechanism and clinical application of diazepam?

Experiment 25   Antiarrhythmic effects of lidocaine

1. Aims

1) Learn the method of making arrhythmia animal model.

2) To observe the antiarrhythmic effect of lidocaine.

2. Principle

Barium chloride can promote Na^+ influx in Purkinje fibers, inhibit K^+ outflow, promote 4-phase automatic depolarization, enhance self-discipline, and induce ventricular arrhythmia. Antiarrhythmic drugs can be divided into four categories. Class I: blocks the sodium channel of myocardium and cardiac conduction system and has membrane stabilizing effect. According to the different blocking effect of drugs on sodium channel, it can be divided into three subclasses, namely Ia, Ib and Ic. Class II: β receptor blockers inhibit the pacing current caused by sympathetic excitation. Class III: drugs for prolonging action potential duration and inhibiting a variety of potassium currents. Class IV: calcium channel blockers. Lidocaine belongs to class Ib anti tachyarrhythmia drug. It is a moderate sodium channel blocker. It can slow down phase 0 depolarization and phase 4 automatic depolarization, reduce self-discipline. Contrary to the effect of barium chloride, lidocaine can be used to treat arrhythmia.

3. Experimental materials

1) Animal: rabbit , 2.0~2.5 kg.

2) Equipments: BL-420 system, mammalian surgical instruments, various intubations, etc.

3) Reagents: 25% urethane solution, 1% barium chloride solution (1 mL/kg), 0.5% lidocaine solution.

4. Procedures and observations

1) Animal Anesthesia: after weighing, 25% urethane solution (4 mL/kg) was injected intravenously into the ear margin.

2) Lead connection: insert the needle electrode under the skin of the corresponding lead limb: red (right upper limb), yellow (left upper limb), green (left lower limb) and black (right lower limb). Each lead is inserted respectively and connected with CH1 channel.

3) The pharmacological experimental module (the effect of drugs on experimental arrhythmia) in BL-420 system was selected to focus on the ECG changes of lead II.

4) After recording a normal ECG, 1% barium chloride (1 mL/kg) was injected intravenously into the ear margin (the dose can be increased if necessary) to observe the changes of rabbit heart rhythm. After arrhythmia, 0.5% lidocaine (1 mL/kg) was injected intravenously for 1~2 min to continuously observe the changes of rabbit heart rhythm.

5. Cautions

1) When barium chloride is injected, the first half dose is injected quickly and the second half dose is injected slowly. At the same time, observe the changes of ECG and stop the drug immediately after arrhythmia.

2) Lidocaine should be diluted to at least 0.5%, and intravenous injection should be slow, otherwise lidocaine poisoning may be caused, resulting in animal death.

6. Questions

Please analyze the pharmacological action of lidocaine and its antiarrhythmic mechanism.

Chapter III   Human Experiments in Medical Functional Experiment

Section 1   Introduction to WebChart-400 system for human experiments

1. Main interface of the system

Choose "WebChart-400" icon to enter the system. When the system is initiated the main interface will appear (Figure 3-1). This system includes 12 experimental options which are recording of ECG, respiration, blood pressure, EEG, heart sound, muscle response, reflex and reflex time, sensory experiment, electric characteristic of eyes and muscle, pulmonary function and urinary experiment, etc. Click on the respective icon to enter the module of aspects mentioned above. Click on "Normal Physiological Parameter" located on the top-left corner, the common physiological parameter will be shown, including blood, liver function, pulmonary function, ECG, heart sound, substances in urine, etc.

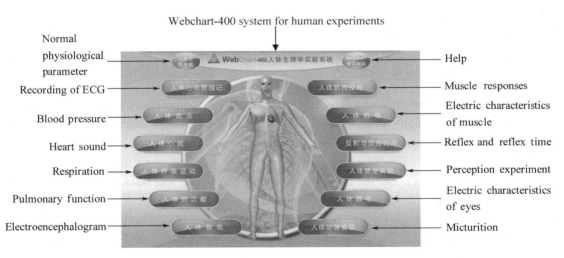

Figure3-1   Main interface of WebChart-400 system

2. Experiment interface

Taking "Recording of ECG" as an example, the processes of starting and conducting an experiment are shown below:

① Click on "Recording of ECG" button, the page as shown in Figure 3-2 will appear:

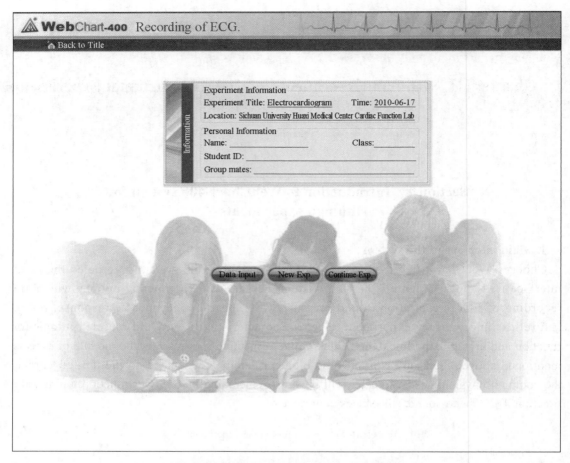

Figure 3-2   Page of starting an experiment

At this page, you can choose different ways to start your experiment. If you are going to conduct a new experiment, please fill in you personal information, then click on the "New Experiment" button. If you want to conduct the experiment you have done before, you can choose "Continue Experiment". This function can be effected when there is an unexpected shutdown of the system. You can retrieve the experiment data with this function, because they are saved in the system cache. You can also choose to import your pervious experiment data to continue the experiment.

② After clicking on the "New Experiment", the following main function menu will appear as shown in Figure 3-3.

Corresponding content will be shown (Figure 3-4) when you click on different buttons, such as "Principle" "Background" "Instrument", etc.

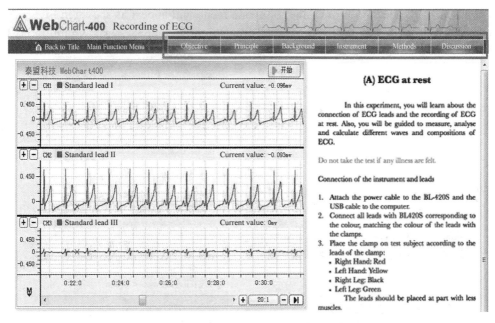

Figure 3-3   Main function menu of experiment

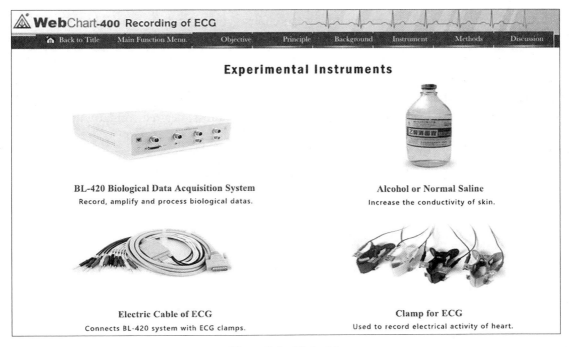

Figure 3-4   Materials

Move the mouse to the "Methods", the following menu will appear as shown in Figure 3-5. Click on " ECG at Rest", related experiment procedures will appear as shown in Figure 3-6.

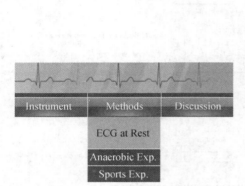

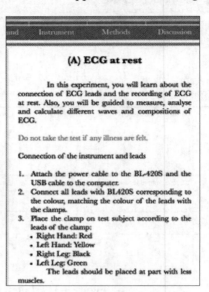

Figure 3-5 The menu used to choose specific experiment module

Figure 3-6 Procedures of recording ECG at rest

According to the procedure shown you can choose corresponding experiment module to complete the experiment.

③ After completing all of the experiment module, click on the "Discussion" to show the interface of experiment report as shown in Figure 3-7. You can adjust the graph obtained to appropriate form. After that, click on the "Save" button. A reminder window will appear to ask you if you want to save the discussion. Also, the save address, desired format will be asked.

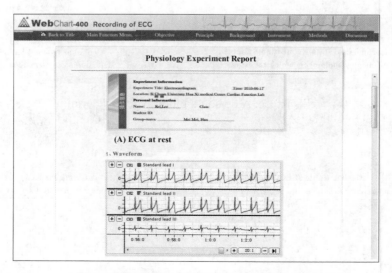

Figure 3-7 Edit page of an experiment report

Finally, an E-version experiment report will be output for you.

Section 2　Classical Human Experiments in Medical Functional Experiment

Experiment 1　Determination of ABO blood types

1. Aims

To determine the ABO blood types/groups.

2. Principles

Blood contains 55% plasma, and 45% cellular elements. There are four types of cellular elements including red blood cells (RBCs or erythrocytes). The surface of red blood cells contains genetically determined antigens called agglutinogen (antigen A and B). Antibodies also called agglutinin (anti-A and anti-B) exist in the plasma.

1) **ABO blood system:** Karl Landsteiner received a Nobel Prize in Physiology or Medicine in 1930 for his discovery of ABO blood system. Figure 3-8 summarizes the characteristics of the four blood types under the ABO blood group. As you can see, these blood types are named after the presence antigens A and B on the surface of the RBCs. The genes that code for these antigens are located on chromosome number 9.

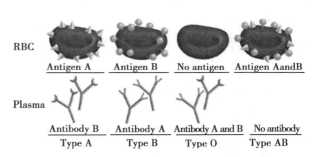

Figure 3-8　The ABO blood system

2) **Rh blood system:** Because the antigen different from antigen A and B was first discovered in Rbesus monkey, it was named Rh factor. This classification is based on the presence or absence of the antigen Rh on the surface of RBCs. If the Rh factor (antigen) is present on the surface of RBC, it is called Rh positive (Rh+). Most of people are Rh+. Rh negative (Rh−) is for those who lack Rh antigen. The genes for Rh factor are found on chromosome 1.

There are two types of blood group systems based on the presence (or absence) of these antigens and antibodies, ABO and blood Rh system. An "A+" person has both antigens A and Rh on his (her) red blood cell surface. A person's blood type is determined by his or her parents' blood type.

3) **Blood type test:** Determination of the ABO group is also called blood grouping, blood typing or blood matching. It is performed by mixing a small sample of blood with antiserum anti-A or anti-B. The presence or absence of clumping (agglutination) is determined by each type of antiserum and blood used. Agglutination reaction is actually an immune response. It indicates a positive reading. In clinical practice, a donor is the person who gives blood, and recipient is the one receives the blood. Universal donors means people with O group blood and their blood can be given to people with any blood group; and universal recipients refer to people with AB group and they can receive blood from people with any blood group.

4) **Cross blood matching test:** Before clinic blood transfusion, cross blood matching test is necessary. Blood typing is a laboratory test which is used to determine the blood group of a person. And the cross blood matching test can be divided into two types. The main crossmatching is carried out by mixing the serum of the recipient and the RBC of donor. The minor crossmatching is carried out by mixing the serum of the donor and the RBC of recipient. If agglutination of RBCs don't occur in both cases, we call cross blood matching is successful, and the blood from the donor can be used for transfusion.

3. Experimental materials

1) Subject: human being.

2) Equipment and reagents: blood typing slides, anti-A serum, anti-B serum, tincture iodine, 75% ethanol, sterile needle, toothpicks, cotton ball.

4. Procedures and observations

1) Prepare a blood typing slide, each half of the slide is labeled with A or B.

2) Add 1~2 drop of anti-A to the side labeled A and 1~2 drop of anti-B to the another side labeled B.

3) Sterilize the finger in tincture iodine and 75% ethanol. Sting finger with a sterile needle.

4) Take the blood with a clean toothpick. Add 1 drops of freshly drawn blood to each half of the slide.

5) Mix them well with a toothpick and tilt the slide back and forth adequately.

6) After 10 min, examine the agglutination. Agglutination indicates a positive test result, labeled+.

7) Record your results (agglutination or no agglutination) and conclusions (blood type) in Table 3-1.

8) Discard the used toothpicks. Wash and save the slides.

Table 3-1　The result of agglutination test

Anti-A serum	Anti-B serum	Blood type
+	−	A
−	+	B
+	+	AB
−	−	O

5. Cautions

1) Use only one toothpick per well to avoid cross contamination.

2) Don't squeeze the finger to draw the blood.

6. Questions

1) Do you know the Nobel Prize in Physiology or Medicine that correlated the blood typing?

2) Who is the first one to find the ABO type system and what is the clinical significance?

3) Which day is the World Blood Donor Day? How was it derived?

4) Is it definitely safe if the main cross blood matching test is negative?

Experiment 2   Measurement of blood pressure

1. Aims

1) To understand the principle of indirect measurement of blood pressure.

2) To measure the systolic and diastolic pressures of brachial artery with a sphygmomanometer.

2. Principles

Blood pressure (BP) is defined as the pressure that the blood exerts against any unit area of the blood vessel walls, and it is generally measured in the arteries. Because the heart alternately contracts and relaxes, the resulting rhythmic flow of blood into the arteries cause the blood pressure to rise and fall during each beat. Thus, you must take two blood pressure readings: the systolic pressure (SP), which is the pressure in the arteries at the peak of ventricular ejection, and the diastolic pressure (DP), which reflects the pressure during ventricular relaxation. Blood pressures are reported in millimeters of mercury (mmHg), with the systolic pressure appearing first; 120/80 translates to 120 over 80, or a systolic pressure of 120 mmHg and a diastolic pressure of 80 mm Hg. Normal blood pressure varies considerably from one person to another. The pulse pressure is the difference between the systolic and diastolic pressure, and indicates the amount of blood forced from the heart during systole, or the actual "working" pressure. The average pulse pressure (PP) for a health adult is about 40 mmHg. The mean arterial pressure (MAP) for each trial can be calculated using the following equation: MAP = (DP + 1/3PP).

Under normal condition, the blood flows in the blood vessels smoothly and no sounds can be heard (Figure 3-9A). The cuff is placed around the arm and inflated to a pressure higher than systolic pressure to occlude circulation to the forearm (Figure 3-9B). As cuff pressure is gradually released, the examiner listens with a stethoscope for characteristic sounds called the Korotkoff sound, which indicate the resumption of blood flowing into the forearm. The pressure at which the first soft tapping sounds can be detected is recorded as the systolic pressure

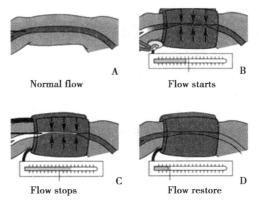

Figure 3-9   The mechanism of indirect measurement of blood pressure by auscultation

(Figure 3-9C). As the pressure is further reduced, the blood flow becomes more turbulent, and the sounds become louder. As the pressure is reduced still further, below the diastolic pressure, the artery is no longer compressed; and blood flows freely and without turbulence (Figure 3-9D). At this point, the Korotkoff sound can no longer be heard. The pressure at which the sounds disappear is recorded as the diastolic pressure.

3. Experimental materials

1) Subject: human being.

2) Equipment and reagents: stethoscope (Figure 3-10), sphygmomanometer (blood pressure

gauge, see Figure 3-10), marker.

4. Procedures and observations

1) Ask the subject to sit in a comfortable position for 5 min, then expose his or her upper arm and keep the upper arm resting on the laboratory table (approximately at heart level if possible).

2) Check whether you can clearly see the mercury scale and make sure you are in line with the scale, make sure that your stethoscope is placed firmly and comfortably in your ears.

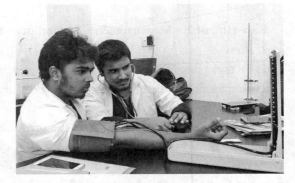

Figure 3-10   Stethoscope and sphygmomanometer

3) The method of measuring arterial blood pressure.

① Palpate the brachial pulse, and carefully mark its position with a felt pen. Take the stethoscope and place its diaphragm over the pulse point.

② The cuff of the sphygmomanometer is placed around the upper arm and fixed approximately 2.5 cm above the cubital fossa, and the chest piece of the stethoscope is placed under it.

③ Rapidly inflate the cuff to approximately 20 mmHg above the estimated systolic blood pressure or 30 mmHg above the pressure required to make the radial pulse disappear.

④ Deflate the cuff slowly (2~5 mmHg per second of mercury) by lightly turning the valve. Listen carefully.

⑤ As soon as the pressure in the cuff falls below the systolic pressure level, sounds can be heard as blood flows through the very narrow artery, and this pressure level indicated by the manometer approximately equals to the systolic pressure.

⑥ When the pressure in the cuff falls to be equal to the diastolic pressure, the sounds suddenly change to a muffled quality, and this pressure level indicated by the manometer equals to the diastolic pressure.

4) Make two blood pressure determinations, and calculate the averages as the final results.

5. Cautions

1) Keep the room quiet and comfortable.

2) Don't talk with the subject.

3) The BP cuff should not be applied over clothing, which means there should be no clothing in the way and nothing that impinges blood flow through the arm (i.e. don't roll the sleeve up to clear the arm and leave it so tight.)

4) The arm should not be higher above the heart level

5) Legs should not be crossed.

6) Select optimal size of the cuff to the subject.

7) The cuff should not be kept inflated for more than 1 min. If you have any trouble obtaining a reading within this time, deflate the cuff, wait 1 or 2 min, and try again. (A prolonged interference with BP homeostasis can lead to fainting.)

6. Questions

1) When performing the Auscultatory-Palpatory technique of blood pressure measurement, if

you feel the radial pulse disappear at 175 mmHg, what should you do next?

2) What will happen to the blood pressure values if the cuff is too big or too small for the subject?

3) Why do we suggest the recipient take off the cloth and expose the arm when taking blood pressure measurement?

4) How to practice the humanistic care in the process of blood pressure measurement?

Experiment 3   Detection of heart sound

1. Aims

1) To practice the auscultatory method of heart sound detection.

2) To identify the characteristics of the first and second sound.

2. Principles

Auscultation of heart sound is performed for the purposes of examining the circulatory system, detecting pathological changes in heart activity. The auscultation is usually performed with a mediate, in many cases, a stethoscope. The most common stethoscope used in auscultation of heart sound is acoustic stethoscope. It operates on the transmission of sound from the chest piece, via air—filled hollow tubes, to the listener's ears. The chest piece is placed on the patient, body sounds vibrate the diaphragm, creating acoustic pressure waves which travel up the tubing to the listener's ears. The result is further analyzed by the health professions.

The two major audible heart sounds in a normal cardiac cycle are the first and second heart sound, S1 and S2. S1 occurs at the onset of the ventricular contraction during the closure of the AV-valves. It contains a series of low-frequency vibrations, and is usually the longest and loudest heart sound. S2 is heard at the end of the ventricular systole, during the closure of the semilunar valves. Typically, its frequency is higher than S1, and its duration is shorter. A third low—frequency sound (S3) may be heard at the beginning of the diastole, during the rapid filling of the ventricles. A fourth heart sound (S4) may be heard in late diastole during atrial contraction.

In summary, the first sound is characterized by a low pitch and a long duration, and the second sound is characterized by a high pitch and a short duration (Table 3-2).

Table 3-2   Comparison between S1 and S2

First sound (S1)	Second sound (S2)
higher frequency	lower frequency
long-lasting	short period
interval of I—II is shorter	interval of II—I is longer

Note: I means AV valves close; II means semilunar valves close.

Auscultation (Figure 3-11) area is the area in which the component of the heart sounds, generated by the vibration of the valve, can be more easily and clearly detected.

Bicuspid valve auscultation area is located at the apex of heart or interior side of the overlap point of the left fifth intercostal space and mid-clavicular line.

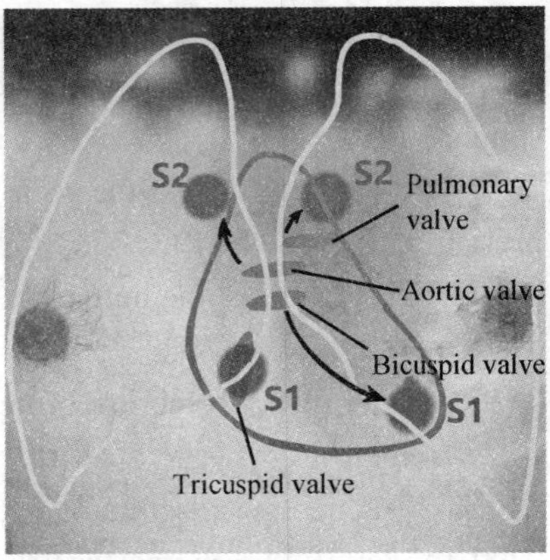

Tricuspid valve auscultation area is located at the right border of the sternum in the fourth intercostal spaces.

Aortic valve auscultation area is located at the right border of the sternum in the second intercostal spaces.

Pulmonary valve auscultation area is located at the left border of the sternum in the second intercostal spaces.

3. Experimental materials

1) Subject: human being.

2) Equipment: stethoscope.

4. Procedures and observations

1) Identify the auscultation areas of the heart sound according to the map.

Figure 3-11   Auscultation areas

2) Place the chest piece of a stethoscope over various areas according to the aforementioned sequence and fit the earpiece into the external auditory canal.

3) While detecting the heart sounds, try to palpate the apex beat or carotid pulse simultaneously.

4) Differentiate the first and second sound by their character i.e. the pitch and the duration, the time interval in between and the relation to the apex beat.

5) Compare the loudness of the heart sounds over various areas.

6) Check the heart rate and its rhythmicity.

7) Calculate the average time for systole and diastole: measure the interval between the first and second heart tones (systole), and then measure the interval between the second and the next first heart tones (diastole), repeat five times to calculate the average time that the heart beats in systole (contracting) and diastole (relaxing).

5. Cautions

1) Keep quite.

2) Locate the right auscultation areas.

3) The bell of the stethoscope should be placed on the participant's chest skin.

4) Inspect the patient's medical history.

5) Touch the heart apex pulsation or carotid artery pulsation when detecting heart sounds, and observe the relationship with the heart sound.

6. Questions

1) Who invented the stethoscope? And what is the mechanism of auscultatory method of heart sound detection?

2) How to distinguish S1 from S2? And what is the significance of identifying S1 and S2?

3) Why do we need to palpate the apex beat or carotid pulse at the same time when we detect the heart sounds?

4) What should you do if you hear heart sounds aside from S1 and S2?

5) How to practice the humanistic care in the process of heart sounds detection?

Experiment 4   Recording of an electrocardiogram

1. Aims

1) To practice the procedure of recording an electrocardiogram on the body surface in human.

2) To understand the mechanisms by which components of a normal electrocardiogram are formed.

3) To learn how to read or analyze a normal electrocardiogram.

2. Principles

Electrocardiograph is the instrument that records the electrical activity of the heart. Electrocardiogram (ECG) is the record of periodic electrical currents in one cardiac cycle spreading to the surrounding tissues spreading to the surface of the body recorded by electrocardiographic apparatus.

A normal ECG is composed of 4 depolarization waves and a repolarization wave (Figure 3-12). Depolarization waves include P wave and QRS complex. The P wave is caused by electrical potentials generated when the atria depolarizes before the contraction begins. The QRS complex (composed of Q wave, R wave and S wave; usually appears as a complex) is caused by potentials generated when the ventricles depolarize before contraction. The T wave, known as repolarization wave, is caused by the potential generated as the ventricle recover from the state of polarization.

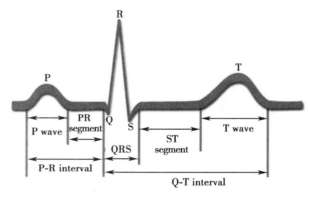

Figure 3-12   The waves and components of a normal ECG

There are some normal ranges of time interval between waves. If the interval greater or lesser than the range, it may suggest some abnormality of the heart contraction. For example, P-Q or P-R interval is the time between the beginning of the P wave and the beginning of QRS complex, which stands for the interval between the beginning of electrical excitation of the atria and the beginning of excitation of the ventricles. The normal interval between two successive QRS complexes in an adult is about 0.83 second, so heart rate is 72 times per minute, or 72 beats/min (60/0.83).

Any change in the pattern of impulse transmission can cause abnormal electrical potentials around the heart and, consequently, alter the shapes of the waves in the ECG. For this reason, most serious abnormalities of the heart can be diagnosed by analyzing the contours as well as the intervals of the waves in the different electrocardiographic leads.

"Lead" means that a combination of two electrodes with the electrocardiograph, there are three kinds of leads, including standard bipolar limb leads, augmented lead and precordial leads (Figure 3-13). "Bipolar limb" means that the ECG is recorded from two electrodes on the surface of the limbs in the body. Electricity always flows from positive to negative. The electrical current should flow from negative to positive in the normal healthy heart. Lead I: positive lead is above the left breast or on the left arm and negative lead is on the right arm. The negative terminal of the electrocardiograph is connected to the right arm via an electrode and the positive terminal to the left arm via another electrode. Lead II: positive lead is on the left abdomen or left thigh and negative lead is on the right arm.The negative terminal of the electrocardiograph is connected to the right arm via an electrode and the positive terminal to the left leg via another electrode. Lead Ⅲ : positive lead is on the left abdomen or left lower lateral leg and negative lead is on the left arm. The negative terminal of the electrocardiograph is connected to the left arm via an electrode and the positive terminal to the left leg via another electrode.

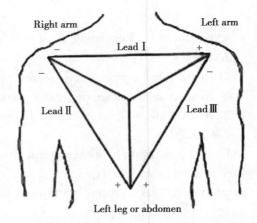

Figure 3-13   The standard limb leads

ECG paper (Figure 3-14) is a grid where time is measured along the horizontal axis and voltage is measured along the vertical axis. The smallest divisions are 1 mm long and 1 mm high. Each small square is 1 mm in length and represents 0.04 s. The larger square is 5 mm in length and represents 0.20 s. 10 mm is equal to 1 mV in voltage.

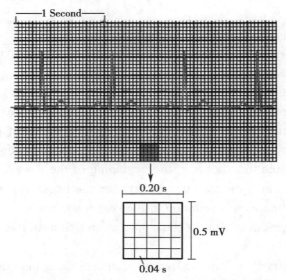

Scale: 25 mm/s, horizontal, 10 mm/mV vertical, little
square = 0.04 s, big square = 0.20 s.

Figure 3-14   The reading of an ECG paper

Heart rate can be easily calculated from the ECG strip. When the rhythm is regular, the heart rate is 300 divided by the number of large squares between the QRS complexes or 60 divided by the P-P interval. For example, if there are 4 large squares between regular QRS complexes, the heart rate is 75 (300/4 = 75).The second method can be used with an irregular rhythm to estimate the rate. Count the number of R waves in a 6 s strip and multiply by 10. For example, if there are

7 R waves in a 6 s strip, the heart rate is 70 (7 × 10 = 70).

3. Experimental materials

1) Subject: human being.

2) Equipments and reagents: electrocardiograph, limb electrodes and precordial leads (Figure 3-15), 75% ethanol cotton ball, saline cotton ball, electrode cream.

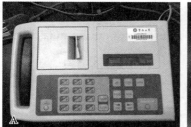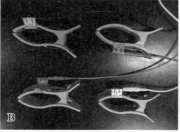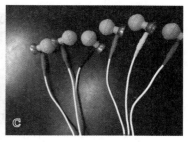

Figure 3-15   The electrocardiograph (A), limb electrodes (B) and precordial leads (C)

(refer to color picture on color pages)

4. Procedures and observations

1) Turn on the electrocardio-graph and warm up for 3~5 min.

2) The subject lies quietly and relaxedly in supine position.

3) Clean the skin with 75% ethanol cotton ball and moisten the skin with saline cotton ball.

4) Connect the electrodes to the ECG leads as follows: There are 12 leads, but we only need 10 electrodes placed with 4 on the limbs and 6 on the chest. Be sure that they are in close contact with the skin.

① The placement of standard bipolar limb leads is as below: red—right arm; yellow—left arm; green—left leg; black—right leg.

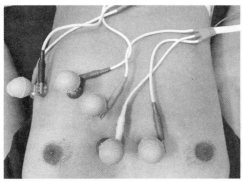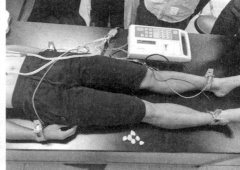

Figure 3-16   The placement of chest leads and limb leads

(refer to color picture on color pages)

② The placement of each chest leads are described as below: V1—red, fourth intercostal, right sternal border; V2—yellow, fourth intercostal, left sternal border; V3—green, equal distance between V2 and V4; V4—brown fifth intercostal, left mid clavicular line; V5—black, anterior axillary line, same level with V4; V6—purple, mid axillary line, same level with V4 and V5.

5) Adjust the amplitude of the deflection of the writing pen in order that a signal of a standard voltage of 1 mV will give a deflection of 1 mm.

6) Record the electrocardiogram manually or automatically.

7) Turn off the power switch. Take off the leads and electrodes from the subject.

8) Read the electrocardiogram.

① Scan the ECG to see if the rhythm is regular.

② Identity the wave components and measure their amplitudes.

③ Measure the P-P or R-R interval. Calculate the heart rate according to the formula: Heart rate = 60/ R-R interval (s).

④ Measure the Q-T interval and ST segment.

5. Cautions

1) Connect the electrodes correctly.

2) Make sure the environment comfortable to reduce or avoid the interference from skeletal muscle contractions.

3) The subject should not be in contact with metal objects (remove wrist and ankle bracelets).

4) Don't talk when taking ECG measurement.

5) Analyse the ECG according to the reading rules.

6. Questions

1) Who invented the Electrocardiograph and who first established the ECG leading method and ECG paper format?

2) What are the differences between ECG and AP of cardiac muscle cells?

3) Could you describe the main findings in ECG when the cardiac muscles are under go ischemia, injury and infarction?

4) How to practice the humanistic care in the process of ECG recording?

Experiment 5　Recording of human respiratory movement

1. Aim

1) To learn how to use the band-type breathing transducer to record the normal respiratory motion.

2) To read the corresponding breathing frequency according to the waveform.

2. Principles

The cells of the human body require a constant stream of oxygen to stay alive. The respiratory system provides oxygen to the body's cells while removing carbon dioxide, a waste product that can be lethal if allowed to accumulate. There are 3 major parts of the respiratory system: the airway, the lungs, and the muscles of respiration. The airway, which includes the nose, mouth, pharynx, larynx, trachea, bronchi, and bronchioles, carries air between the lungs and the body's exterior. The lungs act as the functional units of the respiratory system by carrying oxygen into the body and carbon dioxide out of the body. Finally, the muscles of respiration, including the diaphragm and intercostal muscles, work together to act as a pump, pushing air into and out of the lungs during breathing.

Pulmonary ventilation is the process of moving air into and out of the lungs to facilitate gas exchange. The respiratory system uses both a negative pressure system and the contraction of muscles to achieve pulmonary ventilation. The negative pressure system of the respiratory system involves the establishment of a negative pressure gradient between the alveoli and the external atmosphere. The pleural membrane seals the lungs and maintains the lungs at a pressure slightly below that of the atmosphere when the lungs are at rest. So the air fills in the lungs following the pressure gradient. As the lungs are filled with air, the pressure within the lungs rises until it reaches the atmospheric pressure. At this point, more air can be inhaled by the contraction of the diaphragm and the external intercostal muscles, increasing the volume of the thorax and reducing the pressure of the lungs below that of the atmosphere again.

To exhale air, the diaphragm and external intercostal muscles relax while the internal intercostal muscles contract to reduce the volume of the thorax and increase the pressure within the thoracic cavity. The pressure gradient is now reversed, resulting in the exhalation of air until the pressures inside the lungs and outside of the body are equal. At this point, the elastic nature of the lungs causes them to recoil back to their resting volume, restoring the negative pressure gradient present during inhalation.

External respiration is the exchange of gases between the air filling the alveoli and the blood in the capillaries surrounding the walls of the alveoli. Air entering the lungs from the atmosphere has a higher partial pressure of oxygen and a lower partial pressure of carbon dioxide than the blood in the capillaries does. The difference in partial pressures causes the gases to diffuse passively along their pressure gradients from high to low pressure through the simple squamous epithelium lining of the alveoli. The net result of external respiration is the movement of oxygen from the air into the blood and the movement of carbon dioxide from the blood into the air. The oxygen can then be transported to the body's tissue while carbon dioxide is released into the atmosphere during exhalation.

Under normal resting conditions, the body maintains a quiet breathing rate and depth called eupnea. Eupnea is maintained until the body's demand for oxygen and production of carbon dioxide rises due to greater exertion. Autonomic chemoreceptors in the body monitor the partial pressure of oxygen and carbon dioxide in the blood and send signals to the respiratory center of the brain stem. The respiratory center then regulates the frequency and depth of respiration, returning the gas partial pressure to the normal level.

3. Experimental materials

1) Subject: human being.

2) Equipment: BL-420 system (Figure 3-17), band-type respiratory transducer (Figure 3-18).

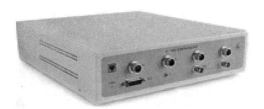

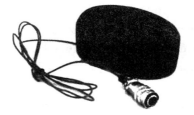

Figure 3-17   BL-420 system   **Figure 3-18   Band-type respiratory transducer**

4. Procedures and observations

1) Devices connection (Figure 3-19): The respiratory transducer is connected to the CH1 channel of BL-420 system.

2) Recording the respiratory movement:

① Ask the subjects to take a sitting position and relax themselves.

② Bind the band-type breathing transducer to the chest of the subject where the most obvious respiratory activity can be observed (Figure 3-20).

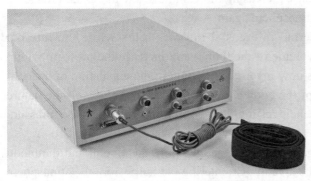

Figure 3-19   Connection of transducer with BL-420 system   **Figure 3-20   The position where the band-type breathing transducer is placed**

③ Click on the start button in the tool bar and start sampling, and the regular respiratory wave in CH1 channel will be seen.

④ Add notes: Enter the subjects in the notes column, then select the button of adding notes.

⑤ Record waveform for 1 min, click the button of stop to end the experiment.

3) Measurement of the respiratory movement:

① Click on button of "slider" and move to the left till the first name label.

② Press the "+" and "−" button on the right of the slider, adjust the waveform to stable position.

③ Click any point in the waveform, the breathing rate will be displayed in the data readout box.

④ Click the left mouse button and choose the data in the data frame, drag and drop the results to corresponding location in the measurable results table (Figure 3-21).

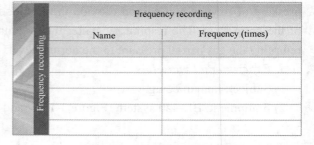

Frequency recording	
Name	Frequency (times)

Figure 3-21   Data recording screen

⑤ Repeat the above steps until all the waveform data are measured.

5. Cautions

1) Keep quite.

2) Find the proper positioning of the subject.

3) The person who feels not good should not receive this test.

6. Questions

1) What factors will change the respiratory frequency and depth?

2) Can activities like thinking and calculating alter the respiratory rate? And why?

Experiment 6　Examination of visual acuity

1. Aims

1) To understand the principle of examining visual acuity with the international chart of visual acuity.

2) To learn how to use the International Vision chart correctly.

2. Principles

Visual acuity is the resolution capacity of the eye or the sharpness of vision, and it is determined by the smallest visual angle needed for one to see words or figures clearly. The viewing angle is the angle defined by the light rays coming from the two margins of the object. The smallest viewing angle at which two distinct points can be discriminated is called the viewing angle limit which is approximately 1 angular minute (1'); this corresponds to about 1.5 mm seen from 5 m for the healthy eye. Visual acuity is the actual viewing angle limit compared to the normal viewing angle limit of 1' expressed in percentage or decimal fraction. Thus, an eye with a viewing angle limit of 1' has a sharpness of vision value of 1 (or 100%), an eye with 2' has a sharpness of 0.5 (or 50%), etc.

The maximal sharpness of vision in an optically perfect eye is determined by the density of photoreceptors on the retina. At the fovea centralis, the cones show a dense, honeycomb-like distribution, and their average distance from each other is 2 μm. We can discriminate between two points, if their images projected onto the retina are located at least at a distance corresponding to one cone diameter. On the peripheral surface of the retina, the rods are located with a similar density, but several rods are connected to the same ganglion cell (convergence), thus the visual acuity here is low. So, visual acuity is the highest at the macula lutea (about 100%); it decreases towards the periphery of the retina.

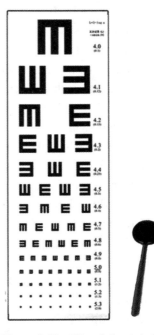

We use international chart of visual acuity to test the visual acuity. There are 14 lines of words in international chart of visual acuity. And the light emitted by every side of the words on eleventh line just form 1' visual angle. So as one see the words clearly in a 5 m distance from them, this visual acuity is normal.

3. Experimental materials

1) Subject: human being.

2) Equipment (Figure 3-22): visual chart, indicated rod and eye-cover board.

Figure 3-22　Visual chart, indicated rod and eye-cover board

4. Procedures and observations

1) Let the subject stand 5 m away from the visual chart.

2) Cover one of the subject's eyes with eye-cover board by himself, and see the chart with the other eye.

3) Let the subject tell if the indicated words can be seen clearly.

4) Do the test from the biggest words on the top line to the bottom one until the line in which the smallest words can just be seen clearly.

5) Repeat procedure 2 to examine the visual acuity of the other eye.

5. Cautions

1) Take standard visual chart which is accepted around the world.

2) Keep required light shedding on the visual chart when doing testing.

6. Questions

1) How to read the standard visual chart and what does it mean when your visual acuity is 1.0?

2) What are the possible causes for near sight? How to prevent the formation of near sight in our daily life?

3) How do you think about the laser treatment of near sight? What is the basic mechanism?

Experiment 7   Examination of blind spot

1. Aims

1) To verify the existence of blind spot in retina.

2) To measure and calculate the scope of blind spot.

2. Principles

The blood vessels supplying the retina have a characteristic distribution. The convergence point of the blood vessels has a somewhat lighter yellow colour than the rest of the retina; this is the optic disc. Because there is no photoreceptor on the optic disc from which the optical nerve comes out and on which there is no vision as lights from outside focus, it is called the blind spot. In temporal direction from the blind spot, a little darker spot called the macula lutea can be found. See Figure 3-23.

The position and scope of blind spot can be determined by its projecting area according to the role of image formation.

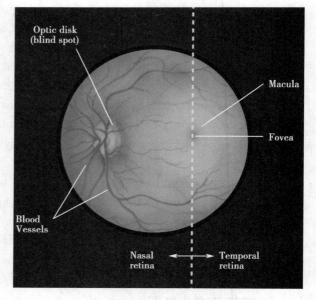

Figure 3-23   The structure of retina under ophthalmoscopy

3. Experimental materials

1) Subject: human being.

2) Equipment: white paper, pencil, small target object, ruler, eye-cover board.

4. Procedures and observations

1) Traditional method.

① Paste a white paper on the wall, and let the subject stand 50 cm away from it. Draw a plus mark on the paper, which is at the same level with the subject's eyes. Let the subject cover one of his eyes with eye-cover board and look at the sign of plus with another fixed eye.

② Slowly move a small black object from the sign of plus to its outer side, and mark the position on the paper as it just can't be seen by the subject. Slowly move the same black object further outer side and mark the position on the paper as it just can be seen again.

③ Move the small target object, a small black object, from the center of two mark points to find the same two kinds of positions in every direction. Connect all the points on the paper consequentially to form an approximate circle, which is called projecting area of blind spot.

④ Calculate the diameter of blind spot and its distance from central fovea in the retina with the following formulas according to the principle of similar triangle.

Distance of blind spot to fovea = distance of projecting area to the sign of plus (+) × 15/500 (mm)

Diameter of blind spot = Diameter of projecting area of blind spot × 15/500 (mm)

2) Using software of Webchart-400 system. (See Figure 3-24)

① Close or obscure the left eye, stand 50 cm in front of the screen, stare at our school's icon (you can replace it with other icon) with the right eye, when the cross symbol moves to the right side, you can see it at first, later it disappears, then it appears again. Ask a person to record the two points and read the distance between them on the scale, and the value stands for the diameter of projection range of your retina blind spot.

② Calculate the blind spot diameter according to the formula: The blind spot diameter calculation formula = detected blind spot projection diameter × (15/500) mm, the general blind spot size is about 1.5 mm. Example: In the open flash, it is 4 when you can see the sign; it is 9 when it disappears. Then, your projection range of blind spot diameter is 5cm, according to the above formula, 50 × 15/500 = 15/10 = 1.5 mm. Of course, if the distance screen is 30 cm, the

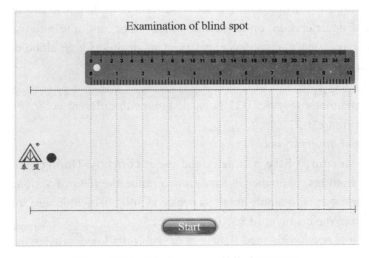

Figure 3-24   Display page of blind spot test

denominator in the formula should be 300.

5. Cautions

1) During the test, the subject's eyes must always follow the "+", and must not move with the small black object .

2) The subject must keep a certain distance from the white paper (normally 50 cm), and can not change it at will.

6. Questions

1) Could you help explain the reasons if someone failed to find his or her blind spots?

2) Do you know which factors can determine the size of blind spot?

3) Why don't you feel the blind spot when you see the object with two eyes?

Experiment 8   Examination of visual fields

1. Aims

1) To understand the concept of visual fields.

2) To know how to use the gauge of visual fields to examine the visual fields of white, red, yellow and green colors in normal persons.

2. Principles

The visual field is the area seen by one fixed eye toward a point directly in front of it. The field of vision is the part of the outer world which is projected onto the surface of the retina by the eyes. In our field of vision, the blind spot is located in temporal direction from the macula, by approximately 1.5° below the horizontal direction, at about 12° ~17° from the center. Due to the anatomical form of the eye and the retina this would be a regular circle or hemisphere, but different structures of the face (the nose, the supraorbital ridge, the cheekbones) mask some parts of the theoretical field of vision.

Examination of visual field is helpful for finding out the functional states of the retina, visual pathway and visual cortex. Visual field problems have a number of causes, including disorders that don't originate in the eye, but in the central nervous system or the part of the brain that deals with vision. The information from the visual field tests help diagnose the following diseases: glaucoma, macular degeneration, optic glioma, brain tumor, multiple sclerosis stroke temporal arthritis central nervous system disorders pituitary gland disorders high blood pressure.

3. Experimental materials

1) Subject: human being.

2) Equipment: perimeter (Figure 3-25), visual signs with different color (Figure 3-26), visual field chart, pencil (Figure 3-27).

4. Procedures and observations

1) Observe the structure of the perimeter and use it correctly. During ophthalmological and neurological examinations, perimeter is used to determine the field of vision. The semicircular metal arc of the perimeter is rotatable about its centre in 360° . The little disc inside the arc can be moved outwards from the centre until 90° (Figure 3-25).

2) Put the gage in a place with good light. Let the subject's lower jaw lag on the jaw supporter and lower edge of eye-socket against the eye-socket supporter.

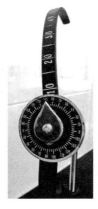

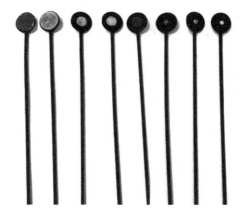

Figure 3-25   Perimeter   Figure 3-26   Visual signs

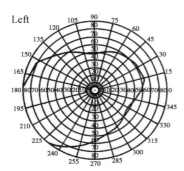

Figure 3-27   Visual field chart

3) Adjust the height of the jaw supporter to make the eye and the central point of the curve frame at the same level. First, the curve frame is placed horizontally; the subject looks at its central point directly with the tested eye and covers another eye with one hand.

4) Move white visual sign from the edge to center on the frame slowly and let the subject tell if white visual sign can be seen at all times. As white visual sign can just be seen, move it back a little and forward again to get the same result. Plot the point on the corresponding longitude and latitude of visual fields. The opposite point can be found and plotted on the chart with the same method.

5) Move the curve frame with a 45° angle, and repeat the test to get two points just seen and plot them on the chart. And do it two more times to get eight points totally on the chart, and connect these points consequentially to form the visual fields of white color.

6) Repeat the test twice to obtain a total of 8 points on the chart, connecting them in turn, and the resulting area was a white field of view.

7)Repeat the above steps to test visual fields of other colors.

5. Cautions

1) Ask the subject to stare at the center of the curve frame of perimeter.

2) Make sure the subject do see the visual sign during testing.

3) Move the color sign slowly when doing the test.

6. Questions

1) How to detect the blind spot with the perimeter?

2) What will happen to the visual fields of a person who has injured the optic chiasma?

3) Is there any difference in size between the black-and-white and coloured (green, blue or red) fields of vision? And why?

Experiment 9　Examination of color blindness

1. Aims

To master the method to examine the color blindness with the visual chart or Stilling-Ishihara plate and make a correct diagnosis.

2. Principles

The photoreceptor cells of the retina are the rods and the cones. The cones are responsible for photopic vision that is for colour vision in daylight. In the central fovea, there are practically cones, their quantity decreases dramatically towards the periphery of the retina. Cones may belong to three groups according to their photopigment type. There are three different kinds of cone pigment existing separately in three different cones. Erythrolabe is the most sensitive to red light waves; chlorolabe is the most sensitive to green light waves; and cyanolabe is the most sensitive to blue light waves. In the retina of colour-blind people, the receptors detecting one of the three basic colours (red, blue, green) are of decreased sensitivity or missing, thus they cannot detect or distinguish certain colours, usually the complementary pairs, like red-green, blue-yellow.

The most common colour perception disorder is red-green colour blindness. According to statistical data, 8% of men and 0.5% of women are colour-blind. The gene coding for the pigment protein of red and green cones is located on the X chromosome; that is why this colour blindness is more frequent among men.

Colour perception is usually examined with Stilling-Ishihara plates (Figure 3-28). These

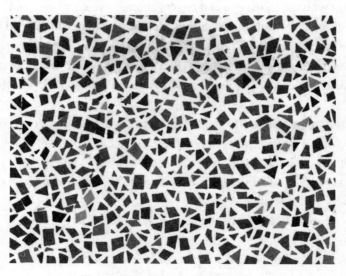

Figure 3-28　Stilling-Ishihara plate

(refer to color picture on color pages)

plates contain a character (letter or number) or a shape in a colour different from that of the background. Both the figure and the background consist of dots to eliminate the contours of the figure. The average size and lightness of the dots is equal for the figure and the background, so the perception of light contrast or pattern cannot help to recognize the figure. Thus, the figure is invisible, or difficult to see, to those who cannot distinguish the colour of the figure from that of the background. The above method to test red and green blindness was invented by Dr. Stilling-Ishihara who is a Japanese, and it was called StillingIshihara blindness measure and currently is the most often used blindness test world widely.

When we do the color blindness examination, the subjects are asked to watch the 8 color plates in Ishihara test to see if they can identify the values. If they can not recognize the color, then they are considered to be color-blind.

3. Experimental materials

1) Subject: human being.

2) Equipment: visual book or chart,Webchart-400 system.

4. Procedures and observations

1) Look at each image and write the number you see on the image in 5 s, then click the "Opinion" button. It will tell you whether you chose the right answer or not and show you the correct answer (Figure 3-29).

2) Click the "Another" button to start the next image test.

3) If the answer is wrong, there automatically appears another picture with the same color for you to identify. If your consecutive answers are still wrong, then the conclusion of "you are red/green/blue blind" will be drawn.

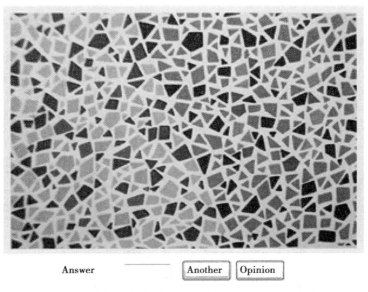

Answer _____   Another   Opinion

Figure 3-29   Displaying page of color blindness test

(refer to color picture on color pages)

5. Cautions

If the computer screen is too large or the pixel is too high, you need to reduce the screen's pixels and make sure there is no screen flashing, or it will blur the entire visual field.

6. Questions

1) Can color-blind patients drive a vehicle? Please explain your answer.

2) Who first discovered the existence of color blindness? How did he realize this abnormal color vision?

3) Why red-green color blindness is far more common in men (8%) than in women (0.5%)?

Experiment 10   The ways of sound conduction

1. Aims

1) To certify and compare air conduction and bone conduction of sound with tuning forks.

2) To understand the simple methods and main principles of distinguishing conductive deafness from nerve deafness in clinical practice.

2. Principles

Sound wave is gathered by the outer ear. The vibration is conducted to the tympanic membrane and three ossicles of middle ear. The middle ears amplify the sound. Sound wave travels to the oval window. The vibration reaches the cochlea fluid and depolarizes the sensory hair cells in the basilar membrane within the organ of Corti. The resulting actions potentials travel along the vestibulocochlear (Ⅷ cranial) nerve to reach the brain. Each region of the basilar membrane vibrates most vigorously at a particular frequency and leads to the excitation of a specific auditory area of the cerebral cortex. Therefore, the different sound pitch is perceived by the brain.

Conductive deafness is caused by the interference with the sound wave reaching the inner ear; sensorineural deafness results from the impairment of hair cells or the damage of the vestibulocochlear nerve.

When the turning fork is striking, the sound is conducted via air and skull. Rinne test (Figure 3-30) compares air conductions with bone conductions. Vibrations perceived through air are heard twice as long as those perceived through bone with normal individual, because the sound wave

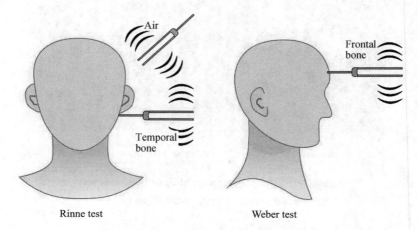

Rinne test   Weber test

Figure 3-30   Rinne test and Weber test

is not absorbed by the tissue. If there is conductive deafness, bony conduction is either normal or slightly enhanced, whereas air conduction is decreased. If there is sensorineural deafness, bone conduction and air conduction are equally suppressed.

Weber test (Figure 3-30) compares bone conduction of two ears. Place a vibrating fork against the center of forehead to let the subject compare the sound loudness in two ears, which are equal in normal persons. Fill a small cotton ball into one ear, and repeat the previous step and ask the subject about the volume of the sound in each ear. For a normal person, his or her filled ear can hear the sound more loudly.

If the sound is louder in the plugged ear, his or her hearing is normal. This is because that in conductive deafness, ambient sound is prevented from getting to the cochlea on the blocked side. This causes the nervous system to amplify sounds on that side by sensitizing cochlear transduction.

3. Experimental materials

1) Subject: human being.

2) Equipment: frequency tuning forks (Figure 3-31), rubber mallet (Figure 3-32), cotton ball.

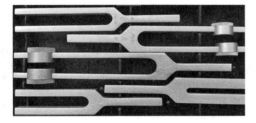

Figure 3-31　Frequency tuning forks　　　　**Figure 3-32　Rubber mallet**

4. Procedures and observations

1) Compare air and bone conductions of one ear (Rinne test).

① Keep silent. Let the subject sit down.

② Strike a tuning fork with the rubber mallet, then place the handle of the vibrating tuning fork (frequency: 512 Hz) against the right mastoid process of the temporal bone (the bone prominence behind the ear) of the subject. The tone of the fork can be heard by him. As it can not just been heard, place the fork in the front of the right ear. The sound can be heard again after a short period of time. See Figure 3-33.

③ Strike a tuning fork with the rubber mallet, then move the vibrating fork in the front of the right ear first until the sound just can't be heard by the subject, and then immediately place it against the mastoid processes of temporal bone. The tone of the fork can't be heard again.

④ So air conduction is better or longer than bone conduction in normal person, which is called Rinne test (+) in clinical practice.

⑤ Fill a small cotton ball into left ear, and repeat steps ② and ③ . Air conduction may be equal to or shorter than bone conduction in this situation, which is called Rinne test (−) in clinical practice.

⑥ Repeat steps ① to ⑤ with the left ear. Record the results on the answer sheet.

2) Compare bone conduction of two ears (Weber test).

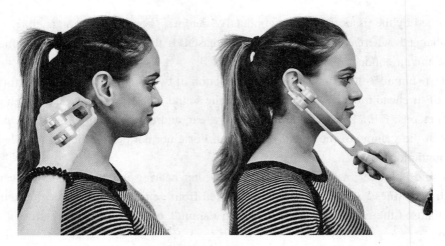

Figure 3-33   Rinne test

① Strike a tuning fork with the rubber mallet and place the tip of the handle on the midline of the subject's forehead. Ask the subject whether the tone is equally loud in both ears. If the sound is heard in the center of the head and equally loud in both ears, his or her hearing is normal, or he or she has symmetrical hearing loss.

② Stimulation of conductive deafness. Repeat step ① with left ear plugged (occluded) with your finger. Describe your results. Repeat step ① with right ear plugged with your finger. Describe your results.

5. Cautions

1) Conduct these tests in a very quiet room.

2) Don't knock the tuning forks on hard objects to avoid damage to the forks.

3) Don't touch the auricle and hair when moving the vibrating tuning fork close to the external auditory canal.

6. Questions

1) What is the Nobel Prize related to the study of auditory organs? What is the clinical application? How is hearing perceived?

2) What are the differences between conductive deafness and sensorineural deafness? How to identify them?

3) What is the mechanism of clinical hearing aids? What are the current research progresses?

Experiment 11   Induction and observation of knee jerk reflex

1. Aims

To induce knee jerk reflex and measure the reflex time.

2. Principles

Reflex is the regular response made by the organism to the changes in internal and external environments under the participation of CNS. It is the basic mode of realizing the function of NS.

A reflex arc is the structural basis and basic functional unit of a reflex. A reflex arc is the smallest, simplest pathway capable of receiving a stimulus and yielding a response. Construction of a reflex arc includes: ① a sensory receptor; ② an afferent or sensory neuron; ③ a nerve center (association neurons); ④ an efferent or motor neuron; ⑤ an effector organ. Reflexes allow a person to react to a stimulus more quickly than would be if conscious thought were involved. The protective value of reflexes is obvious.

Reflex time is the time interval between the application of stimulus and the beginning of reflex action. If the reflex time is just 0.5 ms, then this reflex arc includes only 1 synapse, so this reflex is a monosynaptic reflex. If the reflex time is 1.5 ms, then this reflex arc includes 3 synapses, so this reflex is a polysynaptic reflex.

Knee jerk reflex is a reflex extension of the leg resulting from a sharp tap on the patellar tendon. with the nerve center located in the spinal cord, it is a monosynaptic reflex and the knee jerk reflex test is often used to check for nerve damage in the upper and lower nervous systems.

3. Experimental materials

1) Subject: human being.

2) Equipment: tendon hammer (Figure 3-34), displacement transducer (Figure 3-35), BL-420 system (Figure 3-36).

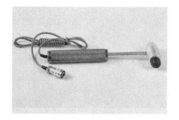 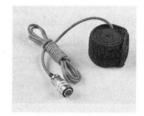 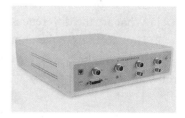

Figure 3-34   Tendon hammer   Figure 3-35   Displacement transducer   Figure 3-36   BL-420 system

4. Procedures and observations

1) Devices connection: the tendon hammer is connected to the CH1 channel and the displacement transducer is connected to the CH2 channel of the BL-420 system.

2) The induction of knee jerk reflex.

① Sit the subject down, put the left leg on the right one, let the left calf relaxes. Check if the left foot can move freely.

② Bind the replacement transducer to the left calf.

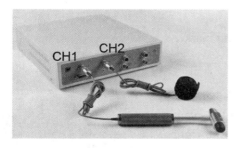 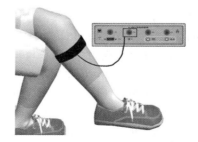

Figure 3-37   Devices connection   Figure 3-38   Binding of the replacement
                                          transducer with BL-420 system

③ Click the start button on the tool bar, you will see two moving data recording lines.

④ Add annotation, input personal information and select it.

⑤ The experimenter strikes the ligament below the left knee cap.

3) Measurement of reflex time.

① Press the slider button, move the waveform to the left till the first name tag.

② Click the slider button, move the waveform to the right till first stimulus signal in CH1 channel. Click the M mark on the lower left corner, drag it to the peak of stimulating signal wave.

③ Move the cursor within the CH1 channel to the right till the first signal peak in CH2, then click the left key.

④ The data displayed in data readout box is the interval from the stimulation to response (muscle contraction).

⑤ Drag the data in data readout box with the left key and drop it to the corresponding position in measurement results form.

⑥ Repeat the steps above, measure all the waveform data.

5. Questions

1) What are the differences between flexor reflex and knee jerk reflex?

2) How to analyse the clinical diagnostic significance of knee jerk reflex?

3) What is the reflex arc of the knee-jerk reflex? Is there any special compared with other reflex arc?

Experiment 12　　Human auditory and visual responses

1. Aims

1) To measure auditory response time through the tendon hammer and displacement transducer.

2) To measure visual response time according to flash signal.

2. Principles

Response time (latency) refers to the interval between the beginning of stimulus and the beginning of response.The length is different from person to person.The time consumed consists of three parts: the time conducting along the sensory nerve; the time the brain processing the information (the longest); and the time the effector producing reaction.

3. Experimental Materials

1) Subject: human being.

2) Equipment: tendon hammer (Figure 3-34), event marker switch (Figure 3-39), BL-420 system (Figure 3-36).

4. Procedures and observations

1) Devices connection (Figure 3-40): The tendon hammer is connected to the CH1 channel (the left one)and the event marker switch is connected to the CH2 channel (the right one) of the BL-420 system.

2) Measure the auditory response time.

① The subject takes a seat and is backs to the experimenter,

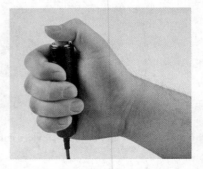

Figure 3-39　Event marker switch

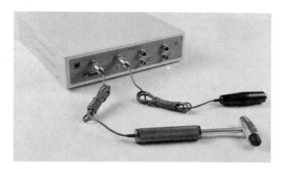

Figure 3-40   The devices connection

holding the event marker switch with the thumb on the button softly.

② Click the button on the tool bar to start recording, and you can see two moving data recording lines.

③ Add annotation to the comment field, then input the subject's name, then choose.

④ The experimenter taps the experimental table with the hammer, the subject presses the event marker switch immediately after hearing the sound.

⑤ Repeat steps ④ , ⑤ for 4 times.

⑥ Press the slider button, move the waveform to the left till the first name tag.

⑦ Click the slider button, move the waveform to the right till first stimulus signal in CH1 channel, click the M mark on the lower left corner, drag it to the peak of stimulating signal wave.

⑧ Move the cursor within the CH1 channel to the right till the first signal peak in CH2 channel, click the left key.

⑨ The data displayed in data readout box is the interval from the stimulation to response.

⑩ Drag the data in data readout box with the left key and drop it to the corresponding position in measurement results screen (Figure 3-41).

Data recording		
	Name	Reaction time (s)

Figure 3-41   Data recording screen

⑪ Repeat the above steps, measure all the waveform data.

3) Measure the visual response time: for the measurement of visual response time, please focus on the screen when the cartoon is played. When you see the red ball, press the left key of the mouse immediately, then you will get your response time. Never press the left button of the mouse before the appearance of the ball. The display screen of measuring the visual response time as shown in Figure 3-42.

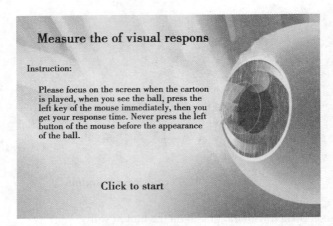

Figure 3-42   The display screen of measuring the visual response time

5. Questions

1) What is the difference between response time and reflex time?

2) Between auditory response time and visual response time, which one is longer?

Chapter IV　Experimental Research of Medical Functional Experiment

With the continuous development of medicine to conform to the urgent demand for innovative talents, medical functional experiment has been developed from simple replication experiment to designed experiment and comprehensive experiment, and more attention is recently paid to training and drilling students' scientific research thinking and scientific innovation ability, so the proportion of innovative experiment has been increased.Innovative experiments generally open to excellent students,after they grasp the basic experimental skills, they design the experiment via literature search for interested research projects under the guidance of teachers. Generally,the experiment will be conducted after feasibility demonstration in opening report, it is likely the integration experiment of morphology-function-molecular biology , its innovation is the first factor to consider, and it is quite difficult.In order to carry out comprehensive and innovative experiments effectively, it is necessary to introduce the experimental research of medical functional experiment.

Section 1　The Basic Principle of Medical Experimental Research

1. Medical experimental research method and experimental design

Medical experimental research methods are scientific methods applied in the field of medical research. It follows a cyclic or iterative process, for instance, when we observe factors that may affect the occurrence of disease or a noted health outcome,we can raise a scientific question from clinical practice or laboratory research or even theoretical speculation; then, we need to identify the important independent and dependent variables, for instance, experimental subjects' exposure to an experimental condition may be a risk factor, it could also be a protective factor or a certain treatment; the outcome may lead to disease or treat disease; we then propose a specific hypothesis to answer specific questions about the relationship between exposure to an experimental condition and the outcome; finally we design an experiment to test if the hypothesis works. The animal experiments include in vivo and in vitro experiments and the human experiment mainly refers to in vivo experiment.An experiment will be then designed to test whether the hypothesis is valid. Experiments include both in vivo and in vitro experiments, and human experiment mainly refers to the in vivo experiment.Therefore, it is very important to do experiments in scientific research, which is a crucial step in scientific research methods, and is applicable to all scientific fields. Firstly, we need to design an experiment.In a narrow sense, experimental design is a well-prepared research plan.The research plan is a description of experimental operations, focusing on problem statements, experimental purposes, and scientific hypotheses.

2. General rules for the experimental design

To design a good experiment, the following rules or methods must be strictly followed.

(1) Experimental group size

To ensure that the statistical result of the experiment is meaningful, we should validate that the amount of subjects in each group is appropriate. The group size should be designed to help us detect a statistically significant difference within experimental group. The number of subjects assigned to each experimental group is often determined by the particular statistical test on the basis of the anticipated magnitude of difference between the expected outcomes for each group.For example, when comparing two groups, the major factors that influence the sample size are:

① The degree of deviation which can be able to detect.

② The degree of variation in the factor of interest.

③ What "p" value you plan to use as a criterion for statistical "significance".

(2) Methods of grouping

The most common way to design an experiment is probably to divide the subjects into two groups, the experimental group and the control group. And then introduce a change to the experimental group and noting to the control group. The researcher must decide how to allocate the samples to these groups.For example, if there are 10 subjects, will all 10 subjects be involved in both conditions (e.g., repeated measures)or will the subjects be split in half and get involved in only one condition each? Basically, there are three types of sample allocation methods

1) Independent measure: Different subjects are used in each condition of the independent variable. This means that each condition of the experiment includes a different group of subjects. This should be done by random allocation, which ensures that each subject has an equal chance of being assigned to one group or the other, and the groups are similar, on average (reducing participant variables).

Independent measures involve using two separate groups of subjects; one in each condition. Such as table 4-1.

Table 4-1　An example of independent measure

Independent variable		Dependent variable
Squat movement (20 s)	Squat movement (40 s)	Changes in blood pressure and respiratory activities
Group 1 (10 students)	Group 2 (10 different students)	

Advantage: Avoid order effects (which refers to the order of the condition being an effect on the subjects' behavior.If a subject is involved in several conditions they may become bored, tired and fed up when they come to the second condition, or becoming aware of the requirements of the experiment.

Disadvantage: More subjects and more repeated measures designs are needed (i.e. more time consuming).Differences between subjects in the groups may affect the results, such as variations in age, sex or social background. These differences are known as subject variables (i.e. a type of extraneous variable).

2) Repeated measure: The same subjects take part in each condition of the independent variable. This means that each condition of the experiment includes the same group of subjects.

Advantage: Fewer people are needed as they take part in all conditions (i.e. saves time). As the same subjects are used in each condition, subject variables (i.e. individual differences)are reduced.

Disadvantage: There may be order effects. Performance in the second condition may be better because the subjects know what to do (i.e. practice effect). Or their performance might be worse in the second condition because they are tired (i.e. fatigue effect). Suppose we use a repeated measures design in which all of the subjects first learn words in loud noise and then learn it noise.

3) Matched pairs: Different but similar subjects are used in each condition. Any important characteristic which might affect performance, such as sex, age, intelligence etc., is considered to match the subjects in each condition. One member of each matched pair must be randomly assigned to the experimental group and the other to the control group.

Advantage: Reduce subject variables because the researcher has tried to pair up the subjects so that each condition has subjects with similar abilities and characteristics. Avoid order effects, and so counterbalancing is not necessary.

Disadvantage: It is impossible to match people exactly, unless identical twins. It is also time-consuming in trying to find closely matched pairs.

(3) Randomization

Randomization is the process of randomly assigning subjects to a control or experimental group. To achieve randomization, one must start with defining populations. A homogeneous population consists of subjects that may not be identical but may share some common characteristics (such as sex, age, weight, etc.). Each subject can be labeled and randomization is then achieved using a random number table or using computer-generated numbers. Subjects can also be randomly assigned to the experimental group using dices or cards.

(4) Replication

If an experiment cannot be repeated to produce the same results, it implies that the original results might have been in error. As a result, it is common for a single experiment to be performed multiple times, especially when there are uncontrolled variables or other indications of experimental error. For significant or surprising results, other scientists may also attempt to replicate the results by themselves, especially if those results would be important to their own work.

(5) Rules of control

Control observations are important parts of any experiment design, particularly when investigating living systems, which are labile. The purpose of a control observation is to determine whether the variable that is directly manipulated by the experimenter is the one that controls the change in response. Apart from experimental variables, there are some factors that can potentially influence the outcome of experiment performed with animals, such as genetic, environmental, infectious agents. In order to minimize the influence of these extraneous variables or to identify the possible presence of unwanted variables, we should arrange control groups of animals that are contrasted directly to the experimental groups of animals. Types of controls include positive, negative, comparative, sham and vehicle controls. One variable that is not under the control of the experimenter is the pass of time. Each observation that you make will happen at a different time, and it is important to know the extent to which differences in responses simply reflect the pass of time. To assess this effect, one can design a control in which a particular measurement is periodically repeated throughout the experiment.

1) **Positive controls:** The so-called positive controls are the groups whose changes will be expected. We usually compare positive control which is already known to produce specific effect with the treatment which is being investigated in the experiment. For example, when testing the effect of new antibiotics upon petri dishes of bacteria, we could use an established antibiotic which is proved to work. If all of the samples fail, except the positive control, it is possible that the tested antibiotics are ineffective.Positive controls are also used to demonstrate that a response can be detected, thereby providing some quality control on the experimental methods.

2) **Comparative controls:** A comparative control is often a positive control with a known treatment that is used for a direct comparison to a different treatment. For example, when evaluating a new chemopreventive drug regime in an animal model of cancer, one would want to compare this regime to the chemopreventive drug regime currently considered as "accepted practice" to determine whether the new regime improves cancer prevention in that model. Comparative control in medicine can be called gold standard. For example, the magnetic resonance angiography (MRA) is the "gold standard" test for aortic dissection, with a sensitivity of 95% and a specificity of 92%.

3) **Negative controls:** The negative control is the process of using the control group to make sure that no confounding variable affects the results, allowing researcher to prove that the results are valid. Negative controls are expected to produce no change from the normal state. In the antibiotic example, the negative control group would be a petri dish with no antibiotic. If all of the new medications work, but the negative control group also shows inhibition of bacterial growth, then some other variable may have an effect on the results. In the toxic example, the negative control would consist of animals not treated with the toxin. The purpose of the negative control is to ensure that unknown variables are not adversely affecting the animals in the experiment, which might result in a false-positive conclusion.

4) **Vehicle controls:** Not all medicine or reagents are water-soluble; the powder may need to be dissolved in specific solvents like widely used ethanol or dimethylsulfoxide (DMSO)which are also called vehicles. In this case, vehicle control is necessary to be set in order to exclude the effects of vehicle itself on the outcomes. The solvents of saline or mineral oil can be innocuous and used in the same way as the tested experimental compound. But for others like ethanol or DMSO which may damage the cells, they need to be diluted to a safe dosage before they are administered. Normally the concentration of ethanol or DMSO should be adjusted to less than 0.5% of the compound solution. When compared with the untreated control, the vehicle control will determine whether the vehicle alone causes any effects.

5) **Sham controls:** a sham control is used to mimic a procedure or treatment without the actual use of the key steps or test substance which may induce changes. A placebo is an example of a sham control used in pharmaceutical studies. Another example is the sham surgery which has been widely used in surgical animal models. Historically, studies in animals allowed the removal or alteration of an organ; using sham-operated animals as control, deductions could be made about the function of the organ. Sham interventions can also be performed as controls when new surgical procedures are developed. When using sham control, we imitate the procedure or treatment of experimental group, but actually we don't execute substantial step which we assume will produce the experimental effect. For instance, studies in animals of the effects of a drug micro-injected into a small defined region of the brain would be expected to be controlled by a matched sham group, treated identically to the experimental group but with vehicle micro-injections. In this case the expected effects of the sham treatment (effects due to anaesthesia, surgery and to incidental, unavoidable damage to brain tissue, and possibly effects of the particular vehicle) can be excluded from the experimental groups.

3. The basic key points of the experimental design

In a broad sense, the rules followed in experimental design and the rules of scientific research planning are basically the same.When designing experiments, we need to carefully design the problems needed to solve, experimental purposes, experimental procedures to verify hypotheses, et al.

(1) Title: effect of an independent variable on a dependent variable.

(2) Experimental variables (independent variables, IV): In the initial stage to learn how to design the experiment, it is better to choose an independent variable for operation.

(3) Appropriate test parameters (dependent variable, DV): Select the test parameters that can accurately assess the effects of the experimental variables.

(4) Hypothesis: what is your guess about what will happen?Write down the conjecture with "if... then...", and clearly write down the effect of the independent variable on the dependent variable. For example, if the independent variable changes in XX, the dependent variable will change in XX.

(5) Determine the optimal methods for sample collection and grouping.

(6) Define the appropriate administration method : If animals need to receive chemical or biological treatment in experiments, the appropriate administration method should be defined. (e.g. diet, gavage, injection, penetration pump, etc.)

(7) Determine the optimal method to obtain test data in the experimental design stage: To conduct statistical test for comparing the differences between experimental groups .

(8) Explain detailed laboratory procedures: There is no need to repeat common sense or general information, for example, there is no need to copy words and graphics from this laboratory manual or textbook, etc. only reference sources are required

(9) Take appropriate preventive measures in advance,if there are known or potential risks.

(10) Consider time constraint: To design experiments that can be finished in an afternoon or 180 min.

Section 2　The Writing and Publication of Research Paper

We spent much time, effort and money in designing a rigorous research plan and implementing it to test the proposed scientific hypotheses; and the final step in all scientific research is to publish research papers to the public. Writing and publish the paper for at least two purposes. First, it spreads scientific achievements and can contribute to the development and progress of science, and secondly, it can promote the career development of individuals. It is very useful, when we try to write papers and publish them in academic journals, to be familiar with some simple principles, which is also the expectation and purpose of this section.

1. Basic structure of scientific papers

Albeit diverse academic journals have their own extraordinary style and requirements, most articles still take after approximately similar parts, which regularly include: title, abstract, introduction, body, discussion and conclusion, references. The short segments of a research paper comprises abstract, introduction, and conclusion. Calling the abstract, introduction, and conclusion segments as the "short" segments means that these three parts should be concise enough to just contain necessary information. The abstract and conclusion sections should be at least detailed, giving the broadest look at the purpose of the experiment and the implications of the results. The introduction should focus on a general statement of the problem to be discussed and the experimental method used to solve that problem, it can be a bit more detailed but not too much.The short sections tell the vital findings of the research work and assure the reader of the incentive to read the whole paper. Normally a reader will firstly take a glance at the abstract to find what really matters in the paper. It the abstract is encouraging, the reader will take a look at the conclusion. If they find it interesting, the reader will then check the introduction to see whether you have recognized what you have done, and afterward they will read the rest of the article for the details.

(1) Title

The title is the part of a paper that is typically perused first and most frequently. Electronic indexing services depend intensely on the precision of the title to enable readers to seek for papers that are important to their exploration. Robert A. Day (1983)characterizes a decent title as "the fewest possible words that adequately describe the contents of the paper". The title shouldn't contain too many irrelative words or too general words; rather, successful titles recognize the fundamental issues of the paper. Main points of the title are listed as following.

A checklist

① Accurate, unambiguous, specific and complete.

② Begin with the subject of the paper.

③ Do not contain abbreviations unless they are well known by the target readers.

④ Grab the eyes of readers.

There are essentially four sorts of title of a research paper, the types, definitions and examples are exhibited in table 4-2.

Table 4-2 Comparision of four sorts of title

Types	Definitions	Examples
Descriptive title	Portray what truly matters to the paper	The effects of 30 min running on the cardio-respiratory exercises
Declarative title	Create an impression about the out-comes exhibited in the paper	30 min running expanded the cardiorespiratory exercises
Interrogative title	Represent a question	Does 30 min of running increase the cardiore-spiratory exercises?
Compound title	Combine a few of the above isolated by colons or question marks	The effects of 30 min running on the cardio-respiratory exercises: increment or diminishing?

(2) Abstract

The purpose of an abstract is to provide readers with a compact outline of the article so the readers can make a speedy choice to lead the entire paper or simply give it up. A good abstract make it workable for the general population who are starting a research project to figure out which article is significant very quickly. An abstract is a rundown of the whole paper, and it typically shows up in small print just beneath the article's title and authors list. The abstract is frequently published independently and distributed more widely than the article itself. As electronic publication databases are turning into the essential methods for searching literature in a specific research area today, the writing of abstracts has become increasingly important.

There are two essential sorts of the abstract. Though the format and content are different, each type of abstract ought to outline what issue is to be dealt with and what are the outcomes and what can be concluded from the results. An informative abstract extract everything from the paper, for example, research goals intended to reach, strategies utilized in solving the issues, results obtained and conclusions drawn. Such abstract is basically a miniature of the structural article and therefore serve as a highly aggregated substitute for the full paper. On the contrary, an indicative or descriptive abstract depicts the content of the paper; it serves as an outline of what is presented in the paper and does not include the goals, methods, results and conclusions in the sequence.

The abstract outlines the whole report, and it contains clues of the wonders to appear, and acts like the "hook" at the start. Although the abstract is the first section of a paper, it is frequently composed last since it is a synopsis of the whole paper.

A checklist

① Question: What is the problem to be solved?

② Motion: Why do we do this research?

③ Solution: What has been done to solve the problem?

④ Results: What is the answer to the problem?

⑤ Implications: What suggestions does the appropriate response imply?

(3) Introduction

In the section of Introduction, we need to answer two vital questions: What is the scientific question that the research attempts to solve, and what is the significance of answering the question? Ordinarily, it regularly starts with a brief summary of previous related research (so-called literature review), a statement of a problem formulated in this research, and a brief description of the experiment designed to solve the problem. The introduction serves the purpose of leading the reader from a general subject area to a particular field of research. In the wake of pursuing this segment, readers will have the capacity to follow the ebb and flow in this research field and comprehend the rest of the paper without reviewing previous publications on the topic. This segment should catch the eyes of readers and persuade them that what you are doing is vital and worth an exhaustive perusing. Although introduction is dependably placed in the first section of main area in a paper, numerous specialists complete it when the paper structure is finished, the experiment has been done and conclusions have been drawn.

A checklist

① Make general statements about the subject.

② Present an overview on current research on the subject.

③ Raise a research question or a problem.

④ Sketch the intention of current work.

⑤ Refine the characteristics and innovation of current research.

(4) Body

The body of a paper consists of two sections of materials and methods and results, it reports on the experiment designed to answer the research question or problem identified in the introduction. Materials and methods tell us how the research question was addressed and results generally depict what was found, which are the two purposes the body serves.

1) **Materials and methods:** This section describes the apparatus and reagents used for the study and the methodologies or experimental procedure applied to answer the research questions; it is very important to give enough information and in an appropriate way that makes it possible for peers to duplicate or reproduce the experiment when applying it to a related problem. Your job in the procedure section is to convince your reader that you carried out an experiment carefully and knowledgeably enough that the reader should take your experimental results seriously. In describing experimental procedures, it is better to regard readers as someone who is inclined to be skeptical about your results and will be picky about your procedure.

A typical description of experimental procedure starts with a list and the description of the equipment. Large pieces of equipment should be identified by manufacturer's name, model, and serial number. A good method section has enough details to allow another investigator to duplicate your experiment. Although it should give enough details for replication, it should not be overly descriptive of nonessential items. If you've made some revision in some seemingly obvious procedures that significantly improves the accuracy of your results, though, make sure you take credit for it.

A checklist

① Provide the main equipment and apparatus required for the experiment.

② Provide a textual list and/or descriptions of equipment.

③ Describe all procedures and arrange them in correct order..

④ List any step taken to reduce experimental uncertainty.

⑤ An appropriate method for administration must be identified.

⑥ Known or potential factors must also be identified and appropriate precautions should be taken to minimize risks from them

2) **Results:** The results present the data obtained from the experiment in a logical order and in various forms including text description, tables, graphs, figures, pictures and even videos. It is recommended that the accepted format be used for all tables, graphs and figures. For example, bar graphs are helpful to compare two or more groups or conditions. The title should clearly explain what is being graphed and never forget to label the units of measure, and organize the data in a meaningful way.

The results section should simply state the factual results without comments and explanations, and interpretation and opinions related to these findings should be included in the discussion section.It is very important to remember that the data tells the fact; try to avoid comments like "Our results prove that the theory is correct", unless you have performed all the possible experimental tests of that theory, or you can never prove a theory.On the contrary, "our results are consistent (or inconsistent)with the theory" is a more acceptable phrase with less rashly assertive.

A checklist

① Briefly describe the data, including the charts.

② Simply state the factual results without comments or explanations.

③ All uncertainties in the experiment are indicated and sample size should be shown.

(5) Discussion and conclusion

The discussion part is sometimes presented as 'Discussion and Conclusion', or simply 'Conclusion'). A conclusion section reviews the experimental purposes and summarizes the implications of experimental results. That is, the fundamental inquiry which was displayed in the introduction ought to be replied by the outcomes in some ways or to some degree. When evaluating your work, never comment an experiment being a "success" or "failure" in the context of agreement with accepted results or theories. Basically, the discussion of the implications of your results should be straightforward; and the discussion of the implications of unforeseen outcomes will show your strength. The conclusion comes at the end as a counterpart to the introduction, so it should give some sense of finality or closure.It will accentuate the deductions from data analysis, portraying them more detailedly than in the abstract and in this manner driving the reader from narrow and/or very specific results to more general conclusions. When evaluating your work, never comment an experiment being a "success" or "failure" in the context of agreement with accepted results or theories.

A checklist

① Briefly present the background information as well as the aims of the study.

② Highlight the most important results; focus on discussing how the results answer the scientific questions raised in the introduction but not recapitulating the results.

③ Compare the results with previously published studies.

④ Indicate the significance and implications of the results and findings.

⑤ Draw conclusions or hypotheses from the results with summary of evidence.

⑥ Point out the limitations of this study. Propose follow-up research questions and suggestions for future improvements.

⑦ Return to the introduction and compared with the original purpose involved in the beginning to form a closed loop.

(6) References

A research is always based on the former research work. If you use the ideas from someone else without acknowledging the source of information, you will be blamed for plagiarism or written falsification which is viewed as a serious offence in the scientific community. Thus, when utilizing other persons' thoughts, opinions, hypothesis or data that are not common knowledge, the right thing we ought to do is to credit them by referring to their related work in segments of Introduction, Body and Discussion; and afterward listing them together in References at the end of the paper.

Distinctive publishers require diverse formats or styles for referring to a paper in the content and for listing references. It is anything but difficult to find the reference organizations or styles online from the website of related journal. Notwithstanding the reference style, the essential principles for the list of references are the same, that is, each listed source must be cited in Introduction, Body and Discussion and each cited source must be listed in Reference.

A checklist

① It is important to check the reference list and make sure that every reference cited in the text is also present in the reference list, and vice versa.

② Uniform the format of references according to the requirements in the journal "Submission Guide".

③ Some tools of literature search and reading can be used to add literature, such as EndNote and NoteExpress.

2. Publish scientific papers in journals

What kind of paper is worth publishing? In O'Connor's opinion, a paper that "records significant experimental, theoretical or observational extensions of knowledge, or advances in the practical application of known principles" is worth publishing.Obviously, in order to prepare a research paper for professional publication, we have to take at least two steps. First, the studies should be designed to answer the research question precisely by doing experiments. Second, the experiments should follow accepted standards and the process of recording the research work be agreed upon in the target community. Even if the reported work is considered to be suitable for submission and worth publishing, a clear, concise and coherent writing style is a basic prerequisite for a paper to be accepted and published. The organization and elaboration of the statement are also the determinates. Most often, it goes many revisions to pass a rigorous peer review process, and it turns out to be very helpful to discuss with others and write the paper while the work is still in progress.

(1) Choose a preferred journal and follow its instructions

After having chosen an appropriate journal for publication, the corresponding author has to edit and submit the paper according to the instructions issued by the journal editor. In order to be familiar with the paper organization, format, and writing style, it is a shortcut to read the papers carefully which was currently published in that journal. To submit the paper via the journal's website or a submission management system is now becoming common and popular. At submission stage, if you don't want to take the risk of being rejected directly, you have to meet all the requirements listed in the instructions. Even if the paper has its scientific contribution and is of high quality, the paper is still likely to be immediately rejected by the editor if any of the following mistakes is made. Here we present some common mistakes at this stage:

① The paper's theme is not within the scope of the journal's subject areas.

② Do not adhere to the paper formatting and layout guidelines (e.g. using the wrong font size, line spacing, page numbering, referencing style, figure and table placement and visual guidelines).

③ Exceed the maximum paper length (word count and/or page count).

④ Be similar to researches already published elsewhere.

(2) External review and peer review

Submitted papers are firstly reviewed by peers of the authors in the respective field's scientific community. This process is hence referred to as peer review, and this is the main mechanism of scientific quality management. The process of peer review involves objective evaluation of the experiment by experts, who give their opinions anonymously. Normally, the editors choose at least three reviewers who are experts in the topic for peer reviewing the paper. Sometimes journals request that the authors offer possible peer reviewers list, especially in the case of highly specialized field. Peer reviewing practices can be blind review in which authors do not know the identity of their reviewers or more seriously double-blind review in which reviewers do not know the author (s)of the paper. Reviewers make comments and give suggestions to the authors for improving the paper. Sometimes they request the author to add new experimental data, which also plays a key role in affecting the editor's decision to deal with the paper. If the work passes peer review, it will be published in a peer-reviewed scientific journal, which indicates the quality of the work are perceived.

A checklist

① Originality of the work, significance of contribution.

② Thematic relevance to the journal's scope of subjects.

③ Coverage of relevant literature.

④ Relevant writing style: clarity of writing, appropriate title and abstract, welldesigned figures and tables, sound conclusion and discussion.

⑤ Appropriate length of the paper relative to its usefulness.

⑥ Characteristics of submitted papers increase the opportunity of acceptance: fair reputation of the author, citation of papers that were published in the journal.

(3) Three outcomes of the review process

After the reviewers have finished reviewing the paper, the editor then collects their comments and makes a decision. Based on the reviewers' recommendations, there are generally three outcomes of the review process of a journal which is sent to the corresponding author by the editor.

1) **Acceptance:** The paper is accepted to be published in the journal directly without revision, which rarely happens.

2) **Revision:** It is more likely that the paper has to be revised. In order to be further considered for publication, the authors have to modify the paper according to the suggestions and comments of the reviewers and the editor. After revising the paper, the author submits the revised manuscript to the editor together with a letter of how the reviewer and editorial comments were addressed. After receiving the revised version, the editor makes an accept or reject recommendation. Sometimes, the paper goes to another reviewing round, which usually involves those reviewers who were most critical about the original submission. Normally, the authors try their best to make the paper comply with the editor's recommendations till it is accepted. Occasionally, if the authors really cannot agree with the reviewers' comments, they may either inform the editor of the disagreement or, give up revision and send the paper to another appropriate journal.

3) **Rejection:** This is actually the most frequent outcome.

The editor usually returns the feedback of the reviewers' comments.Typically, one or more reviewers had serious objections to one of the preconditions mentioned below:

① The paper is out of the journal's scope.

② The paper lacks relevance or significance.

③ The paper has fundamental mistakes.

④ No improvement with regard to previous submissions after revision process.

⑤ Copy phrases, sentences or paragraphs from other people's work. (plagiarism)

In order to avoid rejection and increase the opportunity of publishing your paper, aside from above-mentioned issues, you'd better still keep the following important reminders in mind when you write and submit your paper:

① Follow the style and format required by the submitted professional journals.

② The vast majority of your references should be original research articles, not just reviews or textbooks.

③ Introduction and Discussion are sections where you express your understanding of the topic by selecting and summarizing pertinent information in your own words.Never copy phrases, sentences or paragraphs from other people's work directly even if you do reference the source.

④ Copying from published sources constitutes plagiarism and it will expose the authors to disciplinary action.

Section 3   Experimental Design and Implementation in Medical Functional Experiment

We have already discussed the importance of experiment as one critical step in scientific method cycle in the previous chapter, and described the basic rules to follow when doing scientific research. Still we have learned the information in writing and publishing a research paper in a scientific journal. With all these in mind, it is the right time for us to combine them together to design our own experimental.

Experimental design is a good way to improve the scientific research ability of students from a small group or a team. To design and perform an excellent experiment, normally we need to schedule two lab sessions which are arranged on two consecutive afternoons. Before the first session, the teacher briefly explains the basic methods and principles of experimental design, and provides some alternative topics; then, the students select or decide on a topic, and complete an experiment design report (also known as the pre-lab report) in groups through literature review and the cooperation of group members. In the first introductory session, each group sends student representatives to make a presentation, finally determine the detailed experiment steps through other students' questions and teacher's comments, and get familiar with the available experimental equipment and reagents prepared by the technicians. In the second performing session, the students will conduct a formal experiment according to their experiment design scheme to prove their hypothesis and fulfill the experiment objectives. After this session, the student need to write a full experiment report and submit it on time.

1. The format of the experimental design report/pre-lab report

1) Topic/Title: conceive an appropriate title reflecting factors to be tested and validated.

2) Aim: one or two.

3) Principle: provide background information about the key problem to be resolved or the key hypothesis to be validated.

4) Animal or subject: include the control and test groups.

5) Equipment and reagents: as required.

6) Method/Procedure and observations: list detailed experimental procedures so that others can replicate it if necessary. Include statistical analysis about what data will be gathered and how the data will be analyzed.

7) Caution: indicate all precautions to take for safety and accuracy.

8) Prospective result: anticipate the possible results according to known knowledge.

9) Reference: follow the standard format of certain journal publications and keep constancy.

2. The format of a full experimental report

1) Topic/Title: conceive an appropriate title reflecting factors to be tested and validated.

2) Aim: introduce what is the main purpose of the experiment.

3) Principle: provide with background information about the key problem to be resolved or the key hypothesis to be validated.

4) Animal or subject: include the control and test groups.

5) Equipment and reagents: as required.

6) Methods/Procedure and observations: list detailed experimental procedures so that others can replicate it if necessary. Include statistical analysis showing what data will be gathered and how the data will be analyzed.

7) Results: expressed in detail, using assorted data and statistic graphs.

8) Discussion: based on the results to make reasonable and specific analysis.

9) Conclusion: draw conclusions from results and discussion in concise sentences.

10) Caution: indicate all precautions to take for safety and accuracy.

11) Reference: follow the standard format of certain the journal publications.

3. The format of experimental report in form of journal published paper

Try to write the experimental report as if it is going to be published in a formal journal, and the readers are familiar with the topic. Thus, you need to assume the standard format for a research paper.

1) Cover Page: On the cover page the title of the designed experiment, the authors' names with orders according to their constructions should be included.

2) Abstract: The abstract includes the summary of the question investigated, the methods used, and the principal results and main conclusions. A good abstract allows the intended audience understand the entire report without having to read the rest parts. And this section should be written after you have finished all the other parts.

3) Refer to Section 2 of this chapter for other parts.

Experiment 3　Single Muscle Twitch, Incomplete Tetanus and Complete Tetanus

1. Aim

To observe the relationship between the frequency of stimulation and the patterns of muscular contraction

2. Principle

When an action potential travels along a motor nerve to a muscle cell, it causes a depolarization on the muscle cell membrane. The action potential generated on the muscle cell membrane travels to the centre of the muscle cell, causes the the sarcoplasmic reticulum to release calcium ions which initiate the contractile process. After the calcium level are restored by calcium ion pump the contraction ceased. This whole process is single muscle twitch.

Muscle contraction can undergo a summation process, which means the adding together of individual twitch contractions (single muscle twitch) to increase the intensity of overall muscle contraction (Figure 1). One of the ways of complete this process is frequency summation. Under low frequency of stimulation, individual contraction occurring one after another, which displayed on the left of Figure 1. Eventually as the frequency increases, new contraction will occurs before the previous is over. As a result, the second contraction is partially added to the first one, and thus the contraction strength rises with the frequency. When the frequency continues to rise, it will reaches a critical level that the successive contraction fuse together and the whole muscle contraction appears to be completely smooth and continuous. This phenomenon is called complete tetanus, and the frequencies before complete tetanus is given a name of incomplete tetanus. Tetany occurs based on enough calcium ions are maintained in the muscle sarcoplasm, even between action potentials. Therefore, full contractile state is sustained without allowing any relaxation between the action potentials.

3.Experimental materials

1) Animal: Frogs.

2) Equipment: Electronic stimulator, universal support stand, dissection set for frog, mechanicalelectrical transducer, BL-420 system.

3) Reagents: Ringer's solution.

4. Procedures and observations

1) Making the sciaticgastrocnemius preparation.

2) Connecting the muscle to the input of BL-420 system with a mechanicalelectrical transducer.

3) Putting the stimulating electrodes on the sciatic nerve or muscle directly and keep them contact closely.

4) Using BL-420 system to generate the stimulation to the muscle tissue, adjust the frequency of stimulation. and record the contraction of the skeletal muscle.

5. Results

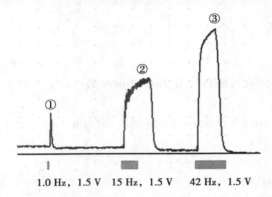

1.0 Hz, 1.5 V   15 Hz, 1.5 V   42 Hz, 1.5 V

① Single twitch; ② Incomplete tetanus; ③ Complete tetanus.

Figure 1   The patterns of muscular contraction with increase of stimulus frequency

6. Discussion

A single muscle twitch is the cycle of contraction, relaxation produced by a single low frequency of stimulation and there are three phases of a single muscle twitch.

The first one is the latent period. In this period, there is no change in length, but the time during which impulse is traveling along sarcolemma & down t-tubules to sarcoplasmic reticulum, calcium is being released into the cytosol that cross bridges begins to cycle and so on. In other words, muscle cannot contract instantaneously. The following one is the contraction phase. Myosin cross bridge cycling causes sarcomere to shorten, tension increases that cross-bridges are swiveling. The relaxation phase is the last one. The calcium ions are actively transported back into the terminal cisternae, the cross bridge cycling decreases and ends, so that the muscle returns to its original length that is decrease of tension. Furthermore, each different muscle has different actual time periods for each phase.

When the frequency of stimulation is increased to the point where the muscle exhibits even shorter contraction-relaxation cycles, but there is still some degree of relaxation after each contraction, so the two twitches will sum. At high frequencies of action potentials, twitches sum to produce a smooth, sustained, maximum contraction called incomplete tetanus.

When the frequency of stimulation becomes fast enough, the contractions fuse into a smooth, continuous,total contraction with no apparent relaxation produces a force approximately 3-5 times a single twitch contraction called complete tetanus.

5. Conclusion

The frequency of stimulation determines the patterns of skeletal muscle contraction and the amplitude of muscle contraction increases with the stimulation frequency.

6. Reference

[1] HALL J E. Guyton and Hall textbook of medical physiology[M]. 13th ed. Philadelphia (PA): Elsevier Science publishers, 2016.

Here we take effects of exercise on cardiovascular and respiratory activities in human subjects for an example to show what a good experimental design looks like. Then you will understand how to design a desirable experiment with the previous described principles and procedures.

Effects of exercise on human cardiovascular and respiratory activity

1. Aims

1) To observe and explain the effects of exercise on cardiovascular and respiratory activities in human subjects.

2) To practice the basic procedures to design an experiment following the basic principles.

3) To learn the methods of recording heart rate, arterial blood pressure and breathing frequency.

2. Principles /Background

The cardiorespiratory system consists of the heart and blood vessels, which works with the respiratory system (the lungs and airways).These body systems carry oxygen to the muscles and organs of the body, and remove waste products and excessive carbon dioxide. Cardiorespiratory system's ability will increase to supply more oxygen to skeletal muscles during sustained physical activity than at rest.

There are lots of indices and measurements to evaluate the functions of the heart, blood vessels and lungs. Considering current experiment should be finished within one afternoon with the limited apparatus, we shall adopt the following indices: heart rate, blood pressure (including systolic pressure, diastolic pressure and pulse pressure) and the respiratory rate.

(1) Heart rate

Exercise uses up the energy derived from oxidizing glucose. Both glucose and oxygen have to be delivered by the blood. This means that the heart has to work harder to pump more blood through the body and it has to beat faster in order to achieve a higher throughput. The heart rate of a human being at rest is about 70 beats/min. During vigorous exercise, the heart rate can increase dramatically (the rule of thumb given for maximal heart rate is 220 beats/min at your age).This will result in an increase in blood flow.

(2) Blood pressure

Along with an increase in heart rate, the force of our heart's contractions also increases while exercising, so more blood is pumped with each beat. This effect increases blood pressure.

However, the blood vessels that supply our muscles dilate, or get larger, during exercise. This enables increased blood to flow to our muscles without putting excess pressure on our blood vessel walls. So when our blood pressure rises during exercise, it is to a much smaller degree than the increase in heart rate. Like our heart rate, our blood pressure returns to resting level a few minutes after we stop exercising.

(3) Respiration rate/Breathing frequency

When we are exercising, the muscle cells in the body will consume more oxygen and produce more carbon dioxide. The lungs will have to work harder to provide oxygen and also remove carbon dioxide. There will be an increase in breathing frequency as the body tries hard to get as much oxygen as possible and to minimize the amount of oxygen debt. This will also happen after exercise as well as when the body has to repay the body's oxygen debt. Respiration rate or breathing frequency is the number of breath per minute when a person stands erect and at rest. A healthy human averages 12~18 breaths per minute while at rest. The respiration rate is considered as abnormal when the reading is more than 25 breaths per minute.

3. Experimental materials

1) Subject: human being.

2) Experimental equipments: sphygmomanometer, stethoscope, timer, stopwatch.

4. Procedures and observations

1) Determine the exercise type and its intensity: Take 3 min step test for example, step on and off the steps or left foot up, right foot up, left foot down, right foot down, using the rhythm of the metronome, begin stepping at 24 step cycles/minute, a total of 72 steps, etc.

2) Assign students into different test groups randomly.

3) Let the subjects sit quietly for 3 min, then take blood pressure, heart rate and respiratory rate before exercise (as baseline/control). The rate is usually measured when a person is at rest and simply involves counting the number of breaths in one minute by counting how many times the chest rises. Get three trails of the respiration rate and take an average.

4) Do exercise at different intensity as planned.

① Ask subjects to do "step on and off" for 20 s (keep the same rhythm), the assigned person immediately measure and record their heart rate (HR), systolic blood pressure (SBP), diastolic blood pressure (DBP) and breathing frequency (BF). 20 min later, the same person measure all the parameters again.

② Ask subjects from the other group to do "step on and off" for 40 s (keep the same rhythm), the same person measure and record their heart rate, arterial blood pressure and breathing frequency immediately and 20 min later.

5) Design the result tables and predict the changing tendency of each parameters.

Table 1   The effects of different degrees of exercise on HR, BP and BF

Student infromation		Pre-Exercise				Exercise for 20 s				Exercise for 40 s			
Gender	Name	HR (times/min)	SBP (mmHg)	DBP (mmHg)	BF (times/min)	HR (times/min)	SBP (mmHg)	DBP (mmHg)	BF (times/min)	HR (times/min)	SBP (mmHg)	DBP (mmHg)	BF (times/min)
Male	Student 1												
	Student 2												
	Student 3												
	Student 4												
Female	Student 5												
	Student 6												
	Student 7												
	Student 8												

5. Prospective results

According to the known theoretical knowledge, the anticipated results could be:

1) The exercise will increase the heart rate. The heart rate will continue to rise in direct proportion to the intensity of exercise until the maximum heart rate is reached.

2) Our blood pressure rises during exercise, but it is to a much smaller degree than the increase in the heart rate. Like our heart rate, our blood pressure returns to the resting level a few minutes after we stop exercising.

3) When we change from the resting state to exercising, the number of breaths we take per minute, immediately responds. Initially, our breathing frequency increases rapidly. After that initial response, or first few minutes, your breathing frequency will level off. However, if we increase the intensity of exercise, our breathing frequency will increase, but not as rapidly as the initial response.

6. Reference

[1] HALL J E. Guyton and Hall textbook of medical physiology[M]. Philadelphia, PA: Saunders Elsevier, 2016.

[2] ZHU D, WANG T H. Physiology textbook[M]. Beijing: People's Medical Publish House, 2013.

The effects of squat-and-straighten-up exercise on respiratory frequency, heart rate and blood pressure in young students

1. Aims

1) To study the measurement and recording method of heart rate and arterial blood pressure, and understand the impact of exercise in the cardiovascular system.

2) To learn the recording method of respiratory frequency, and understand the effects of exercise on the respiratory system.

3) To observe the effects of exercise on respiratory frequency, heart rate and blood pressure.

2. Principles

It is known that the whole body is working in unison during exercise: the heart and blood vessels, the lungs, the muscles, the brain and nerves, and the bones. So we can test exercise effect on any of these organs or systems. For example, exercise brings about short-term changes in the cardiovascular system, breathing (the lungs), and the muscular skeletal system, with messages from the brain as a control or regulatory role. These changes can be measured during and after exercise and the results recorded can be compared to that before exercise.

1) **Anaerobic exercise and aerobic exercise:** exercise requires energy. Aerobic exercise means energy comes from aerobic metabolism in the cells and anaerobic exercise means energy comes from anaerobic glycolysis. In aerobic metabolism, fully oxidating 1 molecule of glucose oxidation can produce 38 ATP, and when anaerobic glycolysis, 1 molecule of glucose produces only 2 ATP.

① Aerobic exercise is the physical activity that uses large muscle groups and causes the body to use more oxygen than it would while resting. The goal of aerobic exercise is to increase cardiovascular endurance. Examples of aerobic exercise include cycling, swimming, brisk walking, skipping rope, rowing, hiking, playing tennis, continuous training, and long slow distance training.

② Anaerobic exercise, which includes strength and resistance training, can firm, strengthen, and tone muscles, as well as improve bone strength, balance, and coordination. Examples of strength moves are push-ups, pull-ups, lunges, and bicep curls using dumbbells. Anaerobic exercise also includes weight training, functional training, eccentric training, interval training, sprinting, and high-intensity interval training increase short-term muscle strength.

2) **Effects of exercise on heart rate:** exercise uses up a lot of energy, which is derived from oxidizing glucose by cells. Both glucose and oxygen have to be delivered by the blood. This

means that the heart has to work harder to pump more blood through the body. So it has to beat faster in order to achieve a higher throughput. Heart rate for a human being at rest is about 70 beats/min. During vigorous exercise, heart rate can increase dramatically, and the maximal heart rate can be calculated by 220 beats/min. This will result in an increase in blood flow.

3) **Effects of exercise on blood pressure:** along with an increase in heart rate, the force of our heart's contractions also increases while exercising, so more blood is pumped with each beat. This effect increases blood pressure. However, the blood vessels will get larger during exercise. This enables the blood flow to our muscles to increase without putting excess pressure on our blood vessel walls. So when our blood pressure rises during exercise, it is to a much smaller degree than the increase in heart rate. Like our heart rate, our blood pressure returns to resting level a few minutes after we stop exercising.

4) **Effects of exercise on respiration:** when we do exercise, the muscular cells in the body will use up more oxygen and produce more carbon dioxide. The lungs have to work harder to provide oxygen and also remove carbon dioxide. The respiratory frequency and depth will increase in order to get as much oxygen as possible and to minimize the amount of oxygen debt. (Oxygen debt means the amount of extra oxygen required by muscle tissue during recovery from vigorous exercise). Respiratory frequency is around 14 per minute at rest and can increase to 32 per minute during exercise.

3. Experimental materials

1) Subject: Human being.

2) Equipments: Stopwatch, stethoscope, sphygmomanometer.

4. Procedures and observations

1) Firstly, Subjects rest for 5 min to ensure that the body is in a state of calmness and relaxation, and others measure and record their respiratory frequency, heart rate and blood pressure.

2) Subjects do 20 squat-and-straighten-up exercise (keep the same frequency), and others immediately measure and record their heart rate, arterial blood pressure and respiratory frequency.

3) After the symptoms return to normal values, subjects do 40 squat-and-straighten-up exercise (keep the same frequency), and others immediately measure and record their heart rate, arterial blood pressure and respiratory frequency.

4) Measurement method in detail.

① **Measure arterial blood pressure indirectly**: The blood pressure cuff is wrapped snugly around the arm just above the elbow and inflated until the blood flowing into the forearm is stopped and no brachial pulse can be felt or heard. Pressure in the cuff is gradually reduced while the examiner listens (auscultates) for sounds (of Korotkoff) in the brachial artery with a stethoscope. The pressure, read as the first soft tapping sounds are heard (the first point at which a small amount of blood is spurting through the constricted artery), is recorded as the systolic pressure. As the pressure is reduced still further, the sounds become louder and more distinct. But when the artery is no longer restricted and blood flows freely, the sounds can no longer be heard. The pressure at which the sounds disappear is routinely recorded as the diastolic pressure.

② **Count breath rate correctly**: To get an accurate measurement before doing exercise, the participant must be at rest (should be still for at least 10 min) before you count the breathing rate. Count the number of times the participant's chest rises and falls during one minute. You can take the measurement three times and average the values to improve the accuracy of your result. You can also count the breath in a 15 s, then multiply the number by 4. This gives a close approximation of breath per minute and is useful in emergency situations.

5. Results

Table 1　The effects of squat-and-straighten-up exercise on cardiopulmonary activities

State	SP (mmHg)	DP (mmHg)	PP (mmHg)	MBP (mmHg)	HR (times/min)	RR (times/min)
Relaxation	106.9 ± 6.52	64.6 ± 8.15	42.3 ± 9.53	78.7 ± 6.19	82 ± 11.35	21.4 ± 3.01
Exercise (20 min)	121.4 ± 11.14	66.7 ± 10.08	54.7 ± 6.66	84.93 ± 9.96	92.5 ± 19.31	29 ± 3.38
Relaxation	106.7 ± 5.62	65 ± 4.84	41.7 ± 4.94	78.9 ± 4.55	83.2 ± 12.2	22.3 ± 3.13
Exercise (40 min)	125.9 ± 7.34	63.2 ± 12.97	62.7 ± 10.69	84.1 ± 10.23	102.4 ± 24.96	32.9 ± 5.92

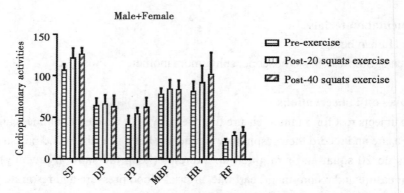

Systolic pressure: SP; Diastolic pressure: DP; Pulse pressure: PP; Mean blood pressure: MBP; Heart rate: HR; Respiratory frequency: RF.

Figure 1　The effects of squat-and-straighten-up exercise on cardiopulmonary activities

Table 2　The effects of squat-and-straighten-up exercise on cardiopulmonary activities in male group

State	SP (mmHg)	DP (mmHg)	PP (mmHg)	MBP (mmHg)	HR (times/min)	RR (times/min)
Relaxation	106.4 ± 8.62	63.6 ± 10.98	42.8 ± 12.17	77.87 ± 8.5	72.8 ± 6.88	19.2 ± 2.48
Exercise (20 min)	114.8 ± 7.76	57.6 ± 3.44	57.2 ± 6.14	76.67 ± 4.42	83.6 ± 15.72	27.6 ± 3.88
Relaxation	108.4 ± 7.09	66.4 ± 4.96	42 ± 4.56	80.4 ± 5.34	75.2 ± 11.97	20 ± 2.76
Exercise (40 min)	123.8 ± 5.53	53.6 ± 6.25	70.2 ± 5.31	77 ± 5.47	90.6 ± 24.06	31.6 ± 6.97

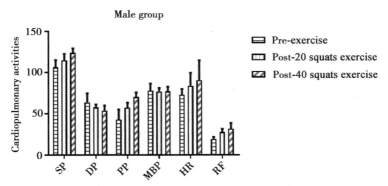

Systolic pressure: SP; Diastolic pressure: DP; Pulse pressure: PP; Mean blood pressure: MBP; Heart rate: HR; Respiratory frequency: RR.

Figure 2   The effects of squat-and-straighten-up exercise on cardiopulmonary activities in male group

Table 3   The effects of squat-and-straighten-up exercise on cardiopulmonary activities in female group

State	SP (mmHg)	DP (mmHg)	PP (mmHg)	MBP (mmHg)	HR (times/min)	RR (times/min)
Relaxation	107.4 ± 3.2	65.6 ± 3.2	41.8 ± 5.74	79.53 ± 1.71	91.2 ± 6.4	23.6 ± 1.5
Exercise (20 min)	128 ± 10.04	75.8 ± 5.08	52.2 ± 6.21	93.2 ± 6.5	101.4 ± 18.46	30.4 ± 1.96
Relaxation	105 ± 2.68	63.6 ± 4.27	41.4 ± 5.28	77.4 ± 2.89	91.2 ± 5.15	24.6 ± 1.2
Exercise (40 min)	128 ± 8.27	72.8 ± 10.63	55.2 ± 9.37	91.2 ± 8.87	114.2 ± 19.7	34.2 ± 4.26

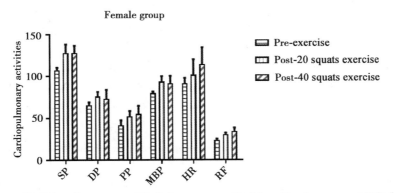

Systolic pressure: SP; Diastolic pressure: DP; Pulse pressure: PP; Mean blood pressure: MBP; Heart rate: HR; Respiratory frequency: RR.

Figure 3   The effects of squat-and-straighten-up exercise on cardiopulmonary activities in female group

6. Discussion

As we know that squat-and-straighten-up exercise is a kind of anaerobic exercise, which produces more lactic acid than aerobic exercise, and will make the muscles experience more fatigue. This may excite the nervous system to increase the cardiovascular and respiratory activity.

(1) Effect of exercise on respiratory rate

From Table 1 and Figure 1, it is easy to find that one of the effects of exercise on the cardiovascular system is an increase in our heart rate. Heart rate will continue to rise in direct proportion to the intensity of exercise until the maximum heart rate is achieved.

When we transit from resting state to exercising state, the number of breaths we take per minute immediately responds. Initially, our respiratory frequency increases rapidly. After that initial response, our respiratory frequency will level off. However, if we increase the intensity of exercise, our respiratory frequency will increase, but not as rapidly as the initial response. During exercise, the tissue in body will consume energy. The energy obtained in normal condition is from aerobic respiration which needs oxygen to undergo a series processes of breaking down the reaction of the glucose. However, when the intensity of exercise increases, more energy is needed. The body will lack of oxygen because the oxygen intake rate is lower than the oxygen consume rate. Therefore, the PO_2 in blood decreases and the PCO_2 and H^+ in blood increases. This condition will stimulate the peripheral chemoreceptor which are carotid bodies and aortic bodies, and the central chemoreceptor which is located in medulla oblongata. Then, it will generate the respiratory centre to promote the pulmonary ventilation which will increase the respiratory rate.

Moreover, when the tissue lacks of oxygen, it will gain the energy from anaerobic respiratory which will produce the lactic acid. Lactic acid will further decease the level of pH which means further increase the H^+ ion level. Therefore, it will further stimulate the peripheral chemoreceptor and central chemoreceptor and then enhance the promotion of pulmonary ventilation thus further increasing the respiratory rate. The more the lactic acid accumulate, the stronger reflex will occur. That is why increasing the intensity of exercise will result in increasing respiratory rate[1].

The final respiratory rate after high intensity exercise is higher than at resting state at the beginning. This is because the lactic acid accumulates in the body, therefore the oxygen debt will occur. Additional oxygen must be needed to metabolize the lactic acid into the glucose to restore all systems to their normal states. Therefore, the respiratory rate will increase for a long lasting period. That is why the final respiratory rate after high intensity exercise is still higher than at resting state at the beginning.

(2) Effect of exercise on heart rate

In all vertebrates, the heart is innervated by a parasympathetic inhibitory system, and a sympathetic excitatory system, while the heart rhythm is regulated entirely by the sinus node under normal conditions. As the body starts to exercise, the skeletal muscle contraction will stimulate the excitation of sympathetic nerves of cardiac muscles. The vagus nerve provides parasympathetic input to the heart by releasing acetylcholine onto sinus node cells. Therefore, stimulation of the sympathetic nerve increases heart rate, while stimulation of the vagus nerve decreases it. The higher the intensity of exercise is, the larger the amount of norepinephrine will be secreted by the sympathetic nerves and thus increase the heart rate. After higher intensity of exercise, the body needs more time to consume the large amount of acetylcholine, which may be due to the limited amount of chemo receptor in cardiac muscle cell. What's more, after the high intensity exercise, the participants' overall heart rate is higher than that is under low intensity exercise, which is because the accumulation of the lactic acid in the muscle leads to the decrease of pH in the blood, and thus causing the heart beats faster than it does under other circumstances.

(3) Effect of exercise on blood pressure

Our mean blood pressure rises during exercising, but the degree of increase in blood pressure is smaller than the increase in heart rate. Like our heart rate, our blood pressure returns to resting level a few minutes after we stop exercising.

According to the figures, we can observe that the systole pressure increases dramatically as the intensity of exercise increases because the demands for blood supply increases. Yet the diastolic pressure decreases as the intensity of exercise increases because of the deposition of lactic acid produced during anaerobic exercise which will dilate the blood vessels and thus decrease the diastolic pressure.

(4) Effect of exercise on the basis of gender difference

Comparing table 2 and 3 and also figure2 and 3, we can find that the effects of squat-and-straighten-up exercise at the same level varies between male group and female group.

Firstly, we can observe that in female group, the heart rate in the first round of exercise (20 squats) and the second round of exercise (40 squats) was higher than male group, which means the ability of ventricular muscle of female is inferior to its counterpart, male. It may reveal the fact that the physical endurance of female is inferior to that of male, thus the female met the maximal heart rate sooner. Secondly, as shown in the table, we can find that the diastolic pressure of male decreases after squat-and-straighten-up exercise at two levels, but in female group, on the contrary, increases.One reason to explain this difference could be that the ability to produce lactic acid in female is weaker than that in male, thus the lactic acid would exert less influence on the blood vessels which mainly determine the value of diastolic pressure by decreasing the total peripheral resistance.

7. Conclusion

Cardiovascular and respiratory activities are increased during exercise due to extra energy demand.

8. References

[1] HALL J E. Guyton and Hall textbook of medical physiology[M]. 13th ed. Philadelphia (PA): Elsevier Science Publishers, 2016.

[2] MARIEB E, HOEHN K. Human anatomy & physiology[M]. 7th ed. New York:Pearson Education,2007.

[3] GOOTMAN P M, COHEN H L, GOOTMAN N. Autonomic nervous system regulation of heart rate in the perinatal period [J]. Pediatric and Fundamental Electrocardiography, 1987(56): 137-159.

[4] DI DONATO D M, WEST D W, CHURCHWARD-VENNE T A, et al. Influence of aerobic exercise intensity on myofibrillar and mitochondrial protein synthesis in young men during early and late post exercise recovery[J]. American Journal of Physiology-Endocrinology and

Metabolism, 2014, 306(9): E1025-E1032.

[5] FISHER J P , ADLAN A M, SHANTSILA A, et al. Muscle metaboreflex and autonomic regulation of heart rate in humans [J]. The Journal of physiology, 2013, 591(15):3777-3788.

[6] ZHU D, WANG T H. Physiology textbook[M]. Beijing: People's Medical Publish House, 2013.

[7] TANAKA H, SEALS D R. Endurance exercise performance in Masters athletes:age-associated changes and underlying physiological mechanisms [J]. The Journal of physiology, 2008, 586(1): 55-63.

Appendix 4   CO generator device and related mechanism

1. CO generator

During this experiment, chemical methods are used to obtain CO. The CO generator is shown in Figure 1. Take 4 mL of formic acid into the tube and then slowly add 2 mL of sulfuric acid. The CO produced is connected with the hypoxia bottle containing mice through a plastic hose (the hypoxia bottle is connected with the air). The reaction principle is as follows:

$$\text{HCOOH} \xrightarrow{\text{H}_2\text{SO}_4} \text{CO} + \text{H}_2\text{O}$$

2. Action mechanism of sodium lime

Sodium lime ($NaOH \cdot CaO$) is a pink particle with the function of absorbing CO_2. The reaction formula is as follows:

$$\text{NaOH} \cdot \text{CaO} + \text{H}_2\text{O} + \text{CO}_2 \rightarrow \text{NaHCO}_3 + \text{Ca(OH)}_2$$

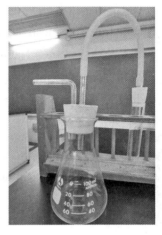

Figure 1   CO generator

3. Detoxification mechanism of methylene blue

Methylene blue is a non-toxic dye. Its oxidation type is blue and its reduction type is colorless. When methylene blue enters the body, the H^+ generated during the dehydrogenation of glucose 6-phosphate are transferred to methylene blue through reduced coenzyme II (pyridine triphosphate nucleoside) to turn it into colorless methylene blue, which can quickly turn $Hb\text{-}Fe^{3+}$ to $Hb\text{-}Fe^{2+}$. Meanwhile, the colorless methylene blue is oxidized to methylene blue. Methylene blue itself is an oxidant. it cannot be turned to colorless methylene blue quickly by coenzyme II if a large amount of methylene blue is used, so that more $Hb\text{-}Fe^{3+}$ will be generated. Therefore, low-dose methylene blue injection should be used in the treatment of methemoglobinemia.

1. Principle

The mouse in airtight flask inhales the oxygen continuously, while the CO_2 exhaled is absorbed by soda lime as indicated by the equation below:

$$NaOH \cdot CaO + H_2O + CO_2 \rightarrow NaHCO_3 + Ca(OH)_2$$

As a result, the pressure in the flask becomes negative, leading to the rise of water in the graduated pipette as well as the fall of water in the graduated cylinder when the flask is connected to the measuring apparatus. The falling volume read from the graduated cylinder is referred to the total amount of oxygen consumed in the bottle, and the oxygen consumption rate by the mouse can be calculated according to the empirical formula shown in page 215.

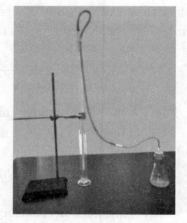

Figure 1   Apparatus for measuring oxygen consumption

2. Methods

1) Pour water into the graduated cylinder to the maximal mark and connect the measuring apparatus to the airtight bottle with rubber tube as shown in Figure 1.

2) Remove the clamp on the rubber tube. When the water in the pipette remains stable, the falling volume read from the graduated cylinder is equal to the total amount of oxygen consumed by the mouse in the bottle.

1. Anesthesia methods of the experimental animals

The basic task of experimental animal anesthesia is to eliminate the pain and discomfort caused by the experimental operation, ensure the safety of the experimental animals, make the animals obey the operation in the experiment, and ensure the progress of the experiment.

1) Commonly used local anesthesia methods: topical anesthesia is a local anesthesia to block the nerve endings on the mucosa surface using the tissue penetration effect. Topical anesthesia is often used in the operation of oral and nasal mucosa, conjunctiva, urethra and other parts.

① Procaine: because of the low toxicity and quick effect,procaine with a concentration of 0.5%~1% is often used for local infiltration anesthesia.

② Lidocaine: because of the quick effect and tissue penetration, lidocaine with a concentration of 1% to 2% is often used for nerve trunk block anesthesia in large animals. Lidocaine with a concentration of 0.25%~0.5% can also be used as local anesthesia.

2) General anesthesia

① Isoflurane is the most commonly used inhalation anesthesia in the laboratory. First, animals are induced anesthesia by isoflurane with a concentration of 2%~3.5% and then maintained anesthesia with appropriate concentration of isoflurane (1.5%~2% for mice and 2%~3% for rats).

② Pentobarbital sodium is injected intravenously at a dose of 30 mg/kg in the rabbit or 50 mg/kg in mouse or rat. The effective time can last for 3~5 h.

③ Urethane is injected intravenously at a dose of 100 mg/kg for rabbit or injected intraperitoneally at a dose of 140 mg/kg for mouse or rat.

When doing anesthesia, using two thirds of the total amount of anesthesia first, and observe the changes of the animal's vital signs closely. If the required depth of anesthesia has been reached, the rest of the anesthetic will not be used to avoid the death of the animal due to excessive anesthesia and breath inhibition.

2. Common used catheterization

1) Tracheal cannula: the rabbit is anesthetized with 25% urethane (4 mL/kg) intravenously in the marginal ear vein and fixed in supine position on the dissecting table for rabbit. Clean the surgical field in the cervical region by removing the fur with scissors. Make a 4~5 cm long longitudinal incision along the middle of the neck. Separate the subcutaneous tissue and muscle layer by layer. Expose and isolate the trachea. Make a T-shaped incision 0.5~1 cm below the thyroid cartilage of the trachea and insert a Y-shape tracheal cannula toward the lung. Fix it firmly with a suture.

2) Carotid artery cannula: the rabbit is anesthetized with 25% urethane (4 mL/kg) intravenously in the marginal ear vein and fixed in supine position on the dissecting table for rabbit. Clean the surgical field in the cervical region by removing the fur with scissors. Make a 4~5 cm long longitudinal incision along the middle of the neck. Separate the subcutaneous tissue and muscle layer by layer, and expose the trachea. Find the carotid artery sheath on the dorsolateral side of the trachea and carefully separate one side of the carotid artery (about 3 cm long). Ligate the distal end with a suture and clamp the proximal end with an artery clamp. The arterial catheter filled with 0.3% heparin sodium solution or a 22G venous indwelling needle is inserted into the artery. Ligate and fix the catheter.

3) Jugular vein cannula:the rabbit is anesthetized with 25% urethane (4 mL/kg) intravenously in the marginal ear vein and fixed in supine position on the dissecting table for rabbit. Clean the surgical field in the cervical region by removing the fur with scissors. Make a 4~5 cm long longitudinal incision along the middle of the neck. Separate the subcutaneous tissue and muscle layer by layer. The jugular vein is located under the skin of the neck and at the outer edge of the sternocleidomastoid muscle can be clearly seen. The subcutaneous fascia on both sides of the jugular vein is separated along the direction of the blood vessel with forceps. Ligate the distal end with a suture. Make a small cut with an ophthalmic scissor and insert the venous catheter. Ligate and fix the catheter.

4) Femoral artery and femoral vein cannula:touch the pulsation of the femoral artery in the groin area first, and then make a 4 cm long incision along the direction of the blood vessel. The femoral artery, vein and nerve are located in the same sheath. Isolation and cannula of the vessels are the same as carotid artery.

Operation video of common used catheterization

Appendix 7　Brief introduction to BL-420N data acquisiton and analysis system

1. Introduction of dominant interface

Dominant interface of BL-420N data acquisition and analysis system (abbreviated to BL-420N system) is introduced in this chapter, which will illustrate four main view area in the dominant interface, respectively are functional area, waveform display area, data file list area, stimulator control area, other information display area. See Figure 1.

View area is a displaying area that has independent functional planning, also it can be loaded into different views. In BL-420N system, all views can be displayed or hidden except the waveform displaying view. The rest of the views can be moved anywhere except for the top of the functional area. The other information display area includes the display measurement result, device information view, channel parameter adjustment view, and channel information view.

Open the software and find the waveform displaying view area. The waveform displaying view is also the dominant view. The upper part is the functional area, and it is divided into experimental data list view area and device's information view area from left part to right part. Please be patient to understand that the dominant interface, which will help you use the software. See Table 1 for the description of the division of main functional area in the dominant interface.

Functional area　Waveform display area

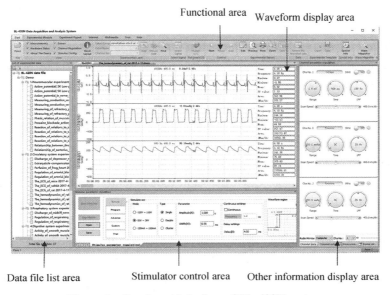

Data file list area　　Stimulator control area　Other information display area

Figure 1　Dominant interface of BL-420N system

Table 1　Division of main view in the dominant interface

Serial number	The name of view area	Function description
1	Functional area	Located at the top of the main interface Showing the main function buttons
2	Waveform display area	In the straight middle area of the main interface Displaying the acquired and analyzed channel data wave forms
3	Data file list area	Located on the left side of the main interface Selecting and opening stored experimental data files quickly
4	Stimulator control area	Located at the bottom of the main interface Adjusting the stimulus parameters and providing the stimulus
5	Other information display area	Located on the right side of the main interface Including the display measurement result , device information view, channel parameter adjustment view, and channel information view

Note:

After entering the BL-420N system, you can see that the dominant interface may be different from the dominant interface in Figure 1, this is because that many views of BL-420N system can be hidden and moved, and the views may be overlapped of each other, causing the dominant interface to change.

If the dominant interface displayed is not the same as the Figure 1 after you entered BL-420N system, no need to worry. Next, we will briefly introduce the operation of the containing view in the dominant interface.

(1) Display and hide the views in the dominant interface

The position of multiple views of system software and displaying status of BL-420N can be changed, this is designed for meet different users' requirements with their different using habits, but this change will cause that the system's dominant interface become Incomprehensible. Nevertheless, as long as you master the law of change, you can easily cope with the change, and you can finish the experiment more easily.

1) Minimizing and restoring functional areas: The functional area is at the top of the dominant interface, and it can be minimized. Click the right mouse button on the classified title position of the functional area, a relevant shortcut menu will pop up, select "minimizing functional areas", the function button below the classified title in the functional area is hidden. If you want to restore the function button hidden, you need to click the right mouse button on the classified title position of the functional area again, and the shortcut menu pop up. After that, select the order of "minimizing functional areas", the minimized functional area has been recovered. See Figure 2.

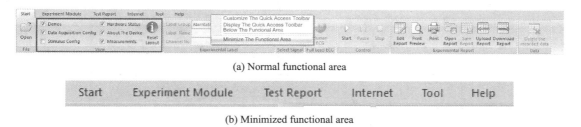

(a) Normal functional area

| Start | Experiment Module | Test Report | Internet | Tool | Help |

(b) Minimized functional area

Figure 2   Function of minimizing and restoring in the top function area of BL-420N system

2) View hiding and displaying

BL-420N system contains multiple views that can be hidden or displayed, except for the main view. The hidden (or displaying) status of these views is shown in the "functional area" → "start" bar category, under "view" selection, as shown in Figure 2 (a). When a box of the "view" that in front of the box has ticked, it indicates that the view is displayed, such as the experimental data list view.

Because the view will be covered in one certain area, even if the view is in the displaying state, it may be neglected by other views and cannot be displayed. If you want to display these covered views, the simplest way is to click the name of the view at the bottom of the view area.

(2) The movement of individual views in the dominant interface

In BL-420N system, all views can be moved and resized as needed, except for the waveform displaying view area and functional area. Each view has two states, one is the docking state next to the edge of the dominant interface of the software, which is also the default state of the view, and the other is the floating state in the form of independent window. See Figure 3 and Figure 4.

1) Switch between docking and floating: Double-click the left mouse button on the view title

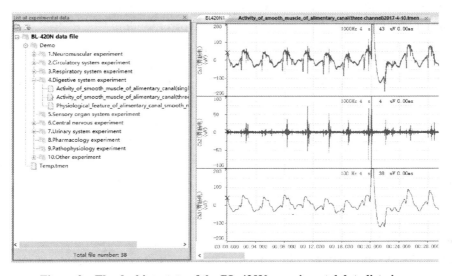

Figure 3   The docking state of the BL-420N experimental data list view

(next to the main view)

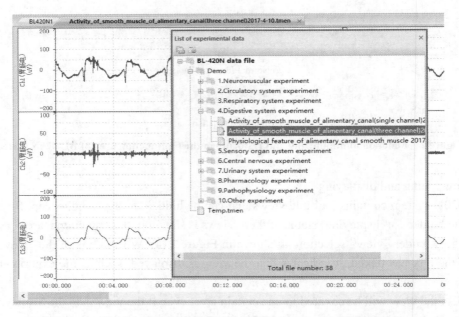

Figure 4　The floating state of the BL-420N experimental data list view
(floating above the main window)

bar to switch between the docking and floating state.

2) Docking and floating movement: Holding the left mouse button on the view title bar, and then move the mouse to the view position as needed.

When the left mouse button is pressed on the view title bar, a docking position reflected in transparency button appears on the dominant interface, as shown in Figure 5. Views can be docked in the main view around. For accurately dock the view, you should move the mouse position to the stop button. When the mouse moves to the stop button, "selecting view" appears in the corresponding position of the main view. When you confirmed the position, the left button of the mouse will stop selecting view, and the view will move to the appointed position. If you do not move the mouse to the stop button, instead of loosening the left mouse button directly in any position, the window is floating at the mouse indicated position.

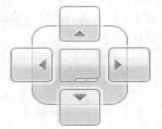

Figure 5　The transparent indicated button of selection view stopping position

The BL-420N system automatically record and save the users' last moving view position, so that all views remain the same location and size the next time you open the software. Therefore, when you move the view, the dominant interface of the software will appear differently from Figure 1.

2. Start experiment

The BL-420N system provides three approaches for starting experiments, respectively are, starting experiments from the experimental module, entering experiments from the signal selection dialog box, or starting experiments from the quick start view. Next, I will briefly introduce the above three ways to start the experiment.

(1) Starting experiments from the experimental module (suitable for teaching students)

Choose the "experimental module" column in the functional area, and then the experiment will be started according to the specified experimental module chosen. For example, select "circulatory" → "extrasystole-compensatory pause", the according experimental module will be triggered and initiated. See Figure 6.

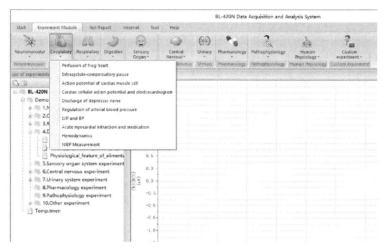

Figure 6   Start by pressing the drop-down button in the experimental module in the functional area.

From experiment module to start the experiment, the system will automatically configure various experimental parameters according to which experimental project that users chose, including: sampling channel number, sampling rate, gain, filtering, and stimulation parameters and so on, it is convenient for users to enter the experiment quickly.

The experimental module is usually configured according to the teaching content, so it is usually suitable for student experiments.

(2) Start experiments from the signal selection dialog box (For scientific research or newly added experiments by students)

Select the "start"   → "select signal" button in the toolbar, and a signal selection dialog box will pop up. See Figure 7 and Figure 8. In the "select signal" dialog box, the experimenter can configure the corresponding experimental parameters for each channel according to their own experimental requirement, and it is the most flexible way to start the experiment.

Select signal dialog box is the most flexible and universal way to start experiments, and it is most applied in scientific research. The flexible configuration of experimental parameters can also be saved as a costumed experimental module in the future BL-420N version, to help researchers quickly start their own experiments.

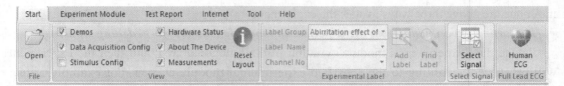

Figure 7   Signal selecting function button in the star bar functional area

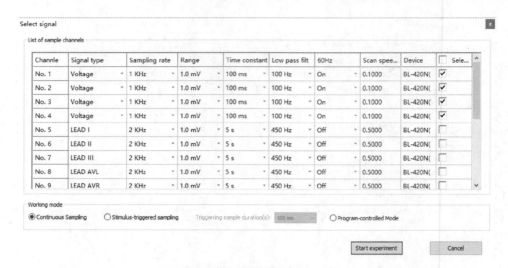

Figure 8   Signal selection dialog box

(3) Start the experiment from the quick start view (For fast opening the last experimental parameters)

You can start the experiment from the quick start button in the start view, or from the "start" button in the "start" menu bar of the function area, as shown in Figure 9. The two methods of quickly starting experiments are exactly the same, and there are two identical start-up approaches to facilitate users' operation.

The experiment will be started quickly when the software runs for the first time. The system will start the experiment in default mode by opening 4 ECG channels at the same time. If the experiment gets started with a quick start since the last step, the system will follow the parameters of the previous experiment and continue the current experiment.

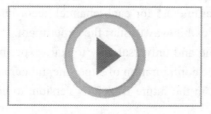

"Start" button in the start view

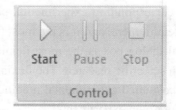

"Start" button in the start menu bar
of the function area

Figure 9   Quickly start button of the experiment

3. Pause and stop experiment

Click the "pause" or "stop" button in "start view", or selecting "pause" or "stop" button in the start menu bar of the functional area, and it can complete the operation of pausing and stopping in the experiment. The two approach towards these two operations are exactly the same, and both of them are provided for the convenience of the user. See Figure 10.

Pausing refers to stop the fast moving waveform during the process of the experiment, for the convenience of observing data analysis carefully from a static image on the screen. The collecting function of the hardware is still on when experimenters choose "pause", but the collected data will not be saved; to start again, the collected data is restored and saved.

"Stop" means that stop the whole experiment and save the data to a file.

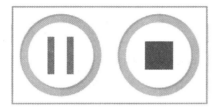 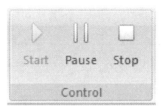

Pause and stop button in the start view   Pause and stop button in the start

menu bar for functional area

Figure 10   Pause and stop controlling button

4. Save data

When click to stop the experiment, a dialog box will pop up in the system asking whether to stop the experiment, if confirmed with that and the system will pop up a "save as" dialog that allows the user to save the name of the data, see Figure 11. The default name of the file is "year_month_day_ Non. tmen". The user can modify the file name of the saving and click "save" to save the data.

5. Data replay

Data replay refers to checking the saved experimental data. There are two ways to open the replay file:

1) Double-click the name of the replay file that you want to open in the "experimental data list" view, as shown in Figure 3.

2) Select "file" in the start menu bar in the functional area → command "open", a file dialog box will pop up and then open the file same as Figure 11, choose to open the replay files in the opening file dialog box, then click "open" button.

BL-420N system can open multiple files simultaneously for replaying, which is able to open up to 4 replaying files at the same time, as shown in Figure 12.

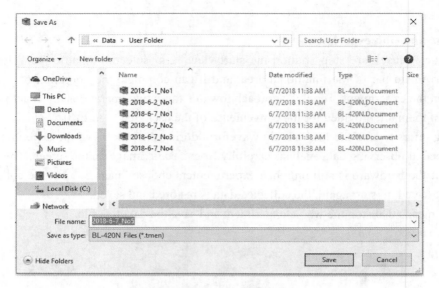

Figure 11　Data saving dialog

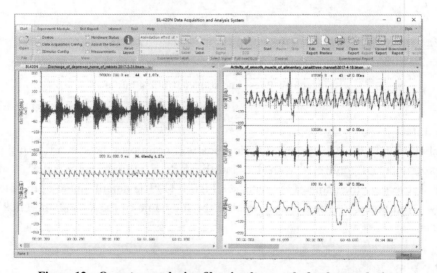

Figure 12　Open two replaying files simultaneously for data replaying

6. Editing and printing experimental reports

When experiment is completed, the user can edit and print the report, which can print directly after editing in the software. In addition, it can also be saved in local files and upload to NEIM-100 laboratory information management system (require independent laboratory configuration). The relevant functions of the experimental reports can be found in the "functional area" → "start" menu → "experimental report" category, which includes 5 common functions related to the experimental report, as shown in Figure 13.

1) Editing experimental reports: Select the editing button in Figure 13, and the system will trigger the editing function of experiment report, as shown in Figure 14. The experimental report editor is identical for editing documents in Microsoft Word, as shown in Figure 14.

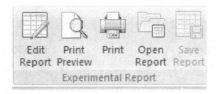

**Figure 13   Relevant functions of the experimental report
in the start menu of the functional area**

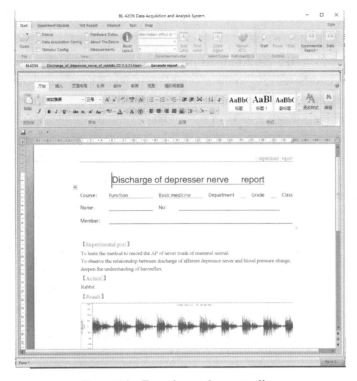

Figure 14   Experimental report editor

Users can enter user name in the experiment report editor, the experiment purposes, methods, conclusions and other information, and it also can choose the waveform from the raw data file, and then paste into the experimental report. In a default mode, the experimental report automatically extracts the waveform of the current screen displaying into the "experimental results" display area.

2) Printing experimental reports: Click the "functional area" → "start" → "experimental report" → "print" functional button to print the currently edited experiment report.

3) Saving experimental reports: Click "functional area" → "start" → "experimental report" → "save" functional button to save the current edited experiment report.

4) Open the saved experimental reports: Click "functional area" → "start" → "experimental report" → "open" functional button to open the saved local experimental report.

Appendix 8   An introduction to HPS-102 human physiology experimental system

1. Main interface

The main interface of HPS-102 human physiology experimental system (abbreviated to HPS-102 system) is composed of "toolbar" and "main work area" as shown in Figure 1. The toolbar collects multiple function buttons such as " open file" , " add tags" , "select signal" and "control " . The main work area is in the middle of the main interface where users can see waveform data, experimental labels, stimulus tag and adjust the waveform in the horizontal or vertical directions. On the right side of the main work area, users can adjust hardware parameter and check instrument connection status. A list of experimental data is docked on the left side. Stimulation and data measurement results can be seen below the main work area. The specific software interface can be expanded by clicking on its corresponding thumbnail.

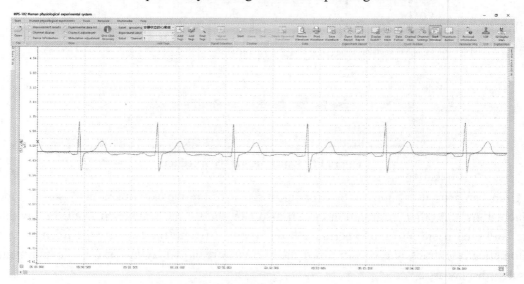

Figure 1   HPS-102 main interface

2. Homepage

The HPS-102 system provides 20 experimental modules by default. Based on human organ systems, these experimental modules are grouped into 10 categories including circulatory system experiments, respiratory system experiments and central nervous system experiments. After launching the HPS-102 system, users will see the grouped modules on the main interface as shown in Figure 2. Each category has varying numbers of experimental modules. The modules contain a combination of experimental overview, experimental methods, quiz and knowledge extension. Besides, experimental parameters such as suggested sampling channel, sampling rates, ranges and filtering setting are provided. Users can start the experiment directly after learning the related knowledge of the experiment.

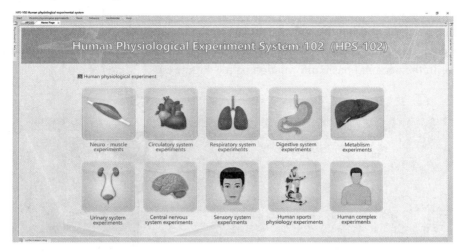

Figure 2　Homepage of HPS-102 system

3. Interface of the experimental modules

Each experimental module mainly contains four sections: experimental overview, experimental methods, quiz and knowledge extension. See the Figure 3. Experimental overview introduces the purposes and principle of the experiment. Experimental methods let users to know the equipment and drugs to be used, preparation before the experiment and observation items. A detailed introduction to the steps of the experiment is provided in this section. The quiz helps to check the students' understanding of the experiment knowledge. Knowledge extension is the expansion on the related knowledge of the experiment. It commonly includes development history, detailed

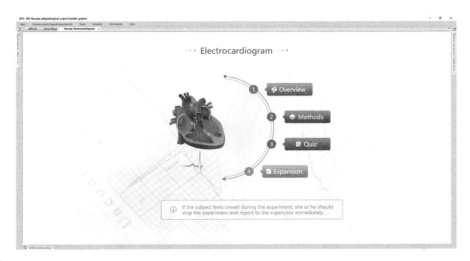

Figure 3　Interface of the experimental modules

principle introduction, clinical applications and references.

4. Interface of the subject's basic information

Basic information of the subject is of great significance for human physiological experiments. In terms of some human physiological indicators, theoretical values can be calculated based on the subject's weight and height, which is meaningful for comparison with experimental data. Users can enter basic information of the subject either prior to the "experimental modules" (See Figure 4) or in the personal basic information page (Figure 5).

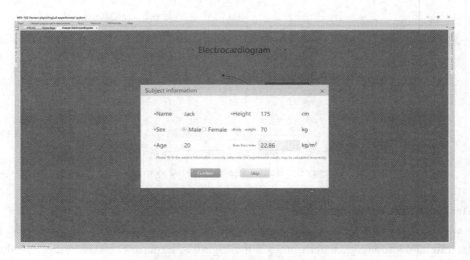

Figure 4   Basic information of the subject

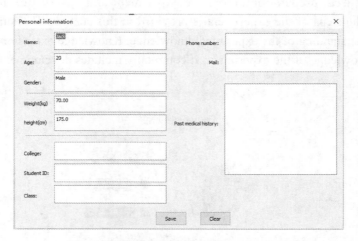

Figure 5   Personal basic information page

5. Interface of the experimental methods

Click the "start" button in the "experimental methods" section and an interface will appear to guide the experiment. See Figure 6. This interface consists of three parts: an navigation area of the experimental lists, a display area of the experimental steps and the experimental control area. In the navigation area, users can switch to any observation item of the experiment. The experimental steps guide the complete experimental process via graphics or videos. In the experimental control area, users can control the experimental sampling through the "start/pause" or "stop" buttons, or switch the experimental steps by the "previous step" or "next step" buttons and edit the experimental report by clicking the "edit report" button.

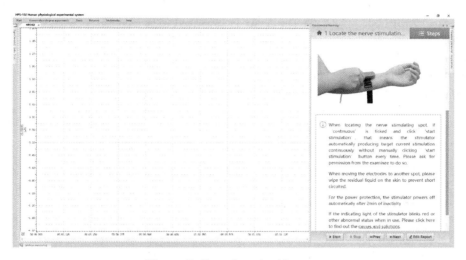

Figure 6   Experiment guide page

参考文献

［1］中华人民共和国国家质量监督检验检疫总局．实验动物 哺乳类实验动物的遗传质量控制：GB 14923-2010［S］.（2010-12-23）［2022-08-02］. http：//c.gb688.cn/bzgk/gb/showGb？type=online&hcno=FEA3D80C9605FAA4BB7CB5F36692925F.

［2］中华人民共和国国家质量监督检验检疫总局．实验动物 微生物学等级及监测：GB 14922.2-2011［S］.（2011-06-16）［2022-08-02］. http：//c.gb688.cn/bzgk/gb/showGb?type=online&hcno=AOEA17DC7258281D7090A05B42C923E2.

［3］秦川．医学实验动物学［M］. 2 版．北京：人民卫生出版社，2015.

［4］秦川．实验动物学［M］.北京：人民卫生出版社，2017.

［5］张汤杰．生理学研究中实验动物的选择［J］.上海实验动物科学，1997. 17（3）：189-190.

［6］何宝国，丁丽艳．蟾蜍的生物学特性及其资源开发与应用［J］.中国畜禽种业，2017. 9：50.

［7］KALISTE E. The Welfare of Laboratory Animals［M］. 2nd ed. Hameenlinna，Finland：State Provincial Office of Southern Finland Social and Health Affairs，2007.

［8］BAYNE K, TURNER P. Laboratory Animals Welfare［M］. Amsterdam：American College of Laboratory Animal Medicine，2013.

［9］王跃春．生理学实验指南及医学研究基础［M］.广州：暨南大学出版社，2018.

［10］HALL J E. Guyton and Hall textbook of medical physiology［M］. 13th ed. Philadelphia（PA）：Elsevier Science Publishers，2016.

［11］DAY R A. How to Write and Publish a Scientific Paper［M］. 8th ed. Philadelphia：ISI Press，2016.

［12］王建枝，钱睿哲．病理生理学实验指导［M］.北京：人民卫生出版社，2017.

［13］胡还忠，牟阳灵．医学机能学实验教程［M］. 4 版．北京：科学出版社，2016.

［14］王建枝，钱睿哲．病理生理学［M］. 9 版．北京：人民卫生出版社，2018.

［15］秦川，谭毅．医学实验动物学［M］. 3 版．北京：人民卫生出版社，2021.

［16］张宝来，路莉．药理学实验指导［M］.北京：清华大学出版社，2020.

［17］叶春玲．药理学实验教程［M］.广州：暨南大学出版社，2007.

［18］肖飞，林熙，刘小文等．基于创新创业理念的"产学研"一体化教学模式在基础医学教育中的研究与实践［J］.教育教学论坛，2020（1）：194-197.

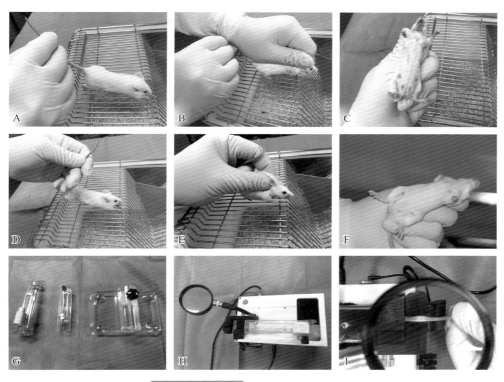

图 2-2/Figure 2-2 小鼠的抓取与固定

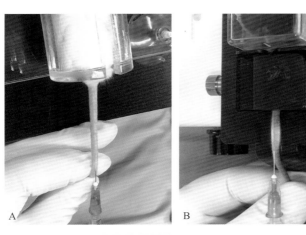

图 2-8/Figure 2-8 小鼠尾静脉注射

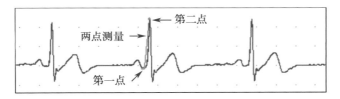

图 2-24/Figure 2-24 两点测量示意图

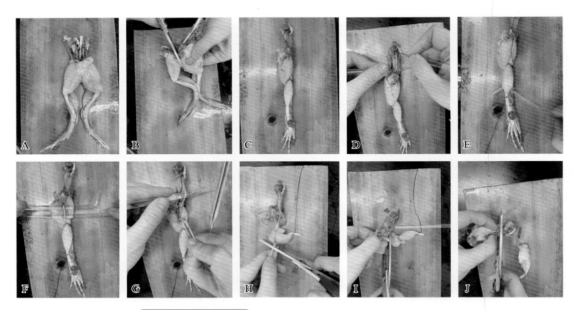

图 2-42/Figure 2-42　制作坐骨神经 - 腓肠肌标本的步骤

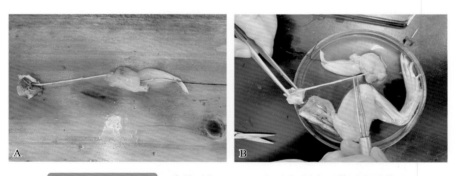

图 2-43/Figure 2-43　坐骨神经 - 腓肠肌标本的组成及其兴奋性检测

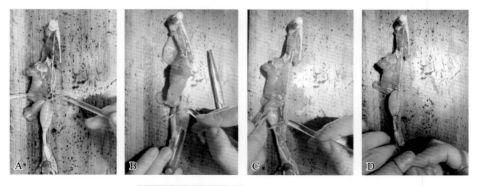

图 2-48/Figure 2-48　坐骨神经的分离

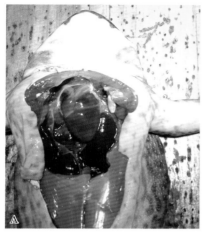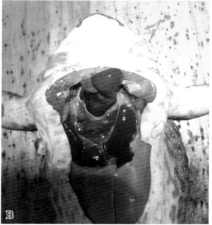

A 腹侧；B 背侧。

图 2-52/Figure 2-52　青蛙的心脏

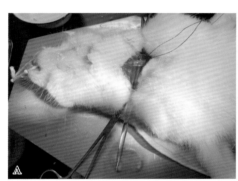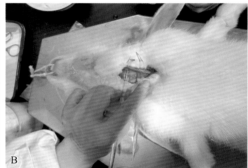

图 2-56/Figure 2-56　迷走神经的分离

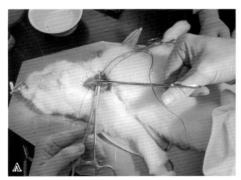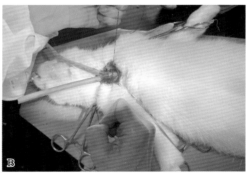

图 2-57/Figure 2-57　气管插管

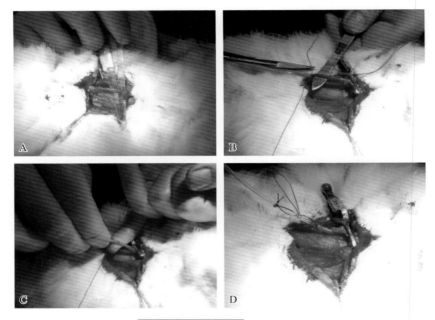

图 2-58/Figure 2-58　动脉插管

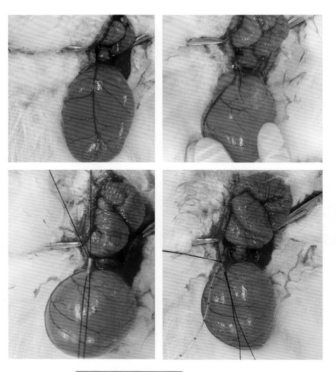

图 2-60/Figure 2-60　输尿管插管

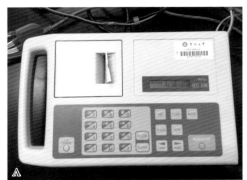
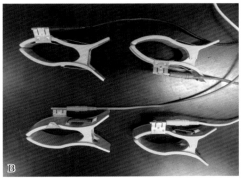
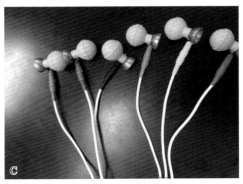

图 3-15/Figure 3-15　心电图仪（A）、肢体导联（B）、胸导联（C）

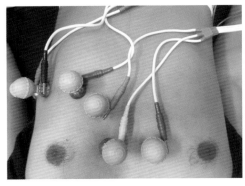
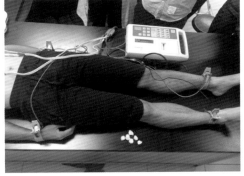

图 3-16/Figure 3-16　胸部导联（左）和肢体导联（右）的放置位置

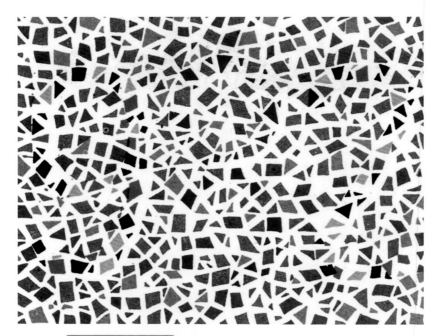

图 3-28/Figure 3-28　　可视化图表（Stilling-Ishihara 平板）

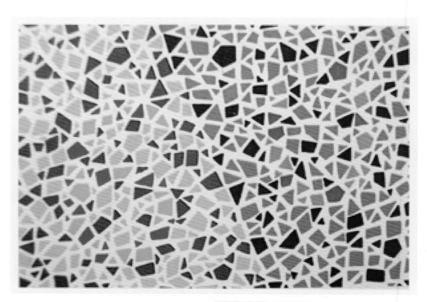

Answer _____　　Another　　Opinion

图 3-29/Figure 3-29　　色盲测试显示界面